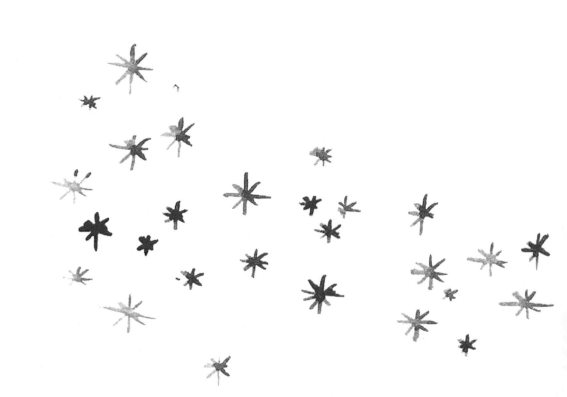

YOUR BODY IS *MAGIC*

WELLNESS STRATEGIES
for A HEALTHY PREGNANCY
and BIRTH

HOPE SMITH

Illustrations by Kimothy Joy

PRAISE FOR YOUR BODY IS MAGIC

"Books like this, which empower and support moms as they go through their own personal journeys with pregnancy, are invaluable. As a mom, businesswoman, and human being, I can't recommend *Your Body Is Magic* enough."

— *Karlie Kloss, supermodel, entrepreneur, and philanthropist*

"Hope is a trailblazer in the birthing/motherhood space, and her book follows the launch of her successful company, MUTHA."

— *Deepak Chopra, MD, author of multiple* New York Times *bestselling books, founder of The Chopra Foundation, and podcast host*

"This is not your mom's book on pregnancy! With wisdom, wit, and raw honesty, Hope Smith has masterfully crafted the *What to Expect When You're Expecting* for our time."

— *Jenny Mollen, actor and* New York Times *bestselling author*

"*Your Body Is Magic* is the perfect companion from conception to early parenthood. Rich in wisdom and real-talk, Hope's passion for all things muthahood is contagious."

— *Carson Meyer, birth doula, birth photographer, and childbirth educator*

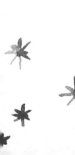

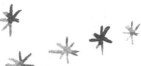

"Hope Smith is a force of nature in everything she does. And it's no surprise that *Your Body is Magic* is just that—MAGIC. This is a must read for any mother, woman, human. You can feel Hope's passion for home births in every word she writes, and though I am a hospital and drug kind of delivery mom, I was inspired and fascinated by her story and her strength. All our bodies are magic."

– Emma Bing, writer, podcast host, and lifestyle editor
for What To Expect

"Wow. This is the modern-day Bible for momhood! There is no tip, no detail, no resource left out of Hope's comprehensive and easy to read guide to pregnancy and birth. Having known Hope from pre-pregnancy to post childbirth, there is no woman I would entrust more for advice (both conventional and unconventional) than her. With the wealth of knowledge imparted in *Your Body is Magic*, I feel more prepared and excited than ever to journey through childbirth again!"

– Christine Chiu, co-founder, Beverly Hills Plastic Surgery,
producer, and philanthropist

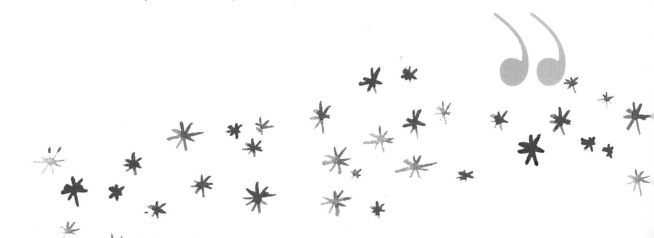

Copyright © 2022 by Hope Smith
Cover design by Jocelyn Foye
Cover copyright © 2022 by HLZZ Books, LLC
Print book interior design by Jocelyn Foye
Illustrations by Kimothy Joy

HLZZ Books, LLC
PO Box 30008
Palm Beach Gardens, FL 33420

First Edition: March, 2022
Library of Congress Control Number: 2022901529

Identifiers: ISBN (trade paperback) | ISBN (ebook)
ISBNs: 9780306924835 (hardcover); 9780306924859 (ebook)

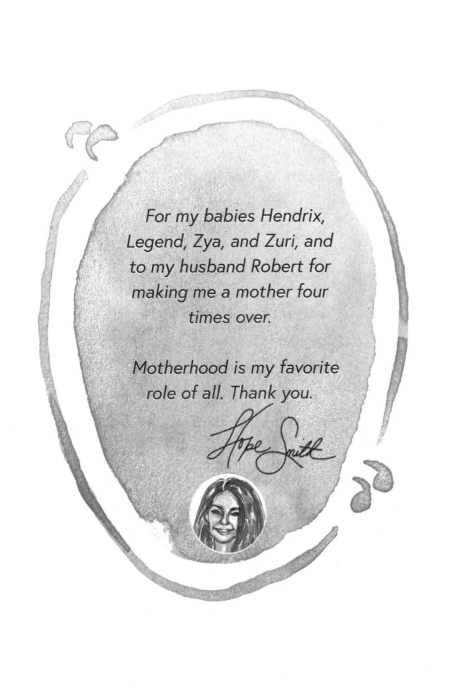

For my babies Hendrix, Legend, Zya, and Zuri, and to my husband Robert for making me a mother four times over.

Motherhood is my favorite role of all. Thank you.

Hope Smith

TABLE OF CONTENTS

FOREWORD

Conceiving, gestating, laboring and delivering a new child into this world is nothing short of a miracle.

As a pediatrician for over 35 years, I have witnessed this moment hundreds of times. The instant a new child is born is profoundly spiritual. Time stops. The world hushes to recognize that something very special has occurred; an entirely new person, unique in every way, has arrived.

This creation of new life is what author Hope Smith celebrates in these pages. The book you're holding in your hands is a tour de force of practical information that she has culled from her personal experiences as a woman who has given birth twice and who oversaw the surrogacy of her two identical twin girls.

With a gentle hand, *Your Body is Magic* guides and encourages new mothers (and fathers too) along the path of gestation (even pre-gestation) through the birth process. The book is chock full of basic and important advice and recommendations, but particularly addresses nutritious foods and vitamins, proper exercise for each stage of gestation, and healthy living like sleep and stress reduction. It's old wisdom for today's mothers.

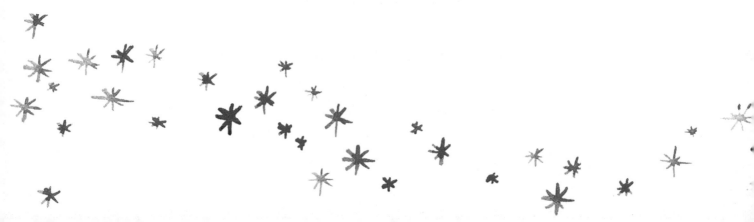

Hope is a cheerleader for motherhood and she writes primarily to nudge every mother toward the healthiest and best pregnancy possible. She also yearns to see that every child born enjoy the advantages of empowered, prepared, and confident parents.

Lovingly constructed, Hope's upbeat take on the process of gestation is highly readable and encouraging. There is something for every soon-to-be mother in this book.

I am frequently asked when I plan to retire. My answer is that I'll know when it's time for me to hang up my stethoscope when I no longer find babies awesome. When the day comes when I walk into the newborn nursery and fail to appreciate the miracle of new life, that will be my signal to move on.

After reading this book, the date of my retirement for me just got pushed waaaaay back!

Robert C. Hamilton, M.D., F.A.A.P.
Santa Monica, California
January 2022

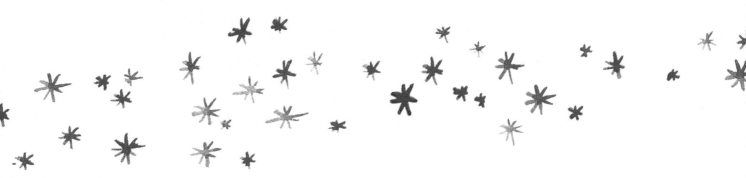

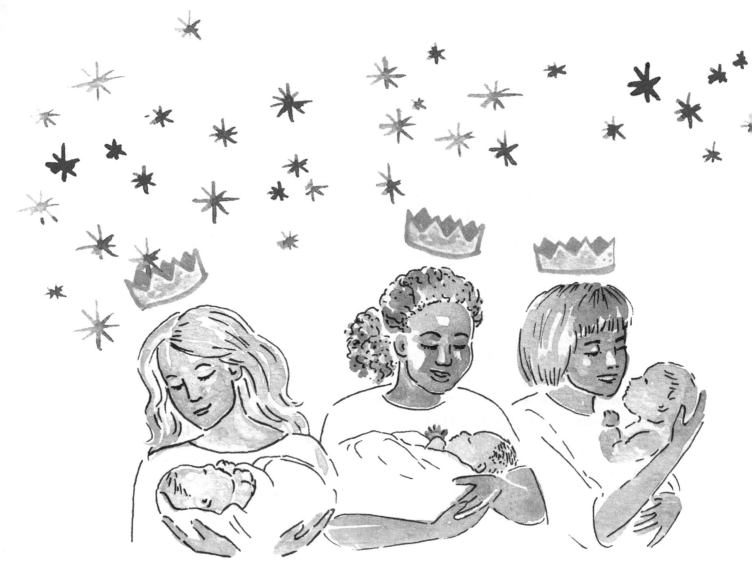

YOU'RE STILL *yourself,*
BUT YOU'RE *more* POWERFUL.
MAGIC, EVEN.

YOU WERE BORN FOR THIS

W hen my husband and I started talking about having kids, I was thrilled by the idea of being a mom. But giving birth? Not so much. I hadn't really given a lot of thought to how I felt about delivering a baby until it became a tangible reality for me. That's when I started thinking back on what I had heard about pregnancy and delivery, and it wasn't pretty.

I realized that, even as a girl, all I had ever heard about pregnancy was how awful it was; how you couldn't sleep, your legs swelled, and your back hurt. And my experiences of birth were just shy of traumatizing: I grew up in a tiny town in Texas, where, whenever a woman had a baby, all her friends and relatives camped out in the hospital waiting room. When I was about six years old, my aunt gave birth to my cousin. I remember being able to hear her screams from the lobby and feeling so worried about her—*what was happening in that room?*—and embarrassed for her—*shouldn't we be giving her some privacy?*

How I saw birth portrayed in movies was even worse. Every film made it seem like women in labor were being tortured, while their husbands nearly fainted (if they were even in the delivery room; more likely, they were handing out cigars in reception).

When I was old enough for my friends to start having babies, and they would talk about how intense their labors were (one said she labored for 36 hours!), all I could think was how awful it would be to have a baby in your vagina for that long. (I didn't yet know that the baby is only in the birth canal when you're ready to push, and that for almost all of labor, the baby is within the uterus; meaning, the vagina really only sees action for a relatively short period of time.)

So when my husband and I began baby talks, it occurred to me that I had never once heard a woman share a positive birth story. And even though I really wanted to have a baby and become a mom, I was scared about giving birth. *Would the baby* actually *come out of me? Would I be able to stand the pain? Would my vagina ever be the same again?*

My mind raced with so many fear-inducing questions that I started to do what I always do when I feel nervous—I began researching.

I started reading the standard pregnancy books. Even though it was fascinating to learn about all the changes the baby went through week by week, these books didn't give me a lot of comfort about what kinds of things *I* was about to go through.

I'm No Hippie, But…

It wasn't until I read *Ina May's Guide to Childbirth* by Ina May Gaskin—a midwife who's been offering women an alternative to hospital births since 1971, when she founded the Farm Midwifery Center near Summertown, Tennessee—that I started to have hope. Her stories of all the different kinds of women who gave birth on that farm showed me that another possibility existed: one where women trusted their bodies, and where a midwife and doula were there to support the mother.

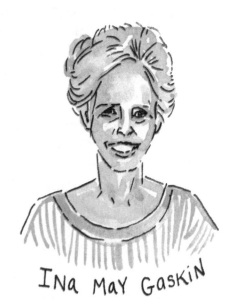

INa MaY GaskiN

The picture it painted was such a stark alternative to the medicalized version of birth that's become the standard of care. These women weren't relying on a doctor to deliver their baby for them; they were active participants in and leaders of their birth experiences. Here at last were the empowering birth stories that I hadn't even realized I'd been craving.

Once I saw that there were more natural approaches to birth, I went on a whole earthy journey. And I was not in any way a hippie, mind you. (Although I grew up in Texas and live in Austin and Malibu now, I moved to New York City when I was 16.)

I devoured every resource I could get my hands on about all the nutrients a mother's body needs to produce a healthy baby, and I started piecing together my own arsenal of supplements to make sure I was getting those vitamins and minerals. I also read up on how synthetic chemicals could compromise my health and my baby's health, and then I began producing my own body butters and skincare creams in my kitchen. (It really is amazing what hormones can help you do!) That's how my skincare brand, MUTHA, was born.

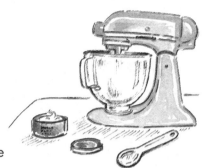

Even though I revered Ina May for her work helping women—and our culture at large—get over their fear of childbirth, I thought to myself about her book, "My friends would never read this." It's way too granola for them.

After all, a lot of my friends opted for scheduled Cesarean births because they wanted to remove some of the unknowns presented by the birthing process. Some of them even scheduled tummy tucks for right after their baby was delivered (in what's known as a 'designer birth'). I understand the desire to turn birth into a medical procedure. But my research showed me that so many of the policies and medicines associated with hospital births and Cesareans can easily lead to worse outcomes for babies and their mothers. It became very clear to me that women aren't being educated about what their bodies are capable of, or supported in trusting their bodies to give birth.

The truth is, a woman's body—your body—is capable of miraculous feats. As I read, I couldn't help thinking that if more women knew just how powerful and wise their bodies were—how, without even thinking about it, you will produce all the right hormones at just the right time to get that baby out—they might be less afraid about giving birth too.

When pregnant, I started investigating all the possible ways I could have the baby. I talked to Ob/Gyns, midwives, and doulas. I visited hospitals and birthing centers. Talking to the midwives and doulas opened my eyes to the fact that birth is a completely normal physical process. It also later inspired me to train to become a doula myself. Ultimately, I decided that I wanted to have the baby at home, because my research showed me that when you are in an environment in which you feel comfortable, your labor tends to go smoother.

> "YOU CAN ABSOLUTELY DO THIS. I WROTE THIS BOOK to HELP you BELIEVE iT."

When I shared my choice with my friends, they said, "Don't be a hero! Schedule a Cesarean birth and let the doctor do the work."

(Just a note here that I use the term 'Cesarean birth' instead of 'Cesarean section' or 'C-section' throughout this book. Whether they are elective or medically necessary, Cesareans are first and foremost a form of birth.)

I know they were only trying to look out for me, and I believe that every woman deserves to have the birth that makes the most sense for her. I do not judge any woman's choices, but I knew that wasn't a route that appealed to me. I wanted to be present in every moment of my child's birth—both because it was the start of his life and because it was the moment I transformed from woman to mother. I wanted to really "be there" for it.

I got a better response to my decision when I posted about my home birth plans on my Instagram account. I started getting messages from women who told me that my choice inspired them to have their babies at home too.

It doesn't mean I didn't have moments of panic—I did! But I realized deep down that I was born for this.

I want you to understand that your body is exquisitely designed to enable you to create and give birth to another human—even if your doctor or midwife has told you you're high-risk because you're over 35, or that you really should lose weight before you get pregnant, or made some other comment that's making you afraid. I love doctors; mine saved my second child's life. But, they have their own timelines and expectations for how a body should work that don't always jibe with what your mind and body need to have a baby.

Ask any of the thousands of women who have given birth in the back of a car on their way to the hospital, and they'll say the same thing: The baby will be born whether your doctor or midwife is there or not. Your doctor or midwife is there to guide and protect you; you're there to deliver the baby. You can absolutely do this. I wrote this book to help you believe it.

HOW TO USE THIS BOOK

This book takes you through the entire pregnancy experience—starting before you conceive, all the way through the first few weeks after the baby arrives. The content comes from a range of disciplines, encompassing the best blend of science and traditional wisdom:

- Research from the American College of Obstetricians and Gynecologists

- Passed-down guidance from my midwife, **Mari Mikel Potter**, and my go-to doula, **Khristina Helmich**, as well as from my own training as a doula

- Prenatal fitness routines from **Brooke Cates** of The Bloom Method

Once you digest the information in these pages, you'll be able to go into your birth well prepared, like a student who's done your homework and is feeling confident that you can handle whatever questions are on the test.

You'll know the road ahead and have a route picked out. And if for any reason you hit a roadblock, you'll know enough about the other paths to remember that you always have options.

Know that I'm not hell-bent on getting you to have a home birth, or even a vaginal birth. Again, I'm not here to make judgments. I only want to help you make informed choices to trust in your ability to give birth to your baby.

They say that it's not just the baby who is born—the mother is too. Having a baby changes the way you think about yourself and the way you see the world. No matter how your baby is born, the experience will show you that you are capable of so much more than you probably ever believed you were. You'll still be yourself, just more powerful. Magical, even. You've always been so; it's just that after giving birth, you'll *know* it's true.

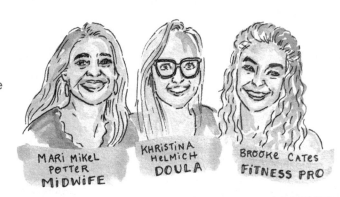

MARI MIKEL POTTER
MIDWIFE

KHRISTINA HELMICH
DOULA

BROOKE CATES
FITNESS PRO

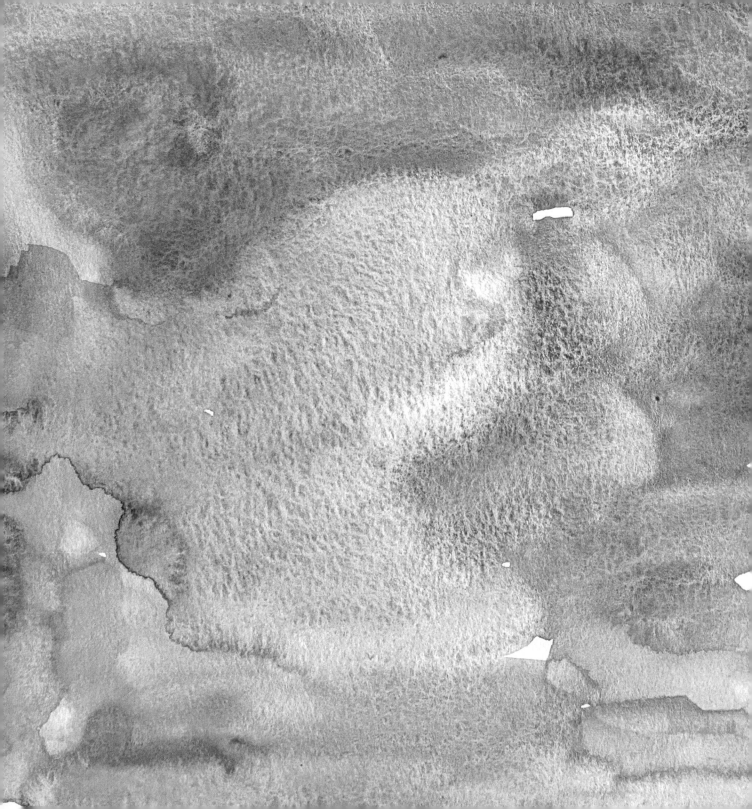

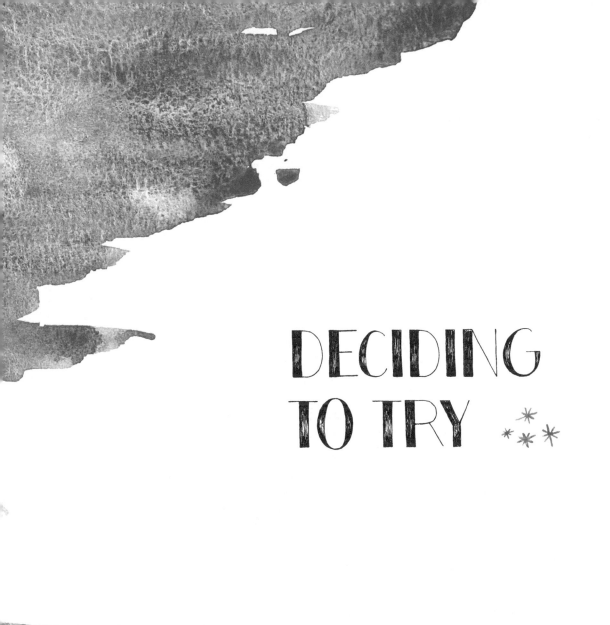

DECIDING TO TRY ✳

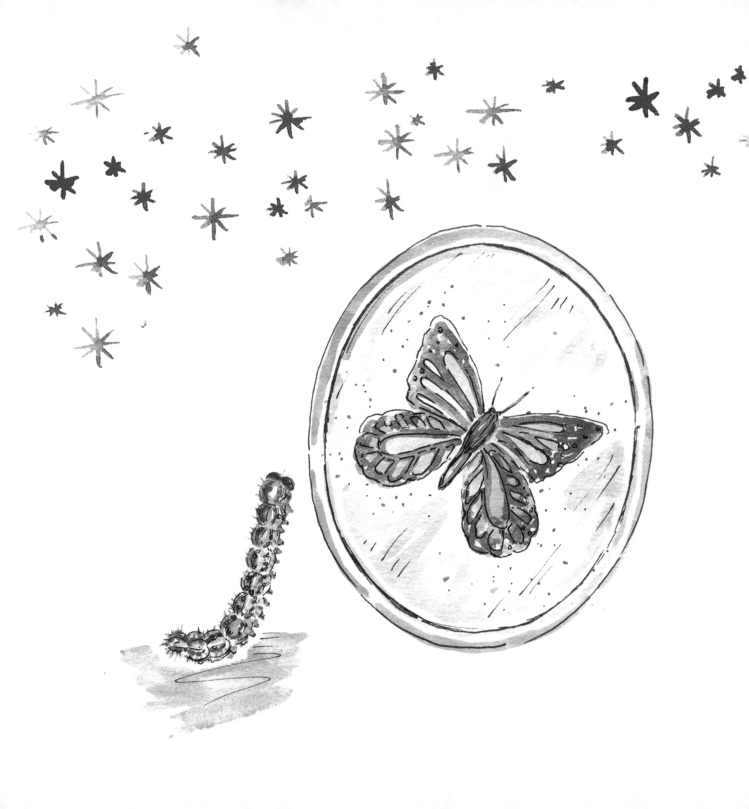

Chapter 1

GETTING YOUR HEAD IN THE GAME

E ven though you're not technically a mother before you're carrying a baby, you start your transition to becoming a mom the moment you decide to try to get pregnant. First of all, after spending your reproductive years trying not to get pregnant, you're suddenly switching teams. Beyond that, it's not just about you any more, or even you and your partner. There's another person whose health and happiness you need to consider, even if at first they're still only an idea.

That's why I wanted to include this stage of prepregnancy in this book. You don't need to be carrying a baby to begin thinking like a mother. It's never too early to start taking better care of yourself and building up your reserves so that you have them to draw on the rest of the way. The more nourished—physically, mentally, and emotionally—you are now, the better off you and your baby will be throughout both of your lives. Getting pregnant presents a huge opportunity to take stock of your life and make positive changes—whether that's caring more about what you eat or how much you sleep, signing up for a yoga class for the first time ever, or evaluating if the place you're living is where you want to raise a child. All of these adjustments start with a shift in your thinking, and that's what this chapter will walk you through.

Knowing Whether It's the Right Time

It's rare that I talk to a friend who tells me she's ready to have a baby. Either she's not *quite* ready yet, or she's been trying to have a baby for a while and it's taking longer than she expected, and now she's way past ready. There's not a lot of middle ground, especially since fewer women are having babies because it's the expected thing to do. It used to be

Signs You're Ovulating

There are four major clues that your ovaries are getting ready to drop an egg:

1) Your vaginal mucus noticeably changes right before ovulation.
There's more of it, typically, and it is usually clear, wet, and stretchy, like an egg white. This is by design—the mucus makes it easier for sperm to swim. After you've ovulated, your mucus production slows down and it becomes thicker, more opaque, and less noticeable.

2) Your resting body temperature rises. You'll likely only notice the rise if you take your temperature in the mornings—before you do anything, like get up to go to the bathroom or reach for your phone—throughout the month so that you can detect changes. Use a sensitive thermometer called a basal body thermometer so that you can accurately determine your temperature, within a tenth of a degree. If you do these things, you'll see that in the days after your body releases an egg, your basal body temperature rises at least two-tenths of a degree higher than before ovulation. To really use this method to best effect, you should write down your temperature every day (or even ask your Ob/Gyn for a graph you can use to chart it) so that you can pinpoint for sure when the change happens.

3) You feel it in your abdomen (maybe). Some, but not all, women can feel ovulation. It's called *mittelschmerz*, or middle pain, because ovulation happens in the middle of your cycle. It's not usually super painful—it feels more like tenderness on one side of your lower abdomen (depending on which ovary is releasing an egg that month). You may have to tune in to your body to feel it. I didn't figure out that the sensation I was feeling was actually ovulation until I was almost 30. But whether you can actually sense it or not, it's happening.

4) You get a boost. You may also notice that you feel more energetic, sexy, and ready to have sex around the time you're ovulating. Go with it!

that if you had gotten married in the last year or two, you were ready, because that's just how it usually happened. Now, with more women waiting to have babies until their career is well established, or because they're still looking for the right partner, or because they just want a chance to settle into adulthood before embarking on motherhood, we do a lot more thinking about when is the right time.

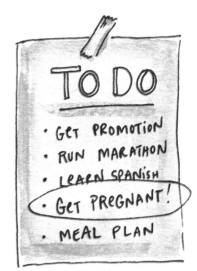

But you know what? Just like it's never a bad time to have a baby, it's never the right time to have a baby. There's always going to be something you still want to accomplish, whether it's being further along in your career, having more money, or waiting until a busy or uncertain time has passed. You'll never have everything perfectly squared away and all the items on your to-do list checked off.

To my mind, the most important consideration to take into account is whether you feel confident about the person you're heading into parenthood with. (That's assuming you're doing it with a partner; many woman choose to have a baby without a partner, and now more men than ever are choosing to do the same, and that's great—then you need to be confident in yourself and your support system.) Because whomever you pick, you and your child are more than likely to be in a relationship of some sort with them for decades to come.

I had my first baby when I was 30, and the only reason I waited as long as I did was because I knew that my past partners weren't the people with whom I wanted to have kids. If you end up not being together, would you still want to co-parent with this person? Are they trustworthy? Reliable? Loving? Committed to doing the right thing, even when it's inconvenient? Because romantic relationships often do end. For the most part, parenting relationships don't.

If you're reading this book, you're thinking about having a baby pretty seriously—way more than a lot of women think about it. Take that as a sign that it's OK to go ahead and start trying. You're not 100 percent in control of the process anyway. It may take longer than you're anticipating; it may not. Now is as good a time as any to start building your trust muscles.

Trusting the Process

Even after you've decided that you're ready to start trying, it can be hard to trust the process. You've heard the stories about how it took months or even years for one of your friends or family members to get pregnant. It can definitely be an emotional roller coaster every month— *Am I pregnant? Am I not pregnant? Will I have a baby this time next year or will I not?*

If you are a person who is used to making up your mind about something and then going out and making it happen, it can be especially difficult for you to not have the final word about when your pregnancy occurs. I know it's easier to say than to do, but you have to let go of your expectations and trust that it is all working out exactly as it should. Your body knows, on a deep level, when is the right time to have a baby, and which egg and sperm combination is the right one to allow to develop into a baby. You've got to let it lead the way. It knows what it is doing. And the more stressed you are, the more of a toll it will take.

I'm sure you've also heard of someone who worked to get pregnant for so long that she eventually stopped trying… and that's when it happened. That's how it went for me. The first time around, my husband and I tried for 18 months. (I believe that I had at least one very early miscarriage—too early even for a pregnancy test to come back positive.) When I still wasn't pregnant, I started to think we might need some medical interventions. So I made an appointment with a doctor to start the in vitro fertilization process. Three days before that appointment, I found out I was pregnant. I fully believe that since I had the appointment on the books, I stopped stressing about when I was going to conceive. And once I relaxed, it happened all on its own. (Well, not totally on its own; my husband had an important role to play! But you get the idea.)

My point is, don't overthink this. Try not to micromanage the process—for example, getting wrapped up in pinpointing the exact moment of ovulation and then trying to have sex within a certain window so that it feels more like something to cross off your list than a potentially life-giving event. The good news is that when you're ovulating, your hormones naturally rise so that just when you're at your most fertile, they give your desire a kick in the pants and help you feel your sexiest. Your body is part of nature, and nature is magic—let it take over and allow the magic to happen.

When exactly am I fertile?

There are only a small number of days in any given cycle when you can feasibly conceive a baby, and those are the five days before you ovulate (because sperm can only live for five days inside your body), the day you ovulate, and the two days after you ovulate (because an egg is only viable for fertilization up to 48 hours after it's released).[1] That's eight days out of 28—not a huge window!

The tricky thing is, you won't necessarily ovulate on the same day of your cycle every month. Typically, it's around Day 14, but that's not a given. You can use the symptoms I list in the sidebar on page 10 to help you pinpoint when those days are. Or, you can get a looser idea of when that window is likely to be just by knowing which day of your cycle you're on.

If you're within six days of when you suspect you're ovulating and you're in the mood, know that you're having sex on a day when you are most likely to be able to conceive. If your cycle is regularly longer then 32 days, know that your period typically starts 14 days after ovulation, so you can count backward from the first day of your period to determine what day you typically ovulate.

Either way, you'll have to track your cycle for a few months to know how many days it is. You'll want to do this anyway, because the first thing a doctor or midwife will ask you is the first date of your last period. (They use this date to calculate how many weeks along you are, as well as your due date.) This way you'll have that information at your fingertips.

You can track your cycle just by writing "Day 1" on your calendar each month on the day when you get your period, then counting the number of days until the next "Day 1." Or, there are some great apps that help you keep tabs on your cycle so that you know what day you're on at all times. My favorites include Clue and Flo.

There is also a good wearable device for this, the Ava Ovulation Tracker bracelet. It tells you, in real time, if it's a fertile day, as well as tracks your skin temperature, resting pulse rate, breathing rate, heart rate variability (how quickly your heart beat normalizes after exertion), and perfusion (the passage of blood through the circulatory system).

Maintaining a Positive Mental Environment

It's so important for your mental and physical health to try and keep your thoughts in a positive place. I know it's easier said than done. While you're trying to get pregnant, it is perfectly OK to excuse yourself from watching the news constantly, or scrolling through Twitter or Instagram if the posts you see there upset you, or even talking to people in your life who love to complain or worry.

Personally, I try to stay positive by making sure that for every negative interaction I have, either inside my own brain or with my kids or my husband, I say or think eight nice things. If my child has exhibited a behavior I need to correct, for example, I try and commend him for four things before I share the one negative, and then follow that up with four other things about him for which I'm grateful.

An 8:1 ratio is pretty high, but it really trains you to keep looking for the good things, so that when something "bad" happens it doesn't get blown up out of proportion in your mind. It keeps you on a more even keel, and that's good for you and everyone around you.

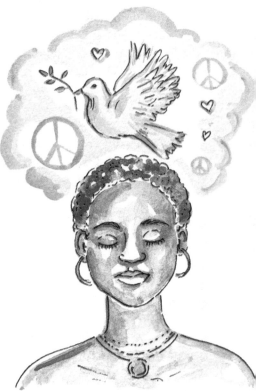

If someone knows you're trying to get pregnant and they start to tell you a negative story about their own pregnancy or somebody else's, it is absolutely within your rights to tell them to stop and explain that you don't have space for that right now, that you don't want any negative seeds planted in your consciousness. So many of us have been told that it's impolite to set boundaries around what other people say and do in our presence, but it's not at all rude to simply comment, "Thank you for wanting to share, but that's not helpful for me."

And make sure that you expose yourself to positive stories about pregnancy, childbirth, and parenthood. Join

"...it's not at all rude to simply comment, 'Thank you for wanting to share, but that's not helpful for me.'"

an online support group—there are so many groups on Facebook and other websites that you can easily find by searching "trying to get pregnant" plus "group." There may even be groups meeting in your town that you can find through a maternity or children's store or even the local birth center or hospital. I made a friend on Instagram who also posted about trying to get pregnant. We both ended up getting pregnant at the same time, and her support was invaluable to me. There are others out there going through the same things you are; you just might have to do a little searching to find them.

Think about who you have in your circle whom you trust to reassure you that everything is unfolding exactly as it should, that your body knows what it's doing, and that everything is going to be OK. Whom do you trust to validate and encourage you? Maybe your mom is a nervous Nellie; even though she means well and loves you, it might be best that you don't talk to her as much right now. Nothing is more important than you feeling your best, and that includes inside your own mind.

I also completely believe in the power of affirmations to keep your thoughts in a healthy place. Affirmations are positive phrases that help you stay focused on what you want instead of worrying about things you don't want to come to pass. You need somewhere to put your attention, whether you're feeling fear in that moment or you're just trying to keep your head in a good place, and affirmations are a great help.

See the sidebar on the next page for trying-to-get-pregnant affirmations. Write them out and hang them up somewhere you'll see them every day. Repeat them to yourself as you fall asleep or while you sit quietly for a few minutes during the day.

Keeping the Faith Despite the Obstacles

There are any number of reasons your pregnancy may be deemed high-risk and cause you to worry. Maybe you're over 35, in which case your doctor or midwife will tell you

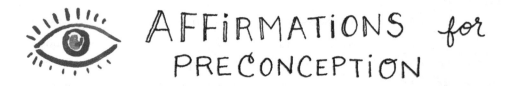

AFFIRMATIONS for PRECONCEPTION

MY BODY KNOWS WHAT IT'S DOING.

I BELIEVE IN MYSELF and IN MY BODY.

MY BODY IS MAGIC.

I TRUST MY ABILITY to GET PREGNANT.

I WILL GET PREGNANT at THE EXACT RIGHT TIME.

that yours will be a 'geriatric pregnancy.' (That's got to be some of the worst branding ever.) Or your doctor thinks you should lose weight because of a BMI calculation, but you know your body and that you're a healthy weight for you. Or perhaps you're a Black woman reckoning with the statistics that women of color have a significantly higher risk of maternal mortality than white women.

   I am not here to tell you that you don't need to be concerned about the statistics. You absolutely do need to be mindful of them. But resist the temptation to think that they mean there is something wrong with your body.

In this case, objective research is your friend. I don't mean talking to anyone with an opinion about whatever particular challenge you might be facing. I mean looking at the data for your specific situation on reputable sites, such as the American College of Obstetricians and Gynecologists (ACOG) or the Midwives' Alliance of North America (MANA). Educate yourself, and then balance the knowledge of your unique position with the trust that you are capable and born to do this.

Healing from Miscarriage

One of the big fears around deciding to try to become pregnant and early pregnancy is the risk of miscarriage. Losing a pregnancy can be devastating. It can make you want to give up. You may try to tell yourself that it's a sign motherhood wasn't meant to be. But one truth about miscarriage that often goes overlooked is that it is normal. Up to 15 percent of all established pregnancies miscarry in the first trimester, and up to five percent in the second trimester. When you consider pregnancies that perhaps the women weren't yet aware of, it's thought that as many as half of all pregnancies end in miscarriage.[2]

We can't know exactly why miscarriages happen, but there is often a beneficial reason for them. Maybe there was something not quite right about the lining of the uterus. Or the genetic profile of the embryo wasn't viable. Here too you've got to rely on your trust in the process that everything you go through will result in the exact right baby for you.

If you experience a miscarriage, or multiple miscarriages, in your process of trying to have a baby, it is perfectly appropriate to give yourself space to grieve. No matter how far along you were, it is a loss. It may feel like a small loss or a devastating one—however you feel, you are entitled to your feelings, and you deserve to take as much time as you need to mourn what might have been.

Honestly, grief is part of parenting that never fully disappears. There are so many little losses along the way, including things that you hoped for that don't end up coming true, whether that's your baby having your eye color or your kid being a math whiz. There are also the losses that come as your kids grow up. With every new stage, as exciting as it is, it also means there's a stage gone by. I remember feeling sad when my son started crawling, because it meant that the days of plopping him on the couch with a few toys were over, even though I was excited for this new phase, too.

In parenting, you have ideas of how things are going to go, but the fact is, they rarely go that way. That's just part of it. Learning to manage your expectations and accept reality is a big piece of how parenthood helps you grow, and it starts as early as preconception.

I experienced this myself when it came time to have my third child and I found out that another pregnancy was not in the cards for me.

Before my first pregnancy, I had a blood test at my annual physical, and the levels of some of my liver enzymes were really high. The doctors didn't know why they were elevated, as I didn't fit the demographics or other criteria of the conditions that might have produced those results. Over the two years that I carried and delivered my first two babies, I had follow-up blood work with no diagnosis. I definitely felt tired, but I thought it was an inevitable part of motherhood.

> "HONESTLY, GRIEF IS PART of PARENTING that NEVER FULLY DISAPPEARS."

During that time, I did my own Googling. My searches finally led me to a rare autoimmune condition that causes the body to attack its organs. Although the only indicators of this condition for me personally were high levels of certain liver enzymes in addition to elevated antinuclear antibodies (ANA) and immunoglobulin G (IgG) levels, it turns out, that's what I had. Luckily for me it was attacking my biliary tract and not my actual liver. It is treatable with periodic infusions of a chemotherapy drug that puts the autoimmune attacks in remission. That was the good news. The bad news was that the treatment can cause birth defects and deplete your B cells, so I wouldn't be able to carry the third baby I had my heart set on.

I felt blessed to have two kids, but I had been saying I wanted three or four children ever since I was a girl. (Be careful of the words you use!) So, I kept asking questions and found out that my eggs were fine, which meant surrogacy was an option.

My point in sharing this story is that no matter what you are facing, you have to be your own advocate. I went to see three doctors, and it took more than three years before I received the correct diagnosis. I could have let that diagnosis be the end of my dream of having another baby. If I hadn't done my own research, I might have gotten pregnant and had a baby who didn't make it. If I had only listened to the doctor, and not advocated for myself, I wouldn't have more kids. But I kept asking questions and found out that my eggs were unaffected.

We ended up using a surrogate, which was a wonderful experience. Although, we were in for a big surprise when the embryo that our surrogate was carrying divided and we learned that were going to have identical twin girls. It was great news, and a total blessing, but it was also shocking—and a little scary. Instead of having three kids in total, we were now going to have four. The news also didn't jibe with my vision of having only one baby in the house. I'd had my first two children back to back, so I was looking forward to being able to focus on one baby. I had to grieve the way I thought things were going to go.

I can tell you from personal experience that the most efficient way through grief is to allow yourself to feel it, and to honor it. Emotions have to come out in some form. If it's not tears it may be anger. If you miscarry, do what feels right to you but treat yourself gently. There will be another cycle when you can try again. Forgive yourself, too, for the loss. When my husband and I were going through the process of having a baby with a surrogate (using my eggs, his sperm, and the IVF process), the clinicians at our reproductive clinic told us that up to half of the embryos they implant—and mind you, these are the strongest, healthiest embryos of the bunch—end in miscarriage.

The good news is that by implementing the nutritional strategies and other tips that I'll cover in the next chapters of this section, you'll give your body more of what it needs to have a viable pregnancy and reduce your exposure to anything that can make the path more difficult.

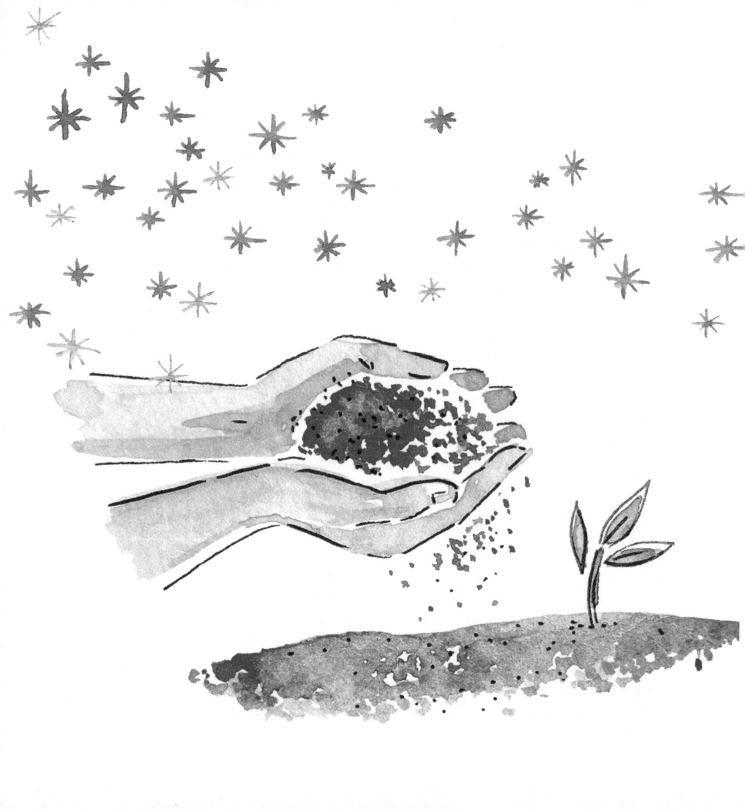

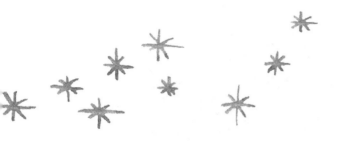

Chapter 2

FERTILIZING THE SOIL

While your body absolutely is magic and will—a lot of the time, all on its own—do what it takes to produce, grow, and deliver a healthy baby, you can certainly help it by giving it plenty of the things it needs to create a new human. If you clean up your diet and become more mindful of your exposure to chemicals and other environmental contaminants, you'll make your body's job a lot easier.

The more nourished you are now, the smoother your conception and pregnancy will go and the healthier your baby will be. A happy side effect of giving your body extra love at this point is that you'll be healthier too The inspiration to take better care of yourself is one of the great byproducts of trying to get pregnant. May as well go with it! Maybe your partner will also get in on the act. This is just one more way a baby changes your life even before they're born, or even in your belly.

So many women get pregnant unexpectedly and don't have the chance to change their diet or their normal routines. Just the fact that you're reading this info, and hopefully implementing it, puts you way, way ahead of the game. Good for you.

Nutrition to Enhance Fertility

It's probably not a surprise that what you eat during pregnancy can influence the health of your baby—not just for the nine months that you're carrying them but for all the years of their life. (I'll talk more about nutrition for each trimester in later chapters.) But what you eat now, even before you're pregnant, can also either help or harm your chances of conceiving.

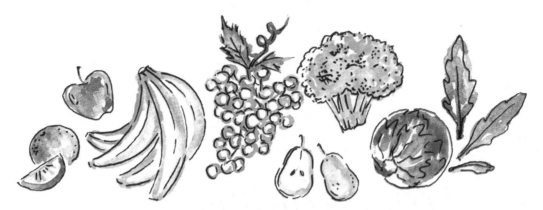

The good news is that you don't have to follow a complicated or challenging diet. Just by carrying out some pretty simple strategies, you'll boost your fertility and give your future baby a solid nutritional foundation.

A team of Harvard researchers reviewed a number of studies on the impact of nutrition on fertility and found that women who followed a "fertility diet" had a 66 percent lower risk of ovulatory infertility (meaning infertility caused by not ovulating or ovulating infrequently or irregularly) and a 27 percent lower risk of infertility due to other causes.[3] But, the "diet" they evaluated wasn't a truly prescriptive eating plan. It was really just common-sense nutrition, with advice including:

- Eat less animal protein, which is high in saturated fat, and more vegetarian sources of protein, such as beans, tofu, nuts, and quinoa;

- Avoid harmful trans fats (like those in chips, cookies, and processed foods) and opt for healthy fats like those found in olive oil, wild salmon, and avocados;

- Put plenty of whole grains on your plate, which are high in fiber;

- And enjoy an abundance of organic fruits and vegetables.

It's your basic healthy eating advice—nothing to stress over. One thing that stuck out to me, though, was that as the researchers analyzed the diets of 18,000 women, they discovered that those who regularly enjoyed full-fat dairy were much less likely to experience ovulatory infertility than those who routinely chose products made with skim or low-fat milk. So although consuming a ton of dairy isn't great for health in general, because it's high in sugar and tends to produce mucous in the body, a little of it is OK, at least when it comes to fertility. Just reach for the whole milk, full-fat yogurt, or half-and-half instead of their low-fat alternatives. Whole milk is a whole food, after all.

Probably the most difficult to implement, yet most helpful, eating for fertility strategy is to cut down on sugar. When you consume sugar, your insulin levels spike. If you eat it regularly—and most people have it a few times a day, because it's in a lot of processed foods and refined grains (like pasta and bread), in addition to the desserts and sweet stuff we tend to associate it with—you flood your system with insulin and your insulin receptors can start to get burned out. If they do, you may develop insulin resistance, which is highly associated with polycystic ovary syndrome (PCOS), a condition that affects roughly five million American women and is a common root cause of infertility.

Simple Ways to Cut Down on Sugar

- Switch to plain yogurt instead of flavored yogurt.

- If you need sweetener in your coffee, try stevia or monk fruit (which don't impact your insulin levels).

- Eat a piece of whole fruit (the fiber, water content, and phytonutrients will lower the impact on your insulin levels) instead of a traditional dessert.

- Drink a glass of water and then go for a walk around the block before you have a sugary snack; sometimes hunger is really dehydration, and it can take a few minutes for your body to register that you're not truly hungry after drinking some water, so taking that quick walk will keep you occupied while your body makes up its mind.

- Cut way back on condiments like store-bought salad dressings, tomato sauces, ketchup, salsas, barbecue sauce, and bottled marinades, as they are typically hidden sources of sugar.

- Snack on nuts and seeds instead of any type of bar—most of which are loaded with sugar.

- Have an egg with avocado slices for breakfast instead of cereal or granola, which are, you guessed it, typically very sugary.

It's also important to note that a low-sugar diet is naturally anti-inflammatory, and that's a good thing. Chronic inflammation seems to fuel many reproductive disorders that interfere with fertility, so getting it under control is key—and diet is one simple way to rein things in. By focusing on consuming fresh fruits and vegetables, lean proteins, and healthy fats, and by avoiding fried and processed junk foods, you'll help reduce inflammation in your body and put out the smoldering fire it causes.

Note that for some people, grains can contribute to inflammation. You may want to consider going gluten-free or eating only traditional gluten-free grains, like millet and buckwheat. The same goes for legumes and dairy products made with cow's milk.

Know that probiotics can also reduce inflammation. In addition to probiotic supplements, you can boost your intake by consuming fermented foods and beverages, such as sauerkraut, miso, kefir, kombucha, and yogurt.

7 Must-Eat Fertility-Boosting Nutrients

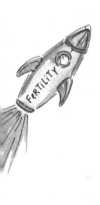

I know I love a list to help me stay on track, so I'm including a rundown of seven important nutrients for fertility. That way, you can more easily keep tabs on whether or not you're getting the nourishment your body needs now—from antioxidants to zinc.

You're likely to be eating these nutrients anyway if you're following the general dietary wisdom I already shared. But I want to go ahead and call them out so that you're aware of the specific vitamins and minerals you need in prepregnancy, and so that you understand how they may help you conceive. You'll also know what foods to make sure are on your list for your next trip to the grocery store.

1. Antioxidants. Free radicals are those unstable atoms in your body that create oxidative stress, which can damage cells and ultimately lead to cancer. Oxidative stress can also mess with female fertility by potentially bringing on reproductive diseases, and it may play a role in unexplained infertility too. Luckily, antioxidants neutralize free radicals, and there are lots of tasty foods that are high in them. In fact, there are some really delicious foods that score off the ORAC charts! What's an ORAC score? The Oxygen Radical Absorbance Capacity, or ORAC, score measures the antioxidant capacity of foods. The higher a food's ORAC value, the more health-boosting, free-radical-busting antioxidants it contains. Some of the highest-ranking foods on the ORAC scale include the spice turmeric, açaí berries, dark chocolate (yes, chocolate, thanks to its cocoa content), and black plums. Other antioxidant-rich foods include:

- *Apples*
- *Pomegranates*
- *Artichokes*
- *Prunes*
- *Beans (red, kidney, pinto, black)*
- *Berries (blackberries, cranberries, strawberries, blueberries, raspberries)*
- *Dark, leafy greens (arugula, spinach, lettuce, kale)*
- *Nuts (pecans, walnuts, chestnuts)*

2. Calcium. A lot of people think of dairy as an ideal source of calcium, but as I've already covered, you really should only eat dairy products in moderation—and when you do eat them, they should be full-fat. Sesame seeds are an even better source of calcium. You can sprinkle them on everything—salads, soups, roasted vegetables. And try tahini, a spread made of ground sesame seeds; mixed with a little miso and lemon juice (and thinned to taste with water), it makes a great dip for raw vegetables.

3. Choline. The amino acid choline helps improve the quality of your follicles, which are what house and release your eggs. In general, the more follicles you have, the better your chances are of becoming pregnant. Once you're pregnant, choline also helps with your baby's brain development. Organic eggs are packed with choline. Just make sure you eat the whites *and* the yolk. Chicken, turkey, and salmon are also healthful sources of this nutrient. You need about 250 milligrams (mg) of choline a day, which you should be able to get through food.

4. Folate. You're going to hear me talk a lot about folate in this book because it is so critical in the prevention of birth defects. But it's also an important factor in fertility: It may help increase levels of the "pregnancy hormone" progesterone in your body and lower your chances of ovulating irregularly. Folate is the natural form of vitamin B9 (folic acid is the synthetic form). These foods are exceptionally high in folate:

- *Citrus fruits*
- *Dairy products and eggs*
- *Dark, leafy greens (kale, turnip greens, spinach, lettuce) and other green veggies (asparagus, Brussels sprouts, broccoli)*
- *Legumes (peas, beans, lentils)*
- *Nuts and seeds*

Note that fresh veggies can lose a lot of their folate content while they sit waiting to be cooked and during the cooking process itself. Try not to store them too long in the refrigerator, and consider eating them raw or cooked only lightly at a low temperature.

5. Iron. This nutrient is another big one for helping reduce your risk of infertility due to problems with ovulation, not to mention for helping you avoid becoming anemic, which can be harmful to both you and your baby. Good sources of iron are:

- *Beets (and their greens) and beet powder*
- *Blackstrap molasses*
- *Butternut squash*
- *Chicken*
- *Dark, leafy greens*
- *Dried fruits: peaches, raisins, apricots*
- *Legumes*
- *Nuts and seeds*
- *Oysters*
- *Rice and wild rice*

In addition to eating the foods listed above, you can also cook in cast iron pots and pans. Doing so can increase the iron content in the foods you're preparing.

6. Omega-3 fatty acids. These healthy fats can help boost blood flow to your reproductive organs, and that stimulates ovulation. Omega-3s may also help regulate all the hormones involved in pregnancy. Wild salmon, sardines, herring, and other cold-water, fatty fish are rich sources, as are yolks from pastured or enriched eggs and grass-fed beef. You can also get a certain type of omega-3 from algae, flaxseed, and walnuts, but this form has to be converted by your body to the forms provided by animal sources (like fish), and it's an inefficient process. So, it's best to eat the salmon and the eggs so long as you're not a staunch vegetarian or vegan. That being said, I'm a big fan of walnuts. Not only are they chock-full of these healthy fats, but they're high in magnesium too. Like omega-3s, magnesium can boost blood flow to the uterus and help your body pump out progesterone.

7. Zinc. This nutrient is absolutely critical for conception. If you're deficient in zinc, your body may not produce good-quality eggs or might produce them more slowly than it normally would. Getting the recommended dietary allowance of zinc is an easy way to keep your reproductive system functioning as it should. Oysters are the most concentrated food source of zinc. If you're not a fan, try eating more legumes, like lentils and chickpeas; whole grains; eggs; and nuts.

Supplements to Enhance Fertility

I definitely recommend meeting as many of your nutrient needs as possible through diet. Meaning, don't think that you can make up for a crappy diet by taking a handful of supplements. But when you're trying to become pregnant, and trying to create the best possible chances for conception—not to mention working to make the healthiest environment for your baby to begin life—I believe supplements are an important part of your routine. The sad truth is that even the freshest organic produce isn't as full of nutrients as it used to be, because factory farming has depleted our soils. That's why supplementation is so important. Just remember, it's not a free pass to eat as much junk food as you want.

I am a huge proponent of taking a prenatal vitamin, even when you are preconception. If you ask me, one prenatal is never enough. Now that I'm in the business of creating nonsynthetic, high-quality skincare products, and have researched adding prenatal vitamins to my line, I can promise you, there's really no way to fit everything you need into one small pill and have it still be first-rate. I think of it this way: Unless you want to have a basic baby, don't take a basic prenatal vitamin! You are going to have to source a few different supplements to cover all your bases. Here's what you should look for:

- Choose a prenatal rich in antioxidants, and that contains nutrients like myo-inositol and N-acetylcysteine, which both increase your ovulation rate, as well as D-chiro-inositol, which supports an appropriate balance of important pregnancy hormones and healthy insulin levels (as I mentioned earlier, high insulin levels can cause problems with pregnancy). I took Ultra-Mins, made by Nature's Plus.

- Also make sure that your prenatal vitamin includes folate, which, remember, is the active form of vitamin B9. The synthetic form, folic acid, isn't bioavailable, meaning your body doesn't easily absorb it. Not to mention, 40 percent of women have a mutation in their MTHFR gene, which keeps them from properly absorbing folic acid. If that's the case for you (you may get a clue that it is if whenever you've taken a B complex you've experienced a flushing sensation in your skin), once you do conceive, it's possible your baby won't get enough folate, which is why you may want to consider taking ample amounts in supplement form. The standard recommendation is for your prenatal to have 400 micrograms (mcg) of folate, but I personally believe you need a prenatal with at least 600 mcg of folate or more. Before my pregnancies, I started taking 800 mcg of folate (note: not folic acid).

- If you are or may be deficient in vitamin B12 (a deficiency vegetarians are more prone to experience, because B12 is mostly only found in animal foods), also make sure you're getting enough through your prenatal or an additional supplement. Taking it together with folate, for roughly three months before conception, may vastly improve

"UNLESS YOU WANT to HAVE A BASIC BABY, DON'T TAKE A BASIC PRENATAL VITAMIN!"

the chances of your baby being born without any neural tube defects. Pregnant and nursing moms need about 2.8 mcg of B12 per day. In fact, the entire family of B vitamins is extremely important for fertility and a healthy pregnancy. If your prenatal doesn't contain adequate amounts of B vitamins, consider a B-complex.

- According to animal studies, coenzyme Q10, also called CoQ10, appears to help improve egg quality in older mice.[4] It may do the same in people: A human trial found that supplementing with CoQ10 resulted in higher fertilization rates, as well as more high-quality embryos. It could also improve ovulation and boost the quantity of ovarian follicles.[5]

- Vitamin C could help address some types of female infertility by promoting ovulation, and one study found that women under 29 who supplemented with vitamin C took less time to get pregnant.[6]

  Before my pregnancies, I took a vitamin C supplement with bioflavonoids, which have some serious antioxidant power (refer back to page 24 for details about antioxidants and fertility).

- In addition to eating more omega-3s before my pregnancy, I supplemented with DHA, a long-chain omega-3 fatty acid. Remember, omega-3s help encourage blood flow to your reproductive organs, stimulating ovulation, and may help regulate pregnancy hormones. DHA, in particular, appears to increase progesterone levels, the hormone that helps regulate the lining of your uterus. In other words, progesterone is essential to pregnancy. Nordic Naturals is a reputable brand of omega-3 supplements.

Of course, you should talk with your doctor or midwife about any supplements that you're taking or plan to take, especially if you're also on conventional hormone or drug treatments for infertility.

Fertility Detox: Chemicals to Avoid

Common chemicals—found in everything from flooring and furniture, to cleaning products, to makeup—can negatively impact your fertility, and your health at large. My doctors told

A Beyond-the-Basics Prenatal Supplement Plan

This is the regimen that Mari Mikel, my midwife, recommended and that I followed. I took all my supplements with food; specifically, I took them when I had eaten about a third of my meal, so that there would already be food in my stomach (to buffer the ingredients and prevent stomach upset) and my digestive enzymes would be flowing (to help break down the pills).

Morning

Vitamin E	400 IUs
Vitamin C (ester C with bioflavonoids)	1000 mg
Probiotics	as directed

(choose one with multiple strains—the more the better)

1 teaspoon ground flaxseed

(sprinkled on your food or in your smoothie, ground fresh right before you eat it so that the fats in the seeds don't oxidize and go rancid)

Lunch

Ultra-Mins	2 tablets
B50	as directed

(has 50 mg of all B vitamins and sometimes folate)

Folate	enough to total 800 mcg

(check to see how much folate your B50 contains)

Dinner

Vitamin E	400 IUs
Vitamin C	1000 mg
Beta-carotene	as directed on bottle
Omega-3s	enough for a minimum of 300 mg DHA

(Nordic Naturals is the official brand of the American Pregnancy Ass.)

Evening primrose oil	1000 mg
Vitamin D	4000 IU

Bedtime

Ultra-Mins	1 tablet

me that my autoimmune condition, which I discussed in Chapter 1, was likely triggered by some toxic exposure. Unfortunately, there are chemicals in so many products and places, like the soil and our water supply, that it would be hard to track down the exact source of your infertility. That means it's best to take a blanket approach and try to remove as many chemicals from your daily life as you can. That said, we do have an idea of which chemicals are some of the top fertility offenders.

Many of the chemicals used in food containers, cleaning products, and personal care products are commonly referred to as endocrine disruptors. That means they can disrupt your hormones, which can negatively impact egg quality and thus your chances of conceiving.

Here are some of the most important chemicals to avoid when you're trying to get pregnant. Of course, it's only possible to do so much. Don't stress yourself out over getting rid of every potentially problematic product in your house and purse. Just do the best you can, and know that every step you take counts.

1. Bisphenol A (BPA). BPA is a plasticizer and is often used in plastic food and beverage containers, including water bottles. It can also be found in the lining of food cans. I'm sure you've heard to avoid this toxic chemical, as it's gotten a lot of press, especially regarding its impact on fertility. Research suggests it can leach from these containers into our food, where it can then find its way into our bloodstream. It's really important that you look for items that are BPA-free or, better yet, use glass or stainless steel products to store your food and carry your water. BPA is also the chemical that makes sales receipts shiny, so avoid handling receipts as much as you can, and clean out the bottom of your purse of any receipts that have collected there. (And when you have kids, don't let them touch receipts or, worse, put them in their mouths!)

2. Polytetrafluoroethylene (PTFE) & polytetrafluoroethylene (PFOA). PTFE is also known as Teflon, and PFOA is used in the process of making Teflon. These chemicals can mess with your menstrual cycle, so say no to Teflon-coated pots and pans; use stainless steel, cast iron, ceramic, or copper-clad pans instead.

3. Parabens and phthalates. These chemicals hide in your personal care products, from your perfume to your shampoo. Parabens can act like estrogen in the body, and when your estrogen is artificially high, your odds of creating healthy eggs decrease. Phthalates can also throw off hormone levels and otherwise negatively impact fertility. (See Chapter 3 for my recommendations of all-natural personal care products, as well as several recipes for making your own skincare products at home.)

4. Pesticides and herbicides. A large number of pesticides and herbicides used in agriculture are suspected endocrine disruptors, and studies link the consumption of high amounts of pesticides through fruits and vegetables with significant reductions in fertility and viable pregnancies. Buy certified organic produce whenever possible. And know that many small farms, although not certified, use organic practices. Visit your local farmers market to talk directly with farmers and ask about how they grow their food. Also avoid using any pesticides and herbicides on your lawn and garden at home. There are lots of natural options that are just as effective at reducing unwanted pests.

To further protect yourself from toxic fertility-busting chemicals, look for all-natural, "green" cleaning products, or make them yourself with things you already have in your pantry, like baking soda and vinegar. (I include a recipe for DIY all-purpose and glass cleaners, as well as share some of my favorite "green" cleaning brands, in Chapter 3.)

And avoid using air fresheners and artificially scented candles in your house, as well as household cleaners containing artificial fragrances; all of these items can emit large quantities of harmful endocrine disruptors into the air. You might also consider using a HEPA filter, which purifies the air and can keep you from breathing indoor pollutants.

Fertility-Harming Habits to Rethink

While yes, your body is programmed to be able to sustain and carry a baby all on its own, there are a couple things you likely do everyday, probably even multiple times a day, that could be getting in the way. Namely: using your cellphone and Wi-Fi, and drinking

What Various Supplements Do

B Vitamins
- Emotional balance
- Nausea prevention
- Protein assimilation
- Muscle and organ development in baby

Vitamin E
- Assistance in skin's ability to stretch
- Softening of ligaments and pelvic floor
- Prevention of stretch marks, varicose veins, hemorrhoids, miscarriages
- Placental attachment and detachment
- Development of baby's reproductive system

Folate
- Neural tube development in baby's spine and skull
- Heart disease prevention for mother
- Liver development in the baby
- Reduction of PMS symptoms

Omega-3s
- Brain and nerve development in baby
- Cancer prevention
- Skin health
- Prevention of Alzheimer's and Parkinson's diseases

Vitamin C
- Iron absorption
- Capillary development
- Immune system function
- Prevention of bruising, nosebleeds, and gum bleeding
- Assistance in creating a strong immune system in baby
- Prevention of stretch marks, varicose veins, hemorrhoids, miscarriages
- Placental attachment and detachment
- Development of baby's reproductive system

Evening Primrose Oil
- Blood pressure reduction
- Pregnancy hormone precursor
- Tissue softening in mother, including uterus, cervix, vagina, and pelvis

unlimited amounts of alcohol and caffeine. I know it may feel like a pretty big sacrifice to cut down on these things; just hear me out before you decide.

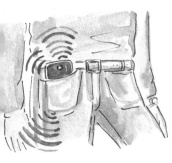

Watch Where You Keep Your Cellphone (and Where He Keeps His Too)

One thing that has a big impact on fertility but isn't yet on most people's radar is exposure to electromagnetic frequencies (EMFs), which are emitted by anything electronic. The EMFs emitted by cellphones, Wi-Fi, smart appliances, cordless phones, and even baby monitors are all microwave frequencies. They have been shown to produce oxidative stress, which, as I talked about earlier in the section on antioxidants, can contribute to infertility.[7]

Even more specifically, though, exposure to EMFs has been shown to reduce sperm count,[8] sperm quality,[9] sperm viability,[10] and sperm motility[11] (the ability of sperm to move). And think about where most men keep their cellphones—in their pockets, right next to their crotch. Really, until the science is more settled, no one should keep their cellphone on their body. But especially when you're trying to get pregnant, convince your male partner to keep his phone out of his pocket. Fertility is a two-person production, and it's widely documented that male sperm counts are declining.

Consider Getting a Flu Shot Now

Once you are pregnant, your immunity can take a little hit, making you more susceptible to the flu. Your health care provider will likely strongly encourage you to get the flu shot (as did my midwife, Mari Mikel—see page 129 for more of her thoughts on why the vaccine is important). The only hitch is that you want to avoid getting the flu shot during your first trimester when your body is so wholly occupied with forming the baby and the placenta. If you're trying to get pregnant during flu season, consider getting the shot now, before you are pregnant, so that you'll already be protected once you conceive. If you miss this window, you may want to wait until the second trimester, when you body has a bit more bandwidth.

Other ways to reduce your EMF exposure:

- Get the Wi-Fi router out of your bedroom (where you definitely don't need it while you're sleeping) and as far away from where you spend most of your time at home.

- Replace cordless phones with regular phones.

- Don't take your cellphone into your bedroom; if that's a habit you can't break, put it on airplane mode before you go to sleep so it can't irradiate you all night while you rest and repair.

- Consider switching from Wi-Fi back to Ethernet cables.

- I'll talk more about this in Chapter 9, but look for a low-EMF baby monitor before you register for one or purchase one.

What About Caffeine?

I love a cup of coffee as much as the next person. And I'm not going to tell you that you have to quit it while you're trying to get pregnant. But it is true that caffeine really isn't good for the baby. My midwife, Mari Mikel, says she can see on an ultrasound how jumpy a baby is whose mom has recently had caffeine. So if you're a caffeine junkie now, you probably want to start to reduce your intake; then when you do get pregnant, it won't be like jumping off a cliff. Turn the page for Mari Mikel's advice on why and how to do it.

Other Lifestyle Changes to Make Now

Pregnancy, labor and delivery, and parenting are all highly physical pursuits. To ensure you have the healthiest pregnancy possible, it's ideal to develop a pregnancy exercise routine and begin following it now, before you even get pregnant. It may have to change some over the course of your pregnancy, and that's okay. But just as you want to give your baby the right foundation from the start through a healthy diet, you also want to ensure that you're strengthening your body right out of the gate too. Plus, exercise creates endorphins, which help your mood and outlook so much.

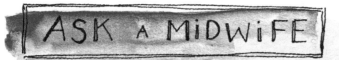

ASK A MIDWIFE

IS IT OK TO DRINK WHILE TRYING TO GET PREGNANT?

from MARI MIKEL:

"Honestly, I think it's mostly fine. The only problem is if you can't be moderate with it; then it's better not to drink at all. But I do think a little bit is very beneficial because it lowers stress hormones, which is why people reach for a drink in the first place! Alcohol is a smooth muscle relaxer. You've got smooth muscle in your gastrointestinal tract, walls of the heart, and walls of the uterus. If you are stressed and you have a drink, it makes your heart feel better, your digestion better, and it relaxes the uterus. In fact, before the drugs we have today, they'd give women alcohol in an IV to slow their contractions down during premature labor.

"My best advice is to start using alcohol medicinally. When you're stressed out, that's the time for a glass of wine. You can have four 4-ounce glasses of wine a month. If it's a special occasion and you want to have two glasses of wine, spread them out over a few hours with plenty of food and drink along the way. If you feel you need more than that, start to experiment with other ways to reduce your stress (like meditation, yoga, exercise, therapy, or even something cathartic like axe throwing)."

If you already exercise, keep it up. If you haven't been getting that much activity, start moving more. It's really common to feel exhausted at the very beginning of pregnancy, so you may find that once you are pregnant you don't have a ton of energy for regular movement—all the more reason to get started now.

You don't have to kill it at an aggressive Cross Fit-type of workout. Taking walks, riding a bike, dancing, gardening, and yoga all count. A little bit of strength training—my favorite strength-training exercises are bodyweight movements like squats and push-ups—can

ASK A MIDWIFE

CAN I DRINK CAFFEINE WHILE I'M TRYING TO GET PREGNANT?

from MARI MiKeL:

"First, let me tell you that I truly love the flavor of coffee and the ritual of it. It's really a special thing. The problem is, caffeine is also super addictive, for you and the baby. I've seen a lot of newborn babies go through caffeine withdrawal: They cry and cry for days after birth because of withdrawal headaches. My baby was one of them. I drank about two cups a day when I was pregnant (this was 45 years ago when no one knew you should wean off caffeine).

"So if you're trying to get pregnant, it's really a good idea to start reducing your dependence on caffeine for everyone's sake. Start cutting down. Because if you get pregnant and try quitting cold turkey, you're going to get headaches at a time when you may already not be feeling all that well.

"To wean yourself off, buy the best all-natural decaf version of whatever it is you like to drink. Initially, replace a quarter of your daily cup with decaf for a week. Then the next week, make it half caffeinated and half decaffeinated. In week three, drink cups that are three-quarters decaf. At this point, you can still have one or two fully caffeinated moments a week. All the other times, switch to decaf. Get to the point where you only have one caffeinated beverage a week. Remember that iced tea and chocolate also have a lot of caffeine, so be mindful of your consumption of those too.

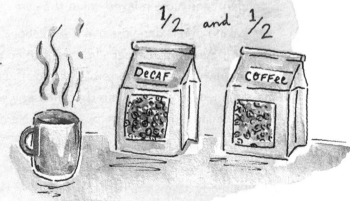

"This way, once the baby is here and you've been up all night and need a pick-me-up to get through the day, you'll be able to have just a half cup of coffee and it will work extremely well!"

go a long way to giving your muscles the power they need to carry a baby and then get the baby out. I love the Lagree Method for the times when I'm not pregnant or recovering from birth, because it covers a lot of exercise bases in a short time. (I talk in depth about specific forms of exercise in Chapter 6—feel free to skip ahead for more inspiration.)

Prepregnancy is also the perfect time to begin building core awareness and strength, and to start caring for your pelvic floor, which, contrary to popular belief, typically needs to be released and lengthened before it can be strengthened. Trust me, you will be so thankful you did. After all, your core is what will help you push your baby out, while your pelvic floor will not only support the weight of the baby but also soften enough to allow them an easy passage. The good news is that you can achieve this needed strength with just two simple breathing exercises: diaphragmatic breathing and the belly pump. These are the two foundational exercises used by Brooke Cates, founder of the Bloom Method, who was my personal trainer when I was pregnant and who taught me—and who has taught thousands of moms-to-be—how to take better care of my core and pelvic floor.

I'm so excited that Brooke has agreed to provide exercises for your entire pregnancy journey, from now until your first checkup post birth. You'll see contributions from her in the chapters to come. For now, to get a jump on your core and pelvic floor training, see Brooke's instructions for diaphragmatic breathing and the belly pump. I think you'll find, like I did, that they will help you not only feel better about these two parts of your body that you either don't like or don't think about all that much, but also feel stronger, more confident, and more relaxed, all at the same time.

Speaking of relaxing, if you're a workaholic, think about how you can start to make room in your life now for the baby you want to come. I think the universe definitely looks not just to our words but also to our actions to see what we're truly ready for. You want to make some space in your life that the baby will be able to inhabit, kind of like you clear off the dining room table before you have a dinner party.

You don't have to make all of these changes at once, so don't let them overwhelm you. Pick one or two changes you'll implement each week, and by the time you're pregnant, you'll already have so many great habits working for you and for your baby.

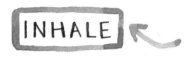

INHALE

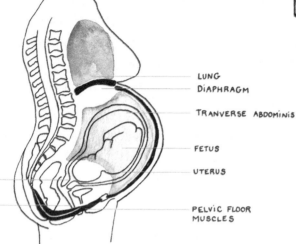

DIAPHRAGMATIC BREATH

LUNG
DIAPHRAGM
TRANVERSE ABDOMINIS
FETUS
UTERUS
CERVIX
VAGINA
PELVIC FLOOR MUSCLES

ACTIVATE LUNGS AND DIAPHRAGM

LENGTHEN TRANSVERSE ABDOMINIS AND PELVIC FLOOR MUSCLES

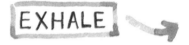

EXHALE

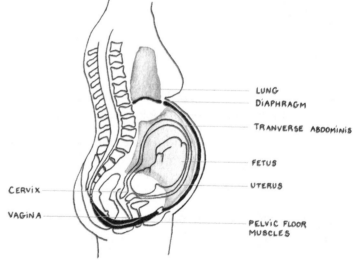

LUNG
DIAPHRAGM
TRANVERSE ABDOMINIS
FETUS
UTERUS
CERVIX
VAGINA
PELVIC FLOOR MUSCLES

TRANSVERSE ABDOMINIS AND PELVIC FLOOR MUSCLES REBOUND TO THEIR NEUTRAL STATE

INTENTIONAL ACTIVATION DOESN'T OCCUR

the BLOOM method

Get Connected to Your Core

The best way to begin to train and tone your core, according to Brooke, is to breathe better. She's got two exercises here to help you do just that—diaphragmatic breathing and the belly pump. Starting with these two exercises is the first step to building your most functional and strongest core ever—something you're definitely going to want to have for birth and beyond. As an added bonus, these two exercises will help you retrain yourself on how to breathe fully, which will help you reduce stress now and steady you when it's time for labor and delivery.

Practice these exercises for a total of five or six minutes a day (so, two to three minutes per exercise). You can do diaphragmatic breathing for one minute, take a break, and then do one minute of the belly pump, alternating for at least five minutes. You can also break it up into two minutes in the morning and three minutes at night.

Diaphragmatic Breathing

Position: Lying supine, sitting, on all fours, or standing

Instructions:

- As you gently inhale, allow your ribcage, abdomen, sides of the body, and back body to expand. Feel the pelvic floor slowly soften as you do.

- Slowly exhale and feel the belly, sides of the body, and back fall back toward the spine and the pelvic floor rise back to its neutral state.

- Don't force anything or intentionally engage any muscles.

- Repeat anywhere, anytime you remember—on the subway, in an Uber, at your desk, lying in bed. If you don't have time or energy for a full workout, this alone can be your core exercise for the day.

Brooke says: "Allow this breath to become your new normal so that you begin to teach the inner core unit how to work together the way it was designed to do. You breathe 20,000 + times a day, so the sky's the limit. It will help reduce your stress as it strengthens your core; it also makes more space for the baby to turn and position themselves head-down when the time is right."

Belly Pump

Position: Sitting on a stability ball or chair, or lying on your back

Instructions:

- As you inhale, expand through your ribcage, abdomen, sides of the body and back body; the ribcage and belly will naturally expand—you may be surprised how far the belly can extend!—and the pelvic floor will soften. You want to allow the belly expansion to be natural; don't force it.

- As you exhale, make an Ssssss sound and begin engaging the pelvic floor muscles as you then start to engage your core as if you were tightening a corset around your torso or hugging the baby, imagining the activation moving up the core from the hip bones, mid-section, ribcage. Take your time and allow your breath and core activation to be slow and controlled.

- Repeat for your chosen duration of time or number of breaths.

From Brooke: "Doing the belly pump decreases the chance of stretch marks because you're teaching the belly to expand and grow gradually, instead of popping later to accommodate the baby. It also lays the foundation for knowing how to use your core in aiding for pushing. And, it helps you practice lengthening and engaging the core and pelvic floor, which prevents the pregnancy-related separation of the abdominal muscles known as diastasis recti, as well as the likelihood of incontinence and uterine prolapse after birth."

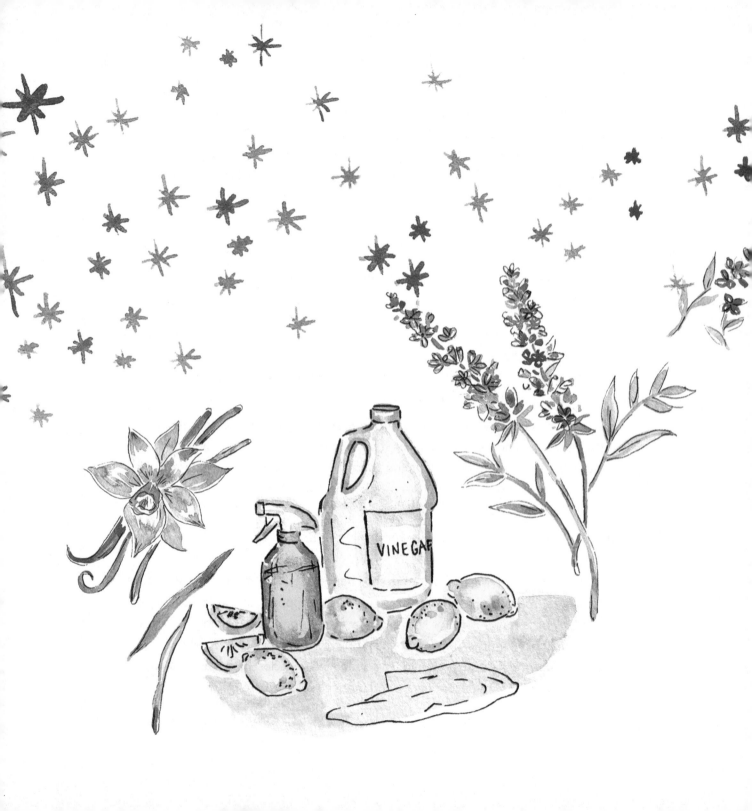

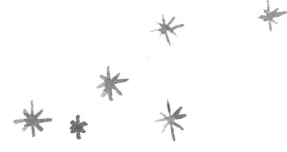

Chapter 3

NATURAL REMEDIES FOR PREPREGNANCY

Throughout the book I'll share my favorite ways to relieve the more challenging parts of the pregnancy journey. At this point, when you aren't pregnant yet, it's less about managing symptoms and more about keeping your mind in a healthy place, so I've included remedies for anxiety and moments of sadness, as well as tips for keeping your sex life feeling like fun (instead of like a baby-making job).

And because so many of the chemicals in household and personal care products can potentially disrupt your delicate hormonal balance, and because doctors told me my autoimmune condition was likely triggered by some chemical exposure, I believe every woman—whether you're seeking to get pregnant or not—needs to reduce the number of chemicals she comes in contact with so that your hormones stay balanced and your body doesn't have to tax itself by spending a lot of energy on detoxing. For that reason, I'm also including recipes for some DIY cleaning and self-care products so you can start reducing your chemical exposure now.

Anxiety

It's completely natural to experience feelings of anxiousness as you're trying to get pregnant. You're embarking on a big endeavor where you aren't in control of the outcome. There are a lot of what ifs. That doesn't mean you have to white knuckle your way through the experience. There are natural ways to lessen anxiety and overall stress; the more relaxed you are, the more you'll be able to navigate whatever twists and turns your journey to motherhood takes.

Cutting down on your caffeine intake, as I covered in Chapter 2, can help because caffeine can make you feel on edge. It's a stimulant, after all, and when you're in the grips of anxiety, your thoughts are generally going a mile a minute. Caffeine can also induce a lot of the same symptoms as anxiety, including nervousness, difficulty sleeping, a fast heart rate, restlessness, and digestive problems. So if you're experiencing a lot of anxiety now, all the more reason to start the caffeine weaning process Mari Mikel suggests on page 37.

There's also a well-established link between anxiety and your gut health. Even very mainstream publications like the *Journal of the American Medical Association* have published papers that suggest that taking probiotic supplements to boost the population of friendly bacteria in your digestive tract can ease anxiety symptoms.[12] Those bacteria play a big role in creating neurotransmitters, such as serotonin, that contribute to mental health. Look for a probiotic supplement that contains the strain *Lactobacillus rhamnosus* or *L. rhamnosus*, because a wealth of evidence suggests that it, in particular, can significantly reduce anxiety.[13]

I also love to use essential oils for anxiety. In a pinch you can inhale their aroma straight from the bottle, although you want to be careful not to get them directly on your skin, as they could burn the sensitive area around your nose. Using a diffuser near you when you work or sleep is another great way to inhale them safely. The best oils for anxiety are clary sage (which isn't safe to use once you're pregnant, as it can stimulate labor; when you're still seeking to get pregnant, it's fine), lavender, ylang ylang, and bergamot. You can use just one or make a blend.

If your anxiety is coming on all the time, find a support group or consider talking to a therapist. Getting some kind of psychological support can help you feel understood and stay positive.

Setting the Mood for Sex

It's fun to try to make a baby... until you get to the point where you start thinking of it like something you have to do. If it takes months or years to get pregnant, sex can stop being anything remotely like fun and can instead become a source of stress and frustration.

You really only have a window of about eight days during the month when you're fertile, so if it's starting to feel like a chore, it can be helpful to save sex for these days. And remember, the days around ovulation naturally make you feel your sexiest, your most energetic, and your most "in the mood." But it can really go both ways here, because having sex when you know you're highly unlikely to get pregnant might take some of the pressure off and help you both enjoy yourselves more. My point is, experiment with your timing so that you can find a frequency that covers your fertility bases without feeling like you've added another task on your to-do list.

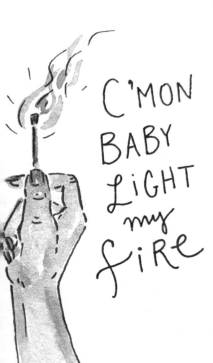

It's easy to treat sex like a job when you're trying to get pregnant, but do what it takes to truly get aroused. Research shows that men produce more sperm after viewing sexy images containing more than one man and a woman (because, researchers theorize, they're trying to prepare themselves to compete with other males and thus will produce more, and more robust, sperm—whatever, guys!)[14], and that women who are more aroused produce more cervical fluid, which is designed to help sperm make their way to the egg.

Finally, talk to your partner about how you're feeling about sex. It's too tempting to keep it inside. Be honest but gentle. It's easy to take things personally when you're talking about sex, but if you don't talk about it, it can also be easy to forget that you're both in this together.

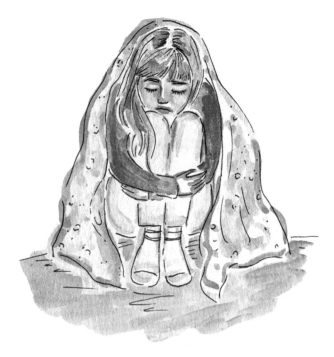

Feeling Sad

If you've suffered one or more miscarriages, or it's taking a lot longer to get pregnant than you thought it would, it's completely natural to experience some big feelings, like loss, sadness, grief, and anger. Fertility challenges and miscarriages hit different women differently. However the journey to pregnancy is affecting you, you've got to let yourself feel these feelings. Honestly, parenthood is a series of mini griefs—as your kid gets older, phases come and go that you wish you could hold onto. What's more, the whole goal of parenting is for them to grow up and become their own people with their own lives. There will be achievements you wish for them that don't come to pass, and hardships you hope they never have to face that do. My point is, being a good parent requires you learn how to process your feelings.

My go-to when I'm feeling all the feels (or feeling blue) is exercise. Getting your heart rate up clears your head; helps bring your hormones, such as insulin, adrenaline, and cortisol, back into balance; and produces endorphins, which boost your mood. Hopefully you're already upping your exercise game, as we covered in Chapter 2. But if you haven't yet and you're reading this section because you're feeling down, let this be the nudge you need to get going.

Again, talking to a therapist can be really helpful, and there are some who specialize in working with women during big life transitions like pregnancy. Journaling is also a great way to get your feelings out and give you some perspective on your thought process.

ASK A MIDWIFE

WHEN CAN I TRY AGAIN AFTER HAVING A MISCARRIAGE?

from MARi MiKeL:

"I always counsel women to have at least two periods before trying to get pregnant again. You want to build your uterine lining back up so that it is strong and healthy for the new baby. That means using birth control for at least two cycles. Give yourself time to heal physically, emotionally, and spiritually so that your heart is in a place of joy. When you are sad or upset there is a whole hormonal state that goes along with that that can imprint on the baby (depending on the baby).

"A lot of women I talk to expect to jump back into trying after a few days, but you have to allow the process to unfold or else your feelings will get stuffed down. Take however much time you need to feel the feelings. And don't listen to the people who say unhelpful things like, 'It's no big deal you were only seven weeks.' For some women, miscarriage isn't that big of a deal and that's completely fine, but for others who had already envisioned the whole life of that child, it's a very tangible and big loss. However you're feeling, don't let anyone negate it, including you."

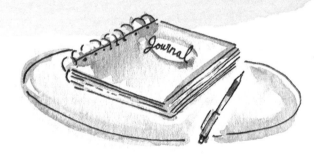

Natural Household and Personal Care Products

It's so easy to make your own cleaning and skincare products, and dare I say, it's fun too, sort of like being a kid and making potions out of stuff you find in the medicine cabinet or pantry. What's more, you can make products that work as well as if not better than what you can find at the store—and for a fraction of the cost. Here are a few of my favorite recipes.

Household Cleaners

All-Purpose Cleaner

This cleaner couldn't be easier to make. You will also need a spray bottle—you can buy a new one (look for a glass version if you can find one) or re-use an empty one that you've washed well with hot water. Using a funnel will make it mess-free.

It works well on any household surface except glass—countertops, toilet seats, walls, floors, tables, even toys.

Ingredients:

- 1 cup water
- ½ cup vinegar
- 2 tbsp baking soda
- Juice of ½ lemon or 15 drops essential oils*

*optional for fragrance

Instructions:

1. Pour the water into a 16-ounce spray bottle.

2. Add the vinegar, then the baking soda, then the essential oils or the lemon juice.

3. Screw the top on and mix by turning the bottle upside down and right side up a few times.

4. When you use the cleaner, mix the cleaner again to redistribute the oils or lemon juice.

There's no need to buy another bottle of that smelly bright blue liquid—this glass cleaner works great. Use with a microfiber cloth for a truly earth-friendly experience.

Ingredients:

- 2 cups distilled (or boiled) water
- 2 tbsp white vinegar
- 10 drops essential oil—use your favorite; I like orange, grapefruit, or lemon for their bright, citrus-y scents

Instructions:

Combine everything in a spray bottle and use as you would a regular glass cleaner.

Note: The first time you make this you may want to add a teaspoon of castile soap to the mixture to remove any residue from the conventional glass cleaner you were using before.

Personal Care Products

According to the Environmental Working Group, the average American woman uses 12 products on her body, which adds up to 168 different chemicals. I love a good skincare product, believe me, but it's really easy to make nontoxic and great-working products yourself—that's exactly how my skincare company, MUTHA, started, with me making various lotions and creams at home. Here, I'll share some of my favorite DIY recipes that I used while pregnant to keep my skin healthy and glowing. If you're like me and interested in turning your kitchen into a full-blown science lab, I have included some recipes that are a bit more advanced and require special ingredients. There are also a few simple ones that you can create with ingredients you have in your kitchen/pantry right now, and they're just as great.

If you're not up for whipping up lotions at home, the Environmental Working Group's Skin Deep database (www.ewg.org/skindeep) is a great resource for finding healthier versions of the personal items you use everyday. They rate everything from sunscreen to face wash in terms of how healthy the item is for both you and the environment. I'm also including a list of my favorite all-natural skincare products in the box on page 55. (Of course, this list includes a couple from MUTHA—I'm nearly as proud of them as I am my own children, and can attest that my team and I put in tons of research to make them the highest quality and the most natural.)

Dual-Purpose Green Tea Toner

Green tea is very high in antioxidants and has many pH-balancing qualities.

Ingredients:

- 1 tsp organic green tea
- 1 cup water
- ¼ tsp raw apple cider vinegar (optional)

Instructions:

1. Bring 1 cup of water to a boil and let it cool to 175 degrees Fahrenheit.
2. Place the tea leaves at the bottom of a cup, and pour the water over the leaves.
3. Cover and let steep for 10 minutes.

Brands that Make High-Quality Nontoxic Cleaners

Making your own cleaning products truly is so easy and satisfying, but you can also buy natural products if you want to save the time and effort. Some of my favorite brands include:

- Supernatural
- Dr. Bronner's
- Method
- Mrs. Meyer's (unscented versions only)
- Seventh Generation
- Bon Ami
- The Honest Company

4. Strain the leaves from the water and allow tea to cool.

5. Add the raw apple cider vinegar if you choose to and stir.

6. On a clean face, apply via a spray bottle or on a cotton round.

7. Apply your moisturizer of choice.

8. Drink the rest and relax.

Hydrating Avocado Mask

The vitamins in avocado are ideal for dry skin. The potassium in bananas will keep your skin soft and hydrated as well, while honey is great for healing wounds and killing bacteria.

Ingredients:

- *¼ banana*
- *¼ avocado*
- *1 tsp organic honey*
- *1 tsp avocado oil*

Instructions:

1. Mash the banana and avocado in a bowl and add the honey and oil. It's easiest to do this with a hand mixer or blender. Otherwise, a fork or whisk will do.

2. Apply to your clean face, neck, and décolletage.

3. Leave on for 15-20 minutes and rinse with warm water. Your skin will be hydrated and glowy.

Fruit Enzyme Exfoliant

This treatment will lighten hyperpigmentation if used regularly. It's normal for it to tingle or sting as the juice dries. This means the acid in the fruit is working by ridding you of your dead skin cells.

Ingredient:

- *3 tbsp raw papaya or pineapple*

Instructions:

1. Use a mortar and pestle to smash the fruit until pulpy.

2. Strain the pulp and collect 1 tablespoon of the juice.

3. Use a cotton ball or cotton round to absorb the juice.

4. Apply to the face, neck, and décolletage in an upward motion.

5. Rinse with cool water after 10 minutes.

Vanilla Bath and Body Oil

This dreamy-smelling oil will leave your skin soft and silky.

Ingredients:

- 3 long vanilla beans
- 1½ cups jojoba base oil

Instructions:

1. Slice the vanilla beans lengthwise and scrape the paste from the pods using the tip of a knife.

2. Chop the empty vanilla bean pods into little pieces and add to a glass jar.

3. Pour the jojoba oil over the vanilla beans and paste.

4. Cover the jar and shake for 60 seconds.

5. Store the jar in a dark place for 2 months—a kitchen cabinet is perfect.

6. Shake the jar every few days for 10 seconds.

7. When the 2 months is up, strain the oil through a mesh strainer or coffee filter (you can even use an old pair of nylon stockings!) and pour into a glass bottle.

8. Add 2 teaspoons to your bath or use on your body as a moisturizer or a massage oil. Use within 2 years.

Note: If the jojoba oil hardens, move the mixture to a warmer spot in your house— like a sunny windowsill—for an hour to soften.

Rosy Lavender Cleanser

Not only does this nourish as it cleanses, it also smells divine.

Ingredients:

- ⅓ cup finely ground oatmeal or oat flour
- 1 tbsp powdered rose petals
- 2 drops rose otto essential oil
- ½ cup finely ground white clay
- 1 tbsp powdered lavender buds
- 5 drops lavender essential oil

Instructions :

1. Put all dry ingredients into a container or glass Mason jar.
2. Cover and shake well to blend.
3. Add the essential oils and shake one more time.
4. Store in a cool, dry place (lasts for six months).
5. When you're ready to use, place 2 teaspoons of the powdered mixture into a small bowl and add 2 teaspoons of water or milk of choice. Stir to blend into a paste and let thicken for 1 minute.
6. Apply cleanser to face, neck, and décolletage, and massage in circular motions for 1 minute.
7. Rinse with warm water.
8. Can also be used as a mask if you let it dry on the skin for 60 seconds after massaging.

Lube

Yes, you can even make your own lubricant! (If you don't want to DIY this one, there are many clean, organic lubes out there—look for options that don't contain glycerin, which could contribute to a yeast infection; parabens, preservatives that are also hormone disruptors; or artificial fragrances, as these tend to be some of the most toxic chemicals in any given product.)

Flax Seed Lube

Flax seeds release a gelatinous substance when boiled (it's their insoluble fiber, which makes them so healthy for your digestion). And it's that substance that gives this lube a high slippery factor. They also release a little oil. Because oil can weaken latex, it's best not to use this lube if you're also using latex condoms.

Ingredients
- 2 cups water
- 2 tbsp whole flax seeds

Instructions:

Put the water and the flax seeds in a small pain and bring to a boil over medium heat, stirring frequently. Once it has reached a boil, reduce heat to a rolling simmer for 20 minutes, stirring occasionally. Strain the flax seeds and store in a glass jar.

My Favorite Natural Skincare Products

MUTHA Body Butter
The ultimate for the prevention of stretch marks

MUTHA Body Oil
Great for post-pregnancy belly!

Farmacy Green Clean Makeup Removing Cleansing Balm

Purito Green Level All in One Mild Pad

Tata Harper Resurfacing Mask

Tatcha Rice Enzyme Powder

Summer Fridays Jet Lag Mask

MUTHA Face Oil

Chantecaille Ultra Sun Protection Sunscreen

MUTHA Deodorant

MUTHA Cell Rejuvenating Essence

MUTHA No. 1 Serum

MUTHA Up All Night Eye Cream

MUTHA Cream and Cream Extreme

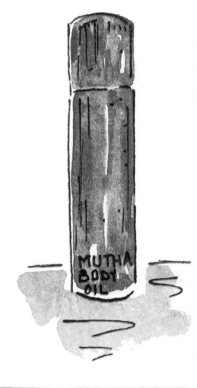

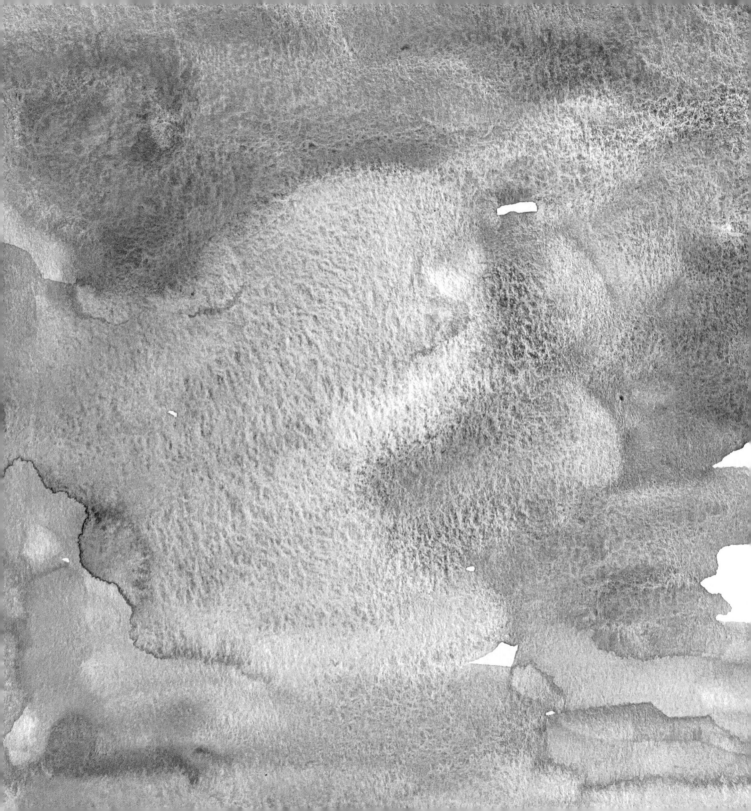

THE FIRST TRIMESTER

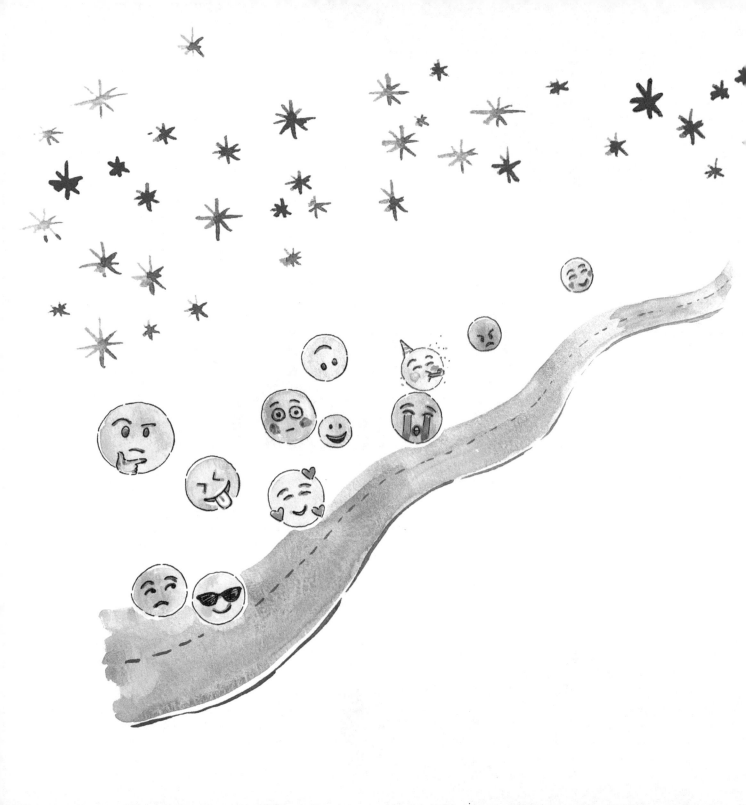

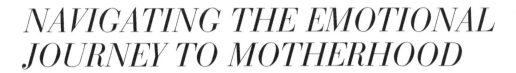

Chapter 4

NAVIGATING THE EMOTIONAL JOURNEY TO MOTHERHOOD

This is it. The second line appeared on the pregnancy test and you are officially carrying a child. It's such an exciting, heady time. Some women get on board with their new reality right away, and others of us take longer. Like most things that involve personal development, we each have our own pace.

Because you are on a journey to not only a new life but also a new version of yourself, it's worth it to take the time you need now to wrap your mind around the fact that you're becoming a mom.

Here's a guide to some of the things I found interesting and/or challenging in those early days and weeks of pregnancy.

Keeping the Secret

A lot of keeping your pregnancy a secret during the first 12 weeks is strictly practical: You're more vulnerable to miscarriage in the first trimester, and as excited as you might be to spread the word, you want to protect yourself from having to share the news of a possible pregnancy loss with people you aren't necessarily emotionally close to. Beyond that, though, one of the nice things about keeping the news of your new pregnancy under wraps for a little while is that it gives you some space to process things before people start asking you questions.

How do you decide who to tell, and when to tell them? I suggest only sharing the scoop with someone you'd be comfortable talking to about a miscarriage. Now, this is changing even as we speak; in the last year or so I've seen so many women I admire talking about a pregnancy loss on social media. They're not just sharing authentically about what's going on with them, they're also seeking to normalize miscarriage, as it is such a common experience yet one that has typically been kept hush-hush. It's really your call. Just know that you don't have to tell anyone before you're ready.

When our surrogate was carrying our girls, I didn't post the news on Instagram until well into the second trimester; I wasn't ready to discuss such a sensitive subject and I also wanted to make sure both babies were healthy. But when I saw a friend in person, I absolutely shared the news—mainly because talking about it helped me process that we were having not just one new baby, but two!

On the other hand, in this first trimester you may not be feeling well. You're probably pretty tired, and because pregnancy can cause your immunity to dip, maybe you've caught a virus, or you've got morning sickness. There may be a couple of people in your closest circle you want to tell so that you have people thinking about you and checking in on you.

I told my mom, my sister, and my best friend when the pregnancy was only a few weeks along. My assistant also knew very early on, because she went with me to the first appointment. If I saw a friend in person and we did the whole "What's going on with you?" download, I told them, because I wanted to be authentic. There's a difference between having people who are close to you know and having everyone on social media in on the secret.

One thing to consider is that the period before the people in your life know about the baby is the only time you have that child completely to yourself. You're walking around with a really big secret, and it can feel really special. I remember being with a friend in a toy store, shopping for a gift for my niece's birthday, and thinking about buying for the babies that I hadn't yet shared were coming. I felt like I was glowing from the inside. Once people know, they'll start asking questions and perhaps asking to touch your belly. For now, try to enjoy having this juicy secret.

What If a Friend Asks Why I'm Not Drinking?

If you're out with friends at this point and someone notices that you're not drinking and asks you if you're pregnant, if you're not ready to share the news you can just say that you're trying. Or you can say that you're doing a detox, which was always my go-to before I was ready to share.

Planning a fun way to announce that you're expecting—either with a social media post or a party—can make it more fun to keep your news a secret until that date.

However, as our understanding of gender is changing, you might want to think about how important it is to you to make the baby's sex the focus of the reveal. After all, the fact that you're creating a new human is pretty miraculous and definitely enough of a cause for celebration—the baby's sex is not the biggest news here. For my first pregnancies, I chose to not find out the sex until the birth. For our surrogacy journey, I posted a picture of our boys, each holding a pink tutu, when I announced that we were having twin girls on Instagram, so it's not like I'm against gender reveals. It's just worth thinking about what it is you want to celebrate—the baby's anatomy, or the fact that you're having a baby? It's entirely your call, so do what feels right to you.

Last but not least, you have to consider when and how your partner wants to share the news too. Talk about it with them and find a time that feels right to you both. With the girls, I was ready before my husband was; he had to dial me back a few times. He's more of a private person, and I respect that. It's vital to remember that it's not just your news; it's also theirs.

Processing the Fact That This Is Real

A moment when it really sank in that everything was about to change was when I was in our house in Austin, Texas, and realized, as if I were seeing the place for the first time, that we live on a cliff. Of course, I'd always known this, but it wasn't until I envisioned an infant toddling over the side of it that I got that our life wasn't really set up for a baby.

Maybe you're looking around your small apartment and wondering where a crib will go, or looking at your dog that you've been devoted to and knowing that he will soon get a lot less attention from you. Whatever your situation, remember that the baby gets nine months to prepare to be born, and you get nine months to grow into your new reality. You will get there.

That being said, if you're looking around and realizing that something about your physical environment has to change, use your new status as a mother to empower you to say, *We have to make this happen.* You have more sway now that you're speaking for two.

Perhaps you have to move. Or get rid of some stuff to make room for a changing table and a crib or bassinet. Or get a bigger car. You may have to lead the way here; you're the one feeling your body change and who has the visceral experience of the shifts that are already happening and will continue to occur. Take any realization like this as an opportunity to get more grounded in your power. My husband wasn't looking at the cliff and thinking about the baby toddling over the side of it. I had to take a stand for why the house wasn't appropriate for us as new parents to small children.

Similarly, when I knew we were going from two kids to four kids, I had a moment of awareness while driving the boys in my car: I looked in the rearview and realized there was nowhere for the girls to go, and that we'd have to get a new vehicle. At dinner one night I looked around our table and started counting seats. Five chairs weren't going to hold us all anymore. While it can be overwhelming to think about how your physical environment may need to change, it's good to start thinking about those adjustments now, before the baby is here, and when you still have time to address them.

> "... USE YOUR NEW STATUS as A *mother* TO EMPOWER YOU to SAY, WE HAVE to MAKE THIS HAPPEN."

Staying Connected to Your Partner

It's frustrating but natural for your partner to not be as in touch with your new reality as you are, since their body isn't experiencing the changes that yours is. You're tired, you're nauseous, you're making sure you take your prenatal vitamins and are watching what you eat, but your partner's probably not. What's oh-so-real for you is still an idea for them.

For my husband, with our first child, it didn't become real to him until I started showing, and then he got a lot more connected to the reality that there was a baby on the way. Once he said, "Let's go get sushi!" Another time he suggested that we meet up with his best friend at a bar after work. And I thought, "Why would I want to do that?" (Although once I switched to a midwife, I learned that it is OK to have sushi—-so long as any fish in your sushi is cooked to kill any bacteria that you may be more susceptible to now and low-mercury.)

I was very sensitive to his comments, so I get if you're upset if your partner is saying things that suggest they're not fully on board with what's going on, too. I suggest not letting things pile up and talking about an issue fairly quickly after it comes up; perhaps not in that exact moment, but the next day. Not weeks later. There's a difference between tabling something until a better time for a conversation and burying it.

I'd bring it up in a really gentle way—couple's therapy has taught me how to tread lightly. (I love going to couple's therapy with my husband. Even when nothing is going on or 'wrong,' it helps you feel closer to each other. You discover how to communicate with one another. And you learn why each of you has the triggers you have—we've all got them—so you can understand where the other person is coming from, especially when otherwise it would seem that their behavior made no sense.)

One of the best things you can do instead of going straight into what they did wrong is to talk about how it made you feel. I would say, "When you do this, I feel like you're not in touch with what's going on with me, and when you invite me to the bar it makes me feel like I'm the only one who's having a child." Versus, "You're so insensitive. I can't believe you! What's the matter with you?" Starting off with blame is highly likely to ensure the message gets taken personally; it never goes anywhere.

Another thing I did to close the gap between our points of view was to download pregnancy apps onto my husband's phone and turn on the notifications so that he would always know what was going on. It's a little sneaky, but it worked great—it helped make the baby more real to him to learn when they had fingernails, or hair, or how big they were. The two apps I used were Sprout and Pregnancy Plus, though new great ones come out all the time.

Put Yourself on an Information Diet

You are growing a new human right now. You want the inside of your body and your consciousness to be as hospitable an environment as possible, and that means you want to be very careful about the kinds of information you're exposed to.

I say stick with books, podcasts, or apps, which are controlled environments, instead of Web searches, which can easily lead you down roads that may make you nervous about something you didn't even realize existed or expose you to horror stories. With these forms of media, you can choose the point of view that speaks to you the most.

When I was pregnant with each of my children, my midwife, Mari Mikel, whose advice is featured throughout this book, suggested that I stop reading the news. She said, "Trust me, if it's big, you're going to hear about it anyway. You don't need to go out looking for things to get upset about right now." I decided that I was going to be blissfully unaware. It wasn't an easy choice to make, as I love checking the headlines on my news app and keeping up with the big stories of the day. I picked the habit—although I like to think of it as a ritual—back up after my kids were out of the newborn phase.

On the other hand, if there was something I was concerned about or didn't know a lot about, I set to researching it. I turned to books first, and then would use just a handful of trusted websites such as the site for the American College of Obstetricians and Gynecologists (ACOG) or the Midwives Alliance of North America (MANA). I wanted to know what to expect if I ended up needing a Caesarean birth, for example. Or, if I heard a term I didn't know, such as placenta previa, I would look it up.

As hungry as I was for information, there were plenty of times when someone with good intentions tried to share a scary story with me about something that had happened to her in pregnancy or labor. I had to give myself permission—and so do you—to say, "Stop right there. That's not helpful for me at this time." You can protect yourself with your words; you don't have to sit there and endure it when a relative or family friend starts telling you all about her difficult delivery. Using your words this way is great training for motherhood, because there will be times when someone is saying something either to or in front of your kids that you don't want them exposed to, and you'll need to ask them to stop.

Addressing Fears as They Arise

As special as this time is, it's also a big opportunity to feel fear—fear about birth, the state of the world, the future state of your vagina… It's really common for your heightened hormones and the bigness of the adventure you're embarking on to occasionally mess with your head.

It's so important to acknowledge your fears, because anything you try to will yourself not to feel or to think about only sticks around longer. Think about who you can trust to share them with—someone who will listen without trying to fix them or piling on fears of their own. And then, you really have to be proactive about not dwelling on them. I'm a huge believer in the power of thought. I believe if you think it, you can create it, both good and bad. When you focus on something you fear, you attract it.

That's why my favorite technique for redirecting your mind away from your fears is using affirmations. I wrote about them in Chapter 1. If you skipped that part because you were

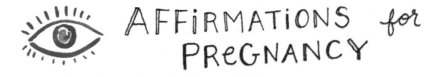

AFFIRMATIONS for PREGNANCY

MY BODY KNOWS WHAT IT'S DOING.

MY BABY and I ARE STRONG and HEALTHY.

MY PREGNANCY is PROGRESSING EXACTLY as IT SHOULD.

I BELIEVE IN MYSELF and IN MY BODY.

MY BODY IS MAGIC.   MY PREGNANT BODY IS BEAUTIFUL.

MY BODY HAS EVERYTHING IT NEEDS to GIVE BIRTH.

THE BABY WILL COME at THE EXACT RIGHT TIME.

I TRUST MYSELF to BE the MOTHER THIS BABY NEEDS.

I PROTECT MYSELF and MY BABY BY MAINTAINING a POSITIVE INTERNAL ENVIRONMENT.

already pregnant when you picked up this book, affirmations are positive phrases that help you stay focused on what you want instead of worrying about things you don't want to come to pass. You need somewhere to put your focus, whether you're feeling fear in that moment or you are just trying to keep your head in a good place, and affirmations are a great way to focus on positive thoughts.

Write them out and hang them up somewhere you'll see them everyday. Repeat them to yourself as you fall asleep, or while sitting quietly for a few minutes during the day.

Fear of being a bad parent

This is so common. So many of us had a childhood that felt traumatic in some way. I had a mother who was very much involved, but I didn't have a father who was regularly there for me. Ever since I was a girl, I knew that I would only have children when I found the right partner—someone who was an inherently good person and who would be in our children's lives for the long-term. It took me a while to find him, but I found him. (That's another example of how what you think and believe creates your reality.) In some ways it's helpful to have a not-great parent, because it shows you an example of what not to do.

Even though I had a great mom, I still had fears that I would mess up motherhood somehow. One thing that got me through those moments was reminding myself that no matter what my husband and I did, every adult feels like their parents messed up in some way. It's impossible to be a perfect parent.

That being said, no one wants to repeat the stuff that scarred you from your own childhood, myself included. Be honest about what you wish you had experienced differently as a kid and work on improving from there. You also need to preemptively forgive yourself for the things you do mess up on. If your parents were yellers, you probably will yell occasionally too because that's what got baked into your brain as "the way to parent." Even if you only yell at the kids one time, because you had that upbringing you'll probably really beat yourself up about it. Just resolve to do better next time, and trust yourself to get support if you need help breaking old patterns, whether that's reading books, taking a parenting class, or seeking counseling.

Whenever you notice this fear creeping in now, use it as an invitation to think about what kind of parent you want to be. Too many people *don't* think about it. It's easy to put off thinking about your parenting beliefs because pregnancy gives you plenty of things to focus on in the moment. Just remember that pregnancy and birth don't last long in the grand scheme of things, but parenting never ends. Take advantage of the time you have now, before your baby is here in this world, to think about your approach to things like how to discipline, and what you want to teach them, and how you'll inspire them to be the best person they can be. Better yet, talk about this with your partner too.

Fear of birth

I had this one, big time. Fear of birth is an actual condition, called tokophobia, and although I was never officially diagnosed, I felt it throughout my life. (In fact, if I hadn't been so afraid of birth, I never would have written this book, because it's what drove me to do so much research about birth and then get inspired to share everything I learned with others.)

In addition to researching, talking to other women who have had positive birth experiences is helpful and empowering. For me, reading Ina May Gaskin's books *Spiritual Midwifery* and *Ina May's Guide to Birth* first exposed me to those positive stories. To this day, I still give Ina May's books to everyone I know when they get pregnant. I have to beg them to keep reading, because the books are very granola and not many of many friends can relate. But birth is a natural physiological process; it's not a medical procedure. Ina May's books are a great introduction to that reality. I hope that you'll read them too!

> BiRTH is A NATURAL PHYSiOLOGiCAL PROcess; IT'S NOT A MEDiCAL PROCEDURE.

Reading those stories inspired me to start iinterviewing midwives, which is how I met Mari Mikel, who has been present at well over 3,000 births. Hearing her stories gave me so much confidence. I also connected with people on Instagram whose feeds were very

Pro-Birth Books, Podcasts, and Documentaries

Books

- *Your Baby, Your Way: Taking Charge of Your Pregnancy, Childbirth, and Parenting Decisions for a Happier, Healthier Family*, by Jennifer Margulis

- *Gentle Birth, Gentle Mothering: A Doctor's Guide to Natural Childbirth and Early Parenting Choices*, by Sarah J. Buckley, M.D.

- *Birth Without Fear: The Judgment-Free Guide to Taking Charge of Your Pregnancy, Birth, and Postpartum*, by January Harshe

- *Spiritual Midwifery*, by Ina May Gaskin

- *Cut, Stapled, & Mended: When One Woman Reclaimed Her Body and Gave Birth on Her Own Terms after Cesarean*, by Roanna Rosewood

- *Born in the U.S.A.: How a Broken Maternity System Must Be Fixed to Put Women and Children First*, by Marsden Wagoner, M.D., M.S.

- *How to Raise a Healthy Child in Spite of Your Doctor: One of America's Leading Pediatricians Puts Parents Back in Control of Their Children's Health*, by Robert Mendelsohn, M.D.

- *Mindful Birthing*, by Nancy Bardacke, CNM

- *Homebirth*, by Sheila Kitzinger

- *Childbirth Without Fear*, by Grantly Dick-Read

- *How Big Is a Placenta Bowl*, by Renee Moilanen

- *The Complete Book of Pregnancy and Childbirth*, by Sheila Kitzinger

- *Gentle Babies: Essential Oils and Natural Remedies for Pregnancy, Childbirth, Infants and Young Children*, by Debra Raybern

Podcasts
- The Birth Hour
- Evidence Based Birth

Documentaries
- *The Business of Being Born*
- *Orgasmic Birth*
- *Micro Birth*

Apps
- What to Expect
- Sprout
- BabyCenter My Pregnancy
- WebMD
- Ovia Pregnancy
- Baby Bump Pro
- Pregnancy+

pro-birth; seeing their examples helped make me feel pro-birth. There are plenty of books, podcasts, and a few documentaries that are helpful too. You want to steep yourself in positive, empowering stories and information.

You may not have the same fear that I did, so you don't have to immerse yourself to the same degree. But raising awareness and education is good for everybody. It's like being an athlete watching footage of previous games: It's confidence building.

Life as you know it is ending

Before I had kids, I didn't think moms were cool, and I never wanted to hang out with them. Once I became one, I didn't see myself fitting in with what I thought moms were. I didn't want to spend my week planning a play date and then getting together. It took me three years to accept my new identity of "mom." It wasn't that I wasn't excited about having kids; I was. I just didn't want to change my habits and activities to revolve around someone else. I was resistant to the idea that I would have anything to talk about with other moms when in actuality, I can now only relate to other mothers and find it hard to have as much in common with friends who don't have the same level of responsibility I now have.

I envisioned still having my same life with my baby on my hip and really didn't realize just how much everything would change—my frame of reference, my priorities, and even my identity. I wish that I had received the guidance to accept my new reality. To be fair, I did have my two boys back to back, and I was really in the weeds for those first three years. Now I fully embrace my identity as a mother... I never would have launched a skincare company inspired by motherhood or written this book! It may not happen overnight, but it will happen. I've fully come to terms with the fact that I now have more in common with other mothers than my pre-baby friends.

It doesn't help that in the newborn phase, and sometimes well into the toddler phase depending on your baby, you're working on little sleep. After all, sleep deprivation is a form of torture, so of course you're not in your right mind. It's a beautiful time, but you're so tired you just don't have a clear head.

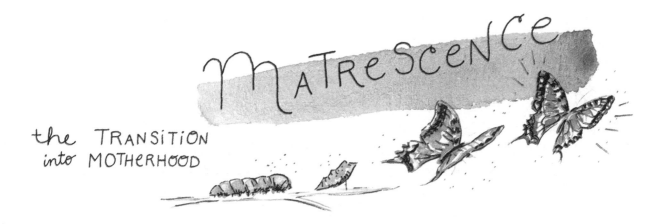

Matrescence

the TRANSITION into MOTHERHOOD

What truly helped me accept my new reality and identity? A TED talk by Alexandra Sacks, M.D., on matrescence—a term coined in the 1970s by medical anthropologist Dana Raphael (who also popularized the term "doula")—that describes the transition you go through when you first become a mother. While you're happy and you love you're baby it's also like you're in the spin cycle.

A lot of matrescence is due to an increase in brain plasticity. This physiological change is designed to help you evolve into your new role; the downside is that other brain functions, like memory and mood, can take a hit at the same time. It's exciting and good to be rewiring your brain, but it can also be disorienting. You forget things. You cry when you're angry and yell when you're sad.

Matrescence is a *huge* transition, bigger even than puberty or menopause, because it involves another creature's dependence on you, and it's only natural to expect that it will be messy and moody. What makes matrescence tougher than it already is though, is that our society expects pregnant and new mothers to be blissfully happy. When your experience doesn't match that expectation, it can be even more bewildering.

It's completely appropriate to also be mourning your identify as a woman without children, to feel like you're at risk of losing yourself. There are parts of you and your life that will naturally fall away. If you're feeling sad about that, it makes sense. Again, talking to a therapist can really help, as can affirmations. You're not just giving birth to a baby, you're giving birth to yourself as a mother too.

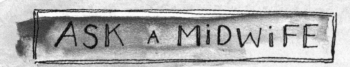

ASK A MIDWIFE

CAN I JUST STAY REALLY BUSY DURING THIS TIME, AND DISTRACT MYSELF FROM THE EMOTIONS I'M EXPERIENCING?

from MARI MIKEL:

"During the first few weeks of pregnancy, you really shouldn't do much of anything. It's so important to let go of stress. Being a workaholic is not conducive to growing a baby and transforming into being a mother. What is happening inside your body in these early weeks of pregnancy are almost beyond our understanding. By the start of the second trimester, the baby is mostly fully formed and is only getting bigger. But now, in the first trimester the baby is essentially creating itself. You're also creating a placenta, an entirely new organ, out of nothing. It's truly astonishing what is going on beneath the surface. That's why you're tired.

"You have to cut yourself some slack and make sure you get as much rest as you feel you need. Cut back on working so hard and pushing on everything. I know how tempting it is to think you've got to get even more done now that a baby is on the way, and how nice it probably sounds to just stay so busy that you don't have to reckon with the fact that your life is changing. But you will have more energy, strength, and stamina in the second trimester.

"You also want to leave plenty of space for joy now. There are super important chemicals that are released when you're in joy that will imprint on the baby's brain and cause the baby to be more joyful. Trying to find more peace creates peaceful people—that includes children and mothers."

What's happening now: First Trimester (Weeks 1-13)

In a nutshell? A whole lot, with you and baby. In fact, the most dramatic changes and development happen in these weeks. Things may get off to a slow start—you're technically not pregnant in weeks one and two; conception occurs in week two. But they really take off after that.

You may not look pregnant at this stage in terms of a noticeable belly, but plenty is going on below the surface. Generally speaking, your blood volume and pregnancy hormone levels (progesterone and estrogen, as well as human chorionic gonadotropin, or hCG, which is what registers on a pregnancy test) surge; your baby transitions from an embryo to fetus; and so much more. As a reminder: Your baby is most susceptible to developmental disorders and birth defects during the first trimester, so it's crucial to take care of yourself now—following the healthy living strategies shared in these first chapters and the advice of your midwife or doctor.

With Baby

From fertilization through week eight, your baby is in what is known as the embryonic stage.

continued on next page

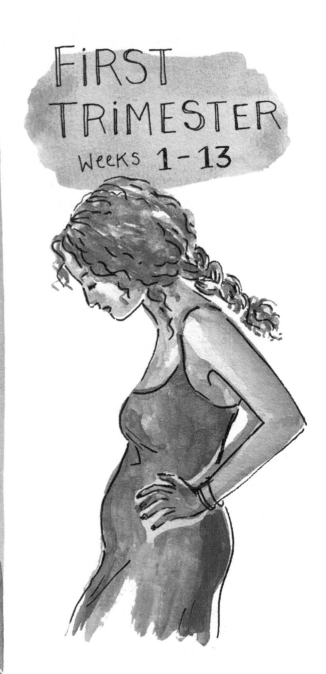

During this time, the amniotic sac and placenta form, your baby's cells multiply rapidly, their organs begin to develop, and their body parts become distinguishable.

- **All systems go.** The neural tube, which becomes your baby's brain and spinal cord, begins to develop now, making your baby most susceptible to neural tube defects, such as spina bifida, now. (This is why you need adequate intake of folate--something you'll hear me talk about later.) Your baby's digestive and circulatory systems begin to develop now too and soon your baby's heart begins to beat.

- **Eye spy.** During this time, your baby begins to shift from looking like a tadpole to more like a human. As their bones begin to develop, their eyes, ears, nose and mouth becoming distinguishable; the foundation is even laid for their baby teeth now. Their arms and legs "sprout" as little buds and eventually become more recognizable as limbs; their fingers and toes form, although they're still webbed.

- **Making a move.** Although you won't feel the activity, since your baby is still very small (only about an inch long), they are on the move, thanks to developing nerves and muscles.

From week nine until birth, your baby is in the fetal stage and is a fetus. By the end of the 12 weeks, all of their major organs are in place. Their arms and legs are fully formed, and they even have their fingernails and toenails. Their genitals have developed, too, although you wouldn't be able to see them yet on an ultrasound. At this point, your baby can weigh up to an ounce, and is about an inch and a half to two inches long.

With You

Of course, every woman is different and experiences the changes of the first trimester in her own way. You may not experience any of the symptoms below or feel any of these shifts, or you may feel them all. They may last a short time, or they may drag on. Some of the possible changes you may feel during the first trimester include:

- **Keep abreast.** Your boobs may become swollen and tender. Your areolas might be larger or darker. And you may notice that the veins in your breasts--as well as your belly and legs--become more noticeable.

- **In a mood.** With all those extra hormones, you may get a little moody. These early pregnancy mood swings can be likened to those many women experience with PMS. One minute you may feel elated, the next anxious, irritable, or weepy.

- **Commode conundrums.** You may have to urinate more frequently as your uterus grows and starts to press on your bladder. Yet you may find you're also constipated; that's because the uterus is also pressing on your intestines and rectum, and because pregnancy hormones tend to slow down digestion. (Prenatal supplements can cause constipation too.) A sluggish digestion can also lead to heartburn and indigestion.

- **Fighting fatigue.** With all the new demands on your body, you may very well feel more tired than normal, even downright exhausted. Don't worry too much, though: You should feel more energized in your second trimester.

- **Infamous "morning sickness."** Yes, you may start to feel nauseous now, and even vomit. That's also thanks to all the extra hormones, particularly oxytocin. It may be called morning sickness, but it can happen any time of day. It can be triggered by certain smells; you may notice you have a heightened, almost superhuman, sense of smell during your first trimester.

- **Expanding waistline.** You likely won't have a baby bump during your first trimester (especially if this is your first baby), but you may notice your clothes feel a bit tighter around your waist, and chest as well.

- **Dealing with dizziness.** Your blood volume increases up to 50 percent over the course of your pregnancy. That's good, because you need a higher blood volume to get vital oxygen and nutrients to your baby. Yet, your blood pressure drops, and your growing uterus can put pressure on blood vessels, both of which can cause temporary dizziness. The good news? Increased circulation can produce a "pregnancy glow."

Early on, you may also experience some light spotting. Happening soon after conception, this is known as implantation bleeding, and it's totally normal. If you're worried, talk with your midwife or doctor.

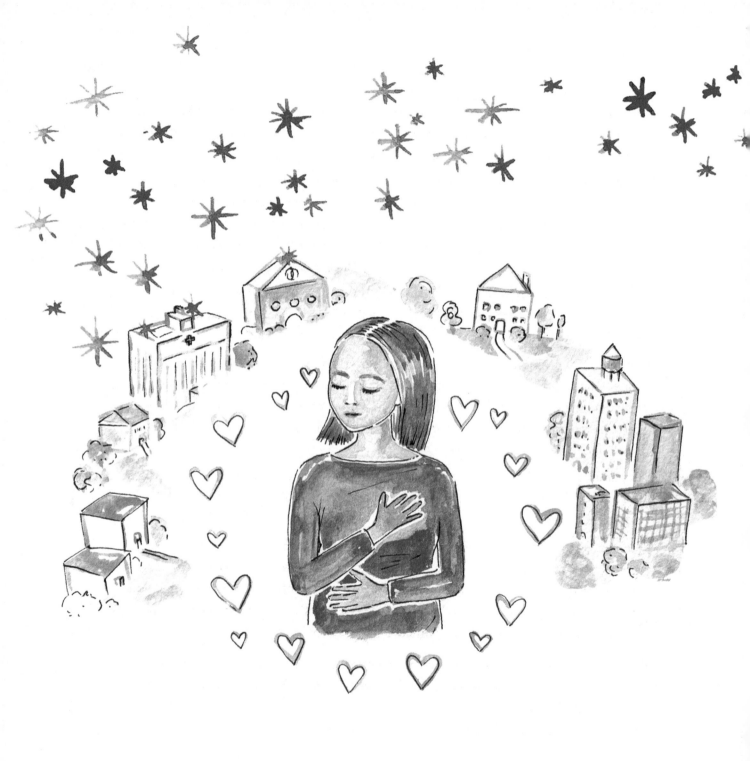

Chapter 5

GATHER YOUR TEAM

Two important things to start thinking about now are: Who is going to be your care provider during your pregnancy, delivery, and postpartum, and where are you going to have your baby?

It may seem like it's early to start answering these questions, but it's really not. I'm including information about health care providers and delivery locations here in this section, because I think it's smart to at least start thinking about these things right out of the gate. As it did for me, it might take you a little time of lived experience, researching, thinking, and talking with your partner to really settle on the best plan and care provider for you. Also, I'm a big fan of having as much support around you as you can from early on in your pregnancy. So I say, start the process now. Especially given the fact that in this first trimester there's so much vital development happening inside your body that you need some extra rest. Researching is great way to 'get things done' while still keeping your stress levels and your energy levels pretty low.

Of course, there's no rule that says you can't switch providers, or change your mind about where you'd like to deliver, as your due date gets closer. That's what eventually happened to me—I started off with an Ob/Gyn and planning a hospital birth, but after doing a lot of research, in my second trimester I decided I wanted to have my baby at home and began working with Mari Mikel as my midwife--a decision that would change not only my birth experience, but also my life.

Thinking about all this now will mean you have the right provider for you by your side from the very beginning of your journey.

Ob/Gyn or Midwife?

When it comes to choosing who's going to be your medical partner for your pregnancy and delivery, you've got two main options: an obstetrician/gynecologist (Ob/Gyn) or a midwife.

Making the decision that's best for you comes down to:

- What's most important to you in terms of medical training, education, and experience

- How you envision your pregnancy and delivery going and where you want it to happen

- The role you'd like a health care provider to play at each step

I want to make it super clear that this is a judgment-free zone. There's no right or wrong choice, only the one that makes the most sense for you. As you think about what you want and who is the best person to help you get it, remember to trust yourself. No matter what provider you choose, you are the one who'll give birth, not your Ob/Gyn, not your midwife, not your partner, not your mother, not your friends. That means your opinion is the most important.

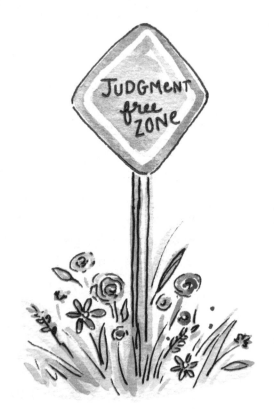

Opting for an Ob/Gyn

You've probably been seeing a gynecologist since you were a teenager—maybe it's even the same gynecologist. But there's a big difference between seeing someone who gives you your yearly exam and helps you figure out your birth control options and choosing someone to help you bring your baby into this world. Even if you've been in the care of an Ob/Gyn for many years, this is a great time to learn a little bit more about what they do and how they're trained.

An Ob/Gyn is a medical doctor, typically an MD but sometimes a DO (a doctor of osteopathy), who specializes in women's health, including general reproductive matters and pregnancy, labor, and delivery. That means they've attended a four-year medical school and spent a minimum of four years in residency, working alongside seasoned doctors and attending to patients before becoming certified. If you've only ever seen your Ob/Gyn for routine Paps, it can be easy to forget that they're also trained surgeons and can perform Cesarean sections. Ob/Gyns can have their own practice, be part of a larger medical group, or work for a hospital.

In general, an Ob/Gyn is more likely than a midwife to use medical interventions for labor and delivery; in other words, to lean towards a less-natural birth (we'll talk more about specific interventions in Chapter 15). This means they may be inclined to induce labor or give IV fluids or medications. Some may even be active proponents of scheduling a Cesarean birth.

That said, it is possible to find an Ob/Gyn who prioritizes natural childbirth and will happily work with you to have a natural delivery. Oftentimes, DOs are more holistic-minded and may be more supportive of natural births; although, that's not always the case.

Keep in mind that even though you may have had a regular Ob/Gyn for years, that doesn't mean they have to be your health care provider for your pregnancy. You want a health care provider you feel comfortable with as a person and whose approach to labor and delivery you agree with. Birth is one of the most important experiences of your life, after all, and your experience in birth will forever change you.

Maybe you've been seeing a male physician but would feel more comfortable having a woman to coach you through labor and delivery. Maybe your Ob/Gyn doesn't deliver at the hospital of your choice (more on that in just a moment—but you basically have to decide where you want to have the baby in order to choose the right provider). Or maybe your Ob/Gyn hasn't focused on delivery, and you'd feel better working with a provider who has more births under their belt. Not all Ob/Gyns are created equal. Asking them the questions on page 82 will help you find the right one if that's the route you choose to go.

Making the Choice for a Midwife

In general, midwives are advocates of natural, vaginal births and are typically more holistic-minded in terms of overall health and wellness than conventionally trained physicians. They may be able to provide you with more individualized care than Ob/Gyns, who can have a high patient load and often favor a more one-size-fits-all approach to the whole process. Like Ob/Gyns, they can assist with pregnancy and childbirth as well as the postpartum period. Many midwives can also help with newborn care. Because midwives have a smaller client load than Ob/Gyns generally have, that translates to more time spent with you, which helps deliver a higher standard of care. They also typically have more training and capacity to address the emotional, nutritional, and spiritual aspects of pregnancy. And research shows that midwifery can improve health outcomes for both mother and baby.

Although midwives most commonly aren't MDs, they do have comprehensive medical education. There are different levels of training and certification. Here are the three primary credentials you'll come across in your search.

- *Certified Nurse Midwives (CNMs)* are registered nurses (RNs) who have additional training in all things pregnancy and childbirth, along with a master's degree in nurse midwifery. They are certified by the national American Midwifery Certification Board (AMCB). They are able to make medical decisions and in some cases prescribe medication; however, they cannot perform Cesareans or assisted vaginal deliveries (like those that require forceps, for example). They are licensed to practice midwifery in all 50 states.

- *Certified Midwives (CMs)* receive the same graduate level of midwifery training as CNMs, but they don't have a degree in nursing and aren't RNs. They, too, are certified by the AMCB, but they are not legally licensed to practice in every state (as I'm writing this, CMs are only licensed to practice in a handful of states).

- *Certified Professional Midwives (CPMs)* are certified by the North American Registry of Midwives. While they must pass exams and tests to obtain certification, their training and level of education can vary. Interestingly, the CPM certification is the only accredited midwife credential that has a requirement for experience with out-of-hospital births. CPMs are also not legally able to practice in all 50 states. As of May 2020, CPMs were legally authorized to practice in 35 states and Washington, D.C. (You can check the MANA website, at www.mana.org, to get the latest updates on which types of midwives are allowed to practice where.)

Just as important—if not more so—than their official training, you want to ask potential midwives about their hands-on experience with births.

One tricky thing about choosing a health care provider is that each one has a different set of delivery locations. So you need to decide who you want to work with and where you want to have your baby at the same time. That's because some hospitals and hospital-associated birthing centers will only work with CNMs, while others will work with CPMs too. If you want to give birth at home, you may want the specialized nursing expertise of a CNM, but not all CNMs perform home births. And again, the CPM credential is the only one to mandate experience with out-of-hospital births. It's a lot to sort through—another reason to start thinking about it now.

Again, another huge consideration in selecting a midwife is that you feel comfortable working with and get along well with the midwife you choose. The questions on page 82 will help you find that person you truly want to include in your pregnancy, labor, and delivery.

Consider Co-Care

It's also possible to work with both an Ob/Gyn you love and trust and a midwife you love and trust. It's called co-care, and some hospitals and birthing centers are built around this type of approach. It seems like the best of both worlds, so long as they have a good working relationship, a clear delineation of responsibilities, and a birthing facility that respects the roles of each.

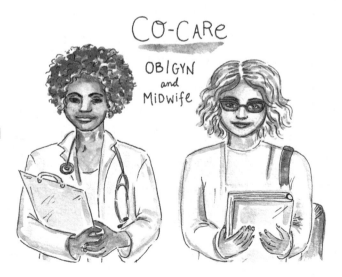

CO-CARE

OB/GYN and MIDWIFE

Questions to Ask Potential Health Care Providers

When you find a care provider who sounds promising it's important to interview them before you decide. How else will you know if they're the one you want to be a part of this process with you? Even if you think you'll stick with your existing Ob/Gyn, interview them, too, as you're unlikely to have asked them all of these questions before. You want to know their answers before you're in labor and perhaps not thinking clearly or feeling empowered enough to ask questions.

Of course, these lists aren't all the questions you may want to ask, but they're a great starting point and can help you feel prepared for your Ob/Gyn or midwife interview.

What to ask an Ob/Gyn:

1. What is your overarching philosophy on and approach to pregnancy, labor, delivery, and postpartum care? What role do you play as my provider during labor and delivery—and beyond?

2. How long have you been practicing, and how many births have you performed in your career?

3. At which hospital or hospitals do you deliver?

4. Do you work with any hospital-affiliated birthing centers? Have you or will you work in partnership with a midwife? What about other support team members, such as doulas?

5. Why might you not be the one to deliver my baby, and what are the odds you will? If you're unable to, who will? What is your availability: between appointments, after hours, etc.?

6. What is your Cesarean rate? What is your rate of assisted deliveries (forceps, vacuum extraction)? What's your episiotomy rate? What's your mortality rate?

7. What's your experience with high-risk pregnancies?

8. What will you do if there is a complication during my labor that is beyond your expertise?

9. What routine procedures do you suggest or require during labor? What routine procedures do you suggest or require for baby right after they're born?

10. How do you approach pain management? What's your view on epidurals?

11. You can also ask any provider outright: Why should I pick you?!

What to ask a midwife/midwife team:

1. What are your credentials? Are you licensed to practice in this state?

2. Tell me about your training.

3. How many years have you been a practicing midwife? How many babies have you delivered?

4. Have you had experience with difficult births? What is your protocol in case of an emergency? What emergency equipment will you bring with you (if attending a home birth)?

5. How many people are on your team? What are their roles?

6. Is there any reason you wouldn't be the midwife to deliver my baby? If you're unable to, who will? What is your availability after hours?

7. What is your Cesarean rate? What's your hospital transfer rate (for home birth midwives)? What's your mortality rate?

8. What happens if my pregnancy becomes high-risk or I experience complications during labor? Do you have a relationship with a hospital or birthing center? Who is your backup?

9. How do you approach pain management during labor and delivery?

10. What is your position on using water (such as a birthing tub) during labor and birth?

11. How do you approach the time right after the baby is born?

12. Why should I pick you?!

You also want to ask with any prospective provider about costs: Do they take your insurance? What are their fees and payment plan options? You can do this with hospitals and birth centers too—ask up front about their fees.

A home-birth midwife, for example, often has an Ob/Gyn that she partners with to be her backup if more medical assistance becomes necessary. And many Ob/Gyn practices have midwives on staff who can be your primary care giver.

Choosing Where You'll Give Birth

This decision is just as important as choosing who your provider will be—you can't really decide who's going to be with you for delivery without also deciding where that delivery will take place.

Just as you want a practitioner you feel comfortable working with, you also want a location where you feel confident and relaxed for your labor and delivery. The main options are a hospital, a birthing center, or at home. Here are some things to consider about each.

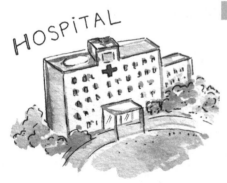

Hospital

Most people default to having a hospital birth because it's a known quantity. With a lot of medical support at the ready, including doctors and nurses trained in a variety of medical areas, as well as a neonatal intensive care unit (NICU) right there in case there's an emergency with your baby, it seems like the safest bet.

Something you may not have considered is that hospitals also have a lot of policies and protocols in place that may or may not be what you want to abide by during your labor. You may have to labor in bed, for example, because policy requires you to have an IV and a fetal monitor at all times. In a hospital, it's also common that any laboring mother be considered a potential surgery patient (in case they decide you need a Cesarean), which can mean you're not allowed to eat or even drink water and have to make do with ice chips.

Some hospitals are teaching hospitals, which means they'll invite residents and other staff who aren't your particular care team to observe your delivery. Even if it's not a teaching hospital, there will be lots of people in and out or your space and lots of people touching and interacting with you throughout the labor and delivery process.

Once the baby's born, the hospital may not allow them to sleep with you that first night. (Although, some hospitals are a designated Baby-Friendly Hospital, which means your baby stays close by right after birth so that you can bond and have a chance to begin breastfeeding right away.)

There are a ton of little things like this you want to take into account when you're deciding where you'll have your baby. For all these reasons, I strongly recommend that you take a tour of potential hospitals and ask a million questions. Take a look and see what the rooms look like and how they feel. Find out if the hospital has an anesthesiologist always on call so you can have an epidural at the appropriate point if that's a route you'd like to take. If a natural birth is important to you, ask about their policies on interventions like IV fluids and whether or not you have to labor on your back, as well as if they work with midwives.

You also want to get an idea of practical things, like which door to enter when you're in labor, and whether single rooms are available or if you'll have to share a room. And you want to ask about their policies for after delivery, on everything from skin-to-skin contact to breastfeeding.

There are also many interventions typically used at hospitals—such as a synthetic form of oxytocin, known as Pitocin, to stimulate labor; IVs; and epidurals—that each have their pros and their cons. I cover these in depth in Chapter 15, so if you're ready to start thinking about this level of detail now, when you're also deciding who will be your care provider and where you'll deliver, go ahead and skip to that chapter. If you're feeling a little overwhelmed by the choices you need to make now, you can wait until you're further along.

As you can see, there's a ton to consider. You want to put as much research into your delivery facility as you would a car or a house purchase!

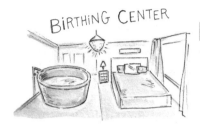

Birthing centers

If you want as natural a birth as possible and aren't a fan of the clinical nature of hospitals (with all the people involved and rules to uphold) but are nervous about a home birth, a birthing center is a good option to consider. In fact, statistics show that in many cases delivering at a birthing center is actually safer than a hospital.

Birthing centers can be stand-alone facilities or they can be affiliated with a hospital. They may have doctors and nurses on staff or be solely staffed by midwives. There may be several options in your city or town, or only one. But in general, birthing centers offer a cozy, private space with some of the creature comforts of home, i.e. a larger bed, comfortable furniture, etc. There are typically fewer rules and restrictions, as well as medical interventions, than in a hospital. And your baby is likely to stay with you from the moment they are born until the moment you leave the facility.

Studies show that only a small percentage of women who give birth at birthing centers end up needing to have a Cesarean, and that their babies are less likely to be delivered pre-term, induced, with the assistance of instruments like forceps, or to be admitted to the NICU. But do keep in mind that while they are just as if not safer than hospitals in many ways, if you have a high-risk pregnancy and are at risk for any pregnancy complications, a birthing center will likely refer you to a hospital.

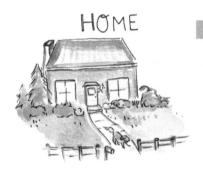

At home

You can also have your baby at home. After all, you'll be in your space that you know and love. You can choose who you want to be there, eat your own food, go at your own pace, and set your own rules. You can be in the tub, or in your own bed. You get to set the mood however you like. There is no bag to pack, and no "going home" ordeal, because you're already there. Also, there are no germs that are foreign to you—while no environment is germ-free, you have already been exposed to every type of germ that's in your house. The same can definitely not be said about the hospital!

Although the American College of Obstetricians and Gynecologists believes that hospitals and birthing centers are the safest settings for births, they definitely don't outright condemn home births. And, they acknowledge that home births can in fact not only be safe but that they're associated with fewer maternal interventions and reduced risk of vaginal tearing and infections.[15] (See the next page for facts about home births.)

How comfortable you feel about giving birth at home depends a lot on how comfortable you feel with your midwife. If you're planning a home birth, add all the questions about their experience with home births and complications to your interview that you need to know to feel safe and secure.

To be a good candidate for a home birth, keep in mind that you should:

- Not have any serious medical concerns or be high-risk in terms of your pregnancy

- Be committed and ready for a natural birth

- Live near a hospital in case of emergency

As with your providers, you'll want to consider the cost of having your baby at home as well. Does your midwife accept insurance? What are the standard fees? What would happen, insurance-wise, if you ended up needing to go the hospital? It's a good idea to get on the phone with your insurance company and ask about different scenarios and figure out if there are in-network restrictions you need to factor into your decision-making.

Another important factor to consider is your race. In America, the horrible truth is that Black mothers are 2½ times more likely to die in childbirth than white mothers. (Interestingly, Latinx women have even lower rates of maternal mortality than white women in America.) There are numerous factors that contribute to this elevated risk, including the stress of being subjected to overt racism, implicit bias, and systemic racism throughout your lifetime, which can take a toll on your health and lead to diabetes and high blood pressure, both of which are risk factors for potentially life-threatening

Home Birth FAQs

Q: Is it safe?

A: Doctors have only been attending at births for about 100 years; before that it was all midwives. Their wisdom on how to deliver breech babies, or switch the position of the mother to relieve pain, or use natural remedies to get a stalled labor going is centuries old (and augmented by their rigorous medical training). Doctors, on the other hand, only know surgery and drugs as options, and these medical interventions all come with side effects and risks of their own.

While no birth is 100 percent risk-free, midwives are trained to handle many complications and are certainly trained to know when you need to be transferred to a hospital—and to make that call quickly and without hesitation.

Researchers who conducted the largest analysis of planned home births to date found that planned home births, among women with low-risk pregnancies, resulted in low intervention rates without an increase in adverse outcomes for mother or baby. Ninety-seven percent of the babies included in the analysis were born full-term at a healthy weight. Only one percent of babies included needed to be transferred to the hospital after birth, and those transfers were typically for non-urgent conditions.[16]

Q: How do I know if my house is fit for a home birth? Can I still give birth at home if I'm in a rental house or rental apartment?

A: Nearly every home can work for a home birth. Contrary to what you may think, you don't actually need a lot of space to have your baby. And since you'll be delivering vaginally and not by Cesarean (unless, of course, there's a medically necessary reason why you need to head to the hospital), you don't need a completely sterile environment. Your house is likely more than clean enough as you keep it, but your midwife will let you know if you need to do anything special in this regard. While you may want to inform your neighbors as to what will be happening if you're in an apartment building—as you might make some loud noises when you're laboring and pushing—ultimately what matters most is just that you feel comfortable in your space. Your midwife will go over important aspects of home births with you in advance, so you'll know what you need to do to prepare your home. But again, typically this isn't about making your space somehow more suitable; rather, it's more about making sure safety precautions are addressed, like knowing how emergency medical team members can access your house or apartment quickly and easily, for example.

Q: What about the mess?

A: It's true, birth isn't mess-free. But it's really not something you need to worry about when it comes to delivering at home. Your midwife can counsel you on how to protect your mattress and floors from blood and other fluids, and they should come prepared with things like absorbent underpads. What's more, your midwife and her team, if she has one, will clean up for you while you're spending time with your little one! You get to focus on being mom and nothing else.

Q: I know I can't get an epidural at home, but is there any way to manage pain?

A: There are tons of non-medical ways to make the experience of childbirth more manageable, pain-wise. For instance, many women find that laboring and giving birth in water provides pain relief. Your midwife is also trained in a wide range of pain-management techniques—breathing, positions, exercises, herbs, homeopathic remedies, and acupressure.

Q: What happens if something goes wrong?

A: Midwives are trained to handle all manner of potential complications and emergency scenarios. Your midwife will come to the birth prepared will all the necessary supplies, including those—from oxygen to instruments to medicines—that can be used if things don't go as planned or in an emergency situation. If for any reason the birth becomes unsafe to continue at home, they will initiate your transfer to a hospital. Again, you'll have made a plan in advance and talked about things beforehand with your midwife, so that you'll feel comfortable about your safety and your baby's safety.

Benefits of Having a Home Birth

- **Greater freedom.** In a hospital, you are typically forced to labor on your back, which slows labor (because when you are upright, gravity helps bring the baby down). With a home birth you are free to walk around, squat, change positions, change rooms, etc. It's about what makes you feel most comfortable!

- **Greater control.** One of the biggest reasons to have a home birth is because you can be in control and participate in your own labor and birth. In a hospital birth, you can't do this because you are often under the influence of heavy pain medications and the doctor makes the final decisions.

- **Faster labor.** In a home birth, you feel the pain but you also feel when it is time to push. In a hospital birth, when you numb the pain, you numb your awareness, sometimes causing the pushing to be more difficult and the labor to be longer. Epidurals typically lengthen labor and pushing because you can't be upright or squat—at home, an epidural is not an option, and you can be in whatever position helps facilitate your birth, which helps things go faster.

- **Faster recovery.** With a home birth, you are able to walk around shortly after delivery. But with a hospital birth, it can take a few days to recover if you took pain medications, and a few weeks to recover if you had a Cesarean birth.

- **Fewer interventions.** In a hospital birth, your baby ingests the medications you ingest. Depending on how much medication you are given, your baby could need to be hospitalized to get the drugs out of their system. Studies have shown that babies who are not exposed to pain medication during labor are more alert and breastfeed better after birth.

- **More empowerment.** There is nothing more profound than being 100 percent in the moment when you see your child for the first time. Experiencing real labor and knowing what your mind and your body are capable of doing is an incredible and irreplaceable thing.

pregnancy complications, such as pre-eclampsia. All forms of racism also show up in the healthcare system, where many doctors and hospital staff don't take Black woman as seriously as they would a white woman, dismissing reports of symptoms and over-estimating pain tolerance, for example. This happens to some extent to all women, frankly, but it's worse for Black women. Every woman deserves to be heard and respected by her care provider. If you are a Black woman, take extra care to find a care provider you trust. Ask to talk to other Black mothers whose babies they've delivered. Ask what their maternal mortality rate is for all mothers and Black mothers in particular. If they can't answer you satisfactorily, keep looking.[17]

Why I Chose a Home Birth

For most of my life, I was the last person to even consider giving birth without drugs. But once I began researching pregnancy—in an effort to tame my fear of birth—and I saw the high rates of interventions, and complications from those interventions happening in hospitals, as well as the good outcomes of home births, I started to reconsider. Also, I knew that I wanted to be comfortable and feel at ease, and hospitals do *not* put me at ease.

When I first started talking about my plans to have a home birth, my friends would tell me, "Don't be a hero. Go to the hospital. Get the meds." But honestly, the thought of the needles, and the high potential for major surgery, and the people coming in and out of the room made me feel like I needed a lot more bravery to go to the hospital.

What really sealed it for me was finding a midwife I trusted implicitly to guide me through the process. Mari Mikel had attended 3,000 births and had such low hospital transfer rates. I felt so at ease thinking about laboring at home with her guidance that I knew I had found the right choice for my family and me. I hope the information in this chapter and this book will help you do the same (feel confident that you've found the right choice for you, that is; I'm not at all attached to whether or not you decide to have your baby at home!).

Here are six other reasons that really compelled me to elect to give birth at home:

1. *Hospitals are for the sick and injured.* A laboring woman is neither. I didn't understand why I would go to the hospital, then, unless complications arose (in which case I would be happy to be transferred).

2. *For low-risk pregnancies, planned midwife-attended home births are just as safe—or can be ever safer—than hospital births.* For women who have no history of birth complications or medical conditions there is no difference in the safety or results when attended by a professional midwife in a home compared to a hospital. In fact, planned home births are associated with reduced rates of obstetric interventions like episiotomies and Cesarean births. Home births also show reduced rates of things like severe perineal tearing and postpartum hemorrhaging.

3. *No stressful drive to the hospital or interruption in labor.* When you are in early labor, many things can stall labor. Transferring or leaving home to head to a hospital is one of them. So many women go to the hospital and by the time they get there and then are checked in, they are no longer progressing and are often sent home. I wanted to be able to stay in the zone throughout all of my labor.

4. *More privacy.* Birth is an intimate event, and not something I wanted to share with strangers. I wanted to be able to tear off my clothes if that's what I felt. I wanted to be able to freely move in and out of the birth tub. And I didn't want a new nurse checking my chart or my cervix every half-hour. Once the birth was over (and we were sure everyone was healthy), I wanted to cuddle up with my husband and baby and relax in my own bed.

> "IN FACT, PLANNED HOME BIRTHS ARE ASSOCIATED WITH REDUCED RATES of OBSTETRIC INTERVENTIONS LIKE EPISIOTOMIES and CESAREAN BIRTHS."

5. ***A comfortable environment.*** A woman's brain and emotions play a huge role in how her birth progresses. Fear, anxiety, and discomfort can slow down labor. And a sterile, unfamiliar environment with bright lights, strangers, and all kinds of medical equipment beeping and dinging isn't calm or comforting. At home, I would be in a familiar place and I could control my surroundings (the lighting, music, bedding). I could wear my own clothes and eat my own food. I wouldn't be ogled or poked by strangers whose shifts might change mid-labor. Once it was all done I could take a shower in my own bathroom and put on whatever clothes I wanted from my own closet. No lumpy hospital beds, bleached-out gowns, weird food, beeping medical equipment, or plastic bins for baby to sleep in.

6. ***Less risk of unnecessary intervention or pressure to medicate.*** I understand that the absence of pain medication might be considered a negative for many women; but for me, it was an advantage. I had time to prepare my mind for an unmedicated birth. I knew from the get-go that I would need to draw from personal resources to get through it because there would be no other ones to draw from. As a consequence I knew I had to do this on my own—and it was one of the most empowering decisions I've ever made.

Another Person to Consider Adding to Your Care Team: A Doula

Full confession: I love doulas so much that I trained to be one. I wish I could wave my magic wand and give every laboring mother a doula—a trained birth attendant who is there to support the mother and help with pain relief, moral support, and practical help (like dimming lights and fetching water). Since I've already thrown a ton of information at you, I'm going to cover doulas in depth in Chapter 8. Stay tuned.

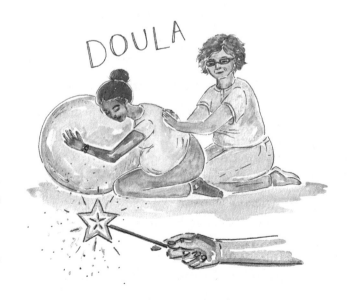

Cesarean Considerations

The Centers for Disease Control states that about one-third of all births in the U.S. are via Cesarean, and estimates that 55 percent of all Cesareans performed in the U.S. are elective.[18]

So if you're considering electing to have a Cesarean birth in a hospital for a non-medical reason, you're certainly not alone. However, before you fully make up your mind, I invite you to consider these facts. I'm not out to dissuade you; I just want you to be as informed as possible when making your decision. Cesareans can absolutely be lifesaving, and some babies are simply unable to be born vaginally. But that doesn't mean they're without risk. I believe as women we have the right and the responsibility to know these risks.

Potential risks to the mother

Compared to a vaginal delivery, moms who have a Cesarean birth are two to four times more likely to die giving birth.

They are also more likely to:

- Develop infections

- Hemorrhage (lose a significant amount of blood) and require an emergency hysterectomy

- Suffer injuries to other internal organs

- Have a complication from anesthesia

- Experience psychological complications, including post-traumatic stress and clinical depression

- Deal with long-term pain, which can last six months or more, including pain from adhesions (internal scar tissue) and endometriosis which can develop as a result of a Cesarean delivery

Potential risks to baby

In general, babies born via Cesarean face more health complications, including:

- Being born prematurely, and all the complications that arise from early delivery, such as respiratory distress, issues with liver function, jaundice, and others

- Respiratory distress in general; Caesareans present a risk of breathing problems even in babies delivered at full-term

- Complications that can be severe enough to involve admission to neonatal intensive care or a special care nursery

- Asthma, allergies, and even type 1 diabetes in childhood

It's also important to note that having a Cesarean birth often means you don't get to interact with your new baby right away, which can impact bonding and attachment as well as breastfeeding (although some hospitals are starting to offer a family-centered Cesarean, where the baby is put on the mother's chest right away so you can bond and begin breastfeeding even before you leave the operating room). What's more, Cesareans increase your odds of infertility as well as other complications for future pregnancies.

You may have heard that having a Cesarean can prevent you from experiencing pelvic floor dysfunction after birth, a cluster of disorders that can bring about problems having a bowel movement and can lead to constipation, the need to urinate frequently, and incontinence. If that's swaying your decision, know that studies don't actually appear to show that it offers any real benefits when it comes to pelvic floor issues, at least not once you've healed from delivery, nor do they suggest it protects you from these issues later in your life. If you have a vaginal birth, you can use the breathing exercises I shared on pages 40 and 41 to strengthen your pelvic floor naturally and reduce your risk of any pelvic-floor-related complications. Resting and lying down a lot in the two weeks after delivery helps your pelvic floor heal better than if you immediately start spending lots of time on your feet (or even sitting up)—more on this in Chapter 23.

If you're adamant about having a natural birth and avoiding a Cesarean delivery but believe you'd prefer to give birth in a hospital, remember to ask the hospitals you're considering about their Cesarean rates. Low rates are considered 15 percent or less.

Home Birth Facts and Figures

If you're on the fence about whether or not to give birth at home, I imagine safety is your biggest concern. But as I mentioned on page 88, according to the largest study of home births to date—published in the peer-reviewed Journal of Midwifery & Women's Health in 2014— planned home deliveries are not only safe in general for women with low-risk pregnancies, they involve far fewer medical interventions than similar hospital births and result in improved outcomes for you and baby (refer to page 257 for a list of interventions typically used during hospital births). Here's a deeper dive into the landmark study's findings.

The study included nearly 17,000 planned home births under midwife care (16,924, to be exact!) and found:

- 94 percent of women in the study had a vaginal birth

- 11 percent of women intending to give birth at home transferred to a hospital, usually because the labor failed to progress; only 4.5 percent of these women needed Pitocin to encourage labor and/or an epidural (typically, those numbers are much higher in standard hospital deliveries: 26 percent and 67 percent, respectively)

- Only 5.2 percent of women had a Cesarean birth (remarkable when you consider that the U.S. national average hovers slightly higher than 30 percent)

- 87 percent of the 1,054 women who attempted a vaginal birth after Cesarean (VBAC) at home were successful in doing so

- 97 percent of babies were carried to full-term, weighing an average of eight pounds when born

- Just 1 percent of babies needed to be transferred to the hospital after birth, most for non-urgent issues; the same goes for moms: only 1.5 percent were transferred postpartum

- Only 1.5 percent of newborns had low Apgar scores, a test given right after birth that provides a quick snapshot of the baby's health

- Almost 98 percent of newborns were at least partially breastfeed at six weeks old; 86 percent were fully breastfed

These findings are incredibly consistent with other studies of planned home births, including a large prospective study published in the *British Medical Journal* in 2005.[19] Notably in that study, more than 97 percent of mothers reported that they were either extremely or very satisfied with the care they received from their midwife. More than 87 percent of mothers and babies didn't require a hospital transfer for any reason, while only 3.7 percent of moms needed a Cesarean. Rates for other medical interventions, such as episiotomy, were also extremely low.

Here are some more interesting facts about birth, home birth, and midwifery in general:

- The percentage of countries providing universal prenatal care that have lower infant mortality rates than the United States: 100 percent

- The percentage of U.S. births attended principally by midwives: 5 percent

- The percentage of European births attended principally by midwives: 75 percent

- Number of midwives practicing in the U.S.: 3,000-4,000 midwives who aren't also trained as nurses; 3,500 certified nurse midwives

- Number of midwives needed in the U.S. to meet European levels: 120,000

- Percentage of babies born worldwide that are delivered by midwives: 80 percent

- Number of countries that have lower maternal mortality rates than the U.S.: 49

- Where the U.S. infant mortality rate falls on a list of the Organization for Economic Cooperation and Development (a group of 36 wealthy countries): 33rd

- Ratio of the U.S. infant mortality rate compared to Japan's: over 3 to 1 (5.8 per 1,000 in the U.S. compared to 1.8 per 1,000 in Japan)

- The U.S. spends more money on health care than any other industrialized country in the world

(Above data is from the World Health Organization)

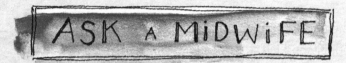

WHAT'S THE DEAL WITH ULTRASOUNDS?

From the very start of your pregnancy, if you're working with an Ob/Gyn, you are likely given an ultrasound exam that allows you to "see" the baby and get one of those little black and white printouts that shows the outline of the baby inside your womb. I know how exciting it is to see your baby, especially for the first time, but there are some things you want to think about before consenting to get an ultrasound at every checkup. I'll let Mari Mikel take this one.

from MARi MiKeL:

"There are occasions when ultrasounds are appropriate and helpful, but in general they are grossly overused in the United States. As you might guess from their name, ultrasounds use a sound wave that's very powerful. It's a little like when you're driving down the highway with the windows up and a person in the backseat rolls down a window; the air pressure can be very uncomfortable on the eardrums of the people in the car in the same way that the sound waves can be very uncomfortable for your baby's eardrums in your womb. You can often see babies put their arms up in front of their heads during an ultrasound. The technician will say the baby's waving, but they're doing it because it doesn't feel good. You can also often see the baby move away from the wand. There is some question about what frequent ultrasounds do to babies' inner ears. Even the 20-week ultrasound, which most providers will tell you is important, is of questionable necessity; they've only been commonly used for about 35 years, and healthy babies were born before then.

"Taking a peek at your baby is valid around 10-12 weeks to help you determine how far along you are and when your due date might be. Later in your pregnancy, an ultrasound is also helpful to know for sure if you suspect you're having twins; to see the baby's position if it is breech or not presenting properly; if you're experiencing unexplained bleeding; or if you've gone past your due date and you need to see how much fluid is in the amniotic sac and the condition of the placenta and baby.

"To my mind, doctors suggest such frequent ultrasounds because they can charge for them (about $250 a pop), and insurance companies don't pay them quite enough for the monthly visits and the delivery; ultrasounds become a convenient way to make the money they need to make with each client. If you have six or seven ultrasounds during the course of your pregnancy—and don't even get me started on 3D ultrasounds—they can make an extra $1,500. But all our medical expenditures aren't necessarily creating better outcomes: The U.S. has now slid to 55th in the world in infant and maternal morbidity, yet we spend $4,000 more than the next closest country per birth.

"Forty percent of my clients don't have ultrasounds at all, and their babies are still born healthy!

"I know most people want to know the sex of their baby, and having an ultrasound can help you determine whether you're having a boy or a girl. Just think long and hard about whether you truly need to know. It might be very special to be surprised."

Back to me again: I personally opted to be surprised with my first two pregnancies, and by the time my babies were born and on my chest the last thing I was thinking about was if it was a boy or a girl. I actually forgot to check until prompted both times.

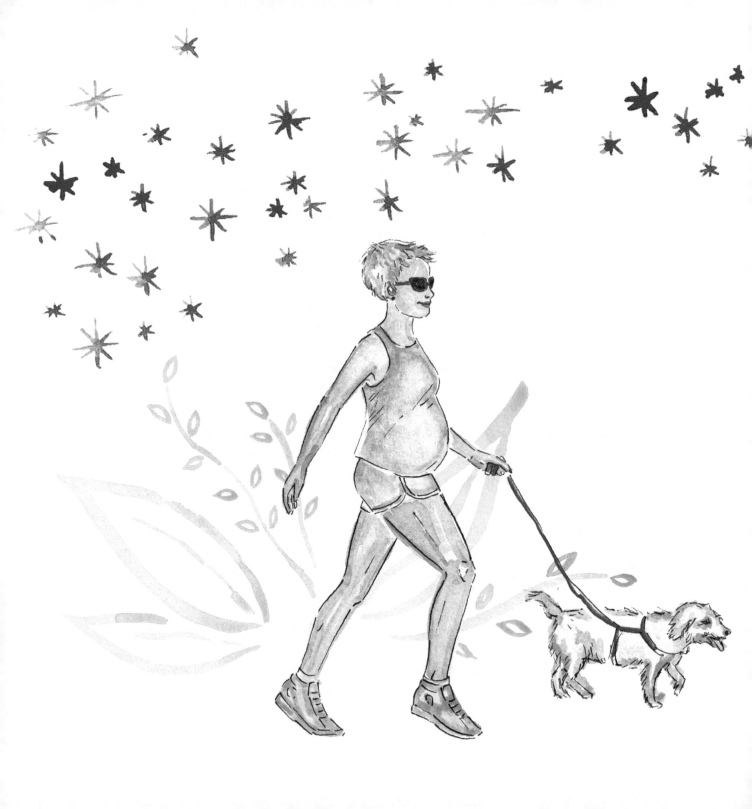

Chapter 6

STAY STRONG WITH FITNESS AND NUTRITION

E ven though there might not be much going on yet in terms of a baby bump, there's a lot happening inside your belly. In fact, the first trimester is the most important time in your baby's development, because all their major systems (skeletal, nervous, cardiovascular, etc.) and vital organs are developing. That's why most birth defects occur during these three months. I'm not saying this to scare you; I'm sharing it to help you get your mind focused on one of the easiest ways to mitigate these odds and to ensure a healthy first trimester for you both: your diet.

Nutrition for This Stage of the Baby's Development

Remember how, in Chapter 2, I stressed that eating for fertility was really just your run-of-the-mill good nutrition advice? The same advice holds true now that you're pregnant. If you skipped Chapter 2 because you were already pregnant when you picked up this book, or you haven't been eating a clean, healthy diet up until this point, now's the time to get serious about nutrition. We'll get in to the specific nutrients that you should focus on in just a bit, but the best way to benefit you and your baby right now is to eat primarily fresh, unprocessed, whole, organic and non-GMO foods—fruits and vegetables, whole grains, legumes, and lean meats.

I know you've heard someone talk about "eating for two" when you're pregnant, implying that you need more calories the minute you conceive. While it's true for your second and third trimesters, you actually don't need to eat any extra calories during your first trimester. Instead, focus on eating delicious nutrient-dense and anti-inflammatory whole

Why You Need to Drink More Water Now Than Ever

As important as choosing healthy foods is, don't forget to hydrate! You need more water than you typically do: While most standard hydration advice will tell you to drink 64 ounces (or eight 8-ounce glasses) a day, now that you're pregnant, you really want to up that to a minimum of 12 8-ounces glasses a day. Your body uses that extra water to create your amniotic fluid, extra blood, the baby and the placenta. It also delivers nutrients and washes away the baby's waste materials and toxins from the environment that you don't want to stick around.

Keep filled reusable water bottles everywhere—on your bedside table, in your bag, by the couch or your favorite chair, and in the car (make sure that the one you keep in the car is stainless steel and not plastic, as chemicals from the plastic can leach into the water, especially when it's left in a hot car). I found a carafe with a glass that doubled as a lid that I loved and used that upstairs in the bedroom, and I got a big water dispenser with a five-gallon tub for the kitchen so that filling up the carafe and my water bottle was so easy, I couldn't not do it. You want to drink so much that your urine is either very light yellow or clear—that's how you know you're getting enough.

It's really best if you can filter your water; a carbon-filter pitcher is great, or maybe your refrigerator has a carbon filter installed if it has an automatic water dispenser. There are so many contaminants in tap water—prescription drugs, chemical fertilizers and pesticides, chlorine, fluoride—and this is such a sensitive time in your baby's development, you want to minimize any chemicals or other toxic substances that might have a negative effect on their health.

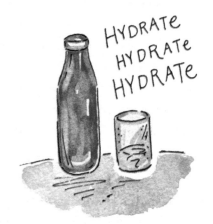

HYDRATe
HYDRATe
HYDRATe

foods and resist the urge to load up on sugary treats or processed snacks because it's "OK" to gain weight when you're pregnant. I always say if it comes in a bag or box, don't eat it. Instead opt for food that's alive and fresh. Of course, you will gain weight while you are pregnant (and there's a breakdown of what comprises that weight gain on page 175), but the majority of those extra pounds aren't fat; they're important things like extra blood supply, your growing uterus, and the amniotic fluid. Binging on foods you might otherwise consider to be off limits just gives your body extra work to deal with the empty calories when it's got a lot more important stuff to focus on now that you're building a baby.

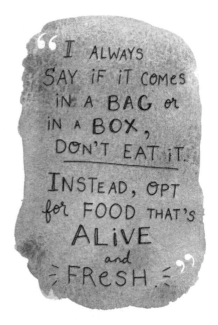

"I always say if it comes in a bag or in a box, don't eat it. Instead, opt for food that's alive and fresh."

You may gain a couple of pounds, or you may actually lose a pound or two during these three months; it's okay either way. Continue to eat the appropriate amount of calories for you and your size and level of physical activity. And keep in mind that you will likely feel better if you have a little extra body fat in early pregnancy, as it will help you have more reserves to carry you through the epic work of growing a baby and a placenta.

I'm not saying don't treat yourself. When I was pregnant with my older son, Hendrix, my favorite thing to eat was meat; I couldn't even look at a salad. This was completely opposite of the way I ate all my life. I had been a pescatarian for 12 years, meaning I hadn't eaten any meat other than fish. But during that pregnancy, I felt like I had to have it, red meat included. For the most part, though, you want everything you eat to deliver nutrients and help you build your baby and nourish yourself—because the baby will take all the nutrients it needs from you, you want to make sure that you eat enough of the good stuff to keep you healthy too.

Speaking of nutrients, all the ones I listed as being good for fertility in Chapter 2 are the same ones that are super important for you to be consuming now. For example, adequate calcium intake will help ensure proper bone, tooth, and nervous system development; ample iodine and choline will aid in healthy brain development and help prevent neural tube defects; and enough zinc will help ensure proper cell division and embryonic development across the board. Iron is also important for your baby's growth and development now. Refer back to pages 25-27 for lists of foods rich in these nutrients. Even though all these nutrients are important, folate is the most crucial for preventing neural tube defects (see the sidebar at the right for more about why folate and omega-3 fatty acids especially deserve your focus during the first trimester).

Folate-Rich Lentil Soup

Lentils are one of nature's perfect foods. For starters, they're great sources of protein, iron, and folate. Plus, they cook quickly and are more digestible than other beans. This flavorful soup is a great one to eat now and all the way through your pregnancy (give it a break in the first few weeks after delivery, as lentils might make your baby gassy if you're breastfeeding).

Ingredients:

- 1 tbsp olive oil
- 1 onion, finely chopped
- 1 garlic clove, crushed
- ½ tsp ground coriander
- ½ tsp ground cumin
- 1 lb fresh tomatoes (seeded and chopped)
- ¾ cup split red lentils
- 5 cups vegetable stock
- Salt and pepper to taste

Instructions:

In a large pan, heat oil then sauté onion and cook until softened, about 5 minutes. Stir in crushed garlic, cumin, and coriander until fully incorporated. Add in tomatoes and lentils. Stir constantly for 4 minutes. Add vegetable stock and bring to a boil, then reduce to let simmer for 30 minutes or until lentils are tender. Add salt and pepper as needed. Use an immersion blender, or carefully transfer to a blender or large food processor and blend until smooth. Rinse your pan and return soup to reheat and serve.

Focus on Folate and Fatty Acids

I said I was going to talk about folate lots in this book, so here I go again. It plays a vital role in the development of your baby's brain and spinal cord. For this reason, it's absolutely critical in the prevention of birth defects, which means the time for you to be eating plenty of folate-rich foods is now. Some of the best sources include:

- Asparagus
- Beets
- Lentils
- Kale
- Spinach
- Black-eyed peas
- Brussels sprouts
- Romaine and other leafy green lettuce
- Avocado
- White rice
- Broccoli
- Orange juice

In general, fresh, colorful, organic vegetables should make up a significant portion of your pregnancy diet. They're anti-inflammatory and have tons of the nutrients I've mentioned here, along with fiber—which will keep you regular—and are also a healthy source of carbohydrates. Healthy carbs are important to include in your diet; they support gut health and contribute to a healthy thyroid and healthy adrenal gland. Note that "below-ground" vegetables, or starchy veggies, like potatoes and sweet potatoes, are okay but in moderation. Don't go crazy on them, because your body metabolizes them into glucose, aka sugar. And since the hormones that rise during pregnancy can affect your insulin production (insulin is the hormone that regulates blood sugar levels), you want to avoid eating too many glucose-producing foods.

The omega-3 fatty acids EPA and DHA are also critical for your baby's developing brain. Wild salmon is chock-full of these nutrients. You can also find these omega-3s in fortified eggs, the yolks of pastured eggs, and other seafood. For details about what's safe to eat and not safe to eat from the sea, see the Safe Seafood box on pages 196-197. Because omega-3s are so important, especially now while your baby's brain is developing, I suggest taking a fish oil supplement that's been purified (so that any contaminants in the fish, such as mercury, are removed)—see the box on page 109 for dosage information.

Green Folate Smoothie

A smoothie is such a great way to eat your fruits and veggies—it's a whole-food meal that only takes 5 minutes to make! This smoothie helps you get your greens and your folate; the almond butter helps it keep you full until lunch.

Ingredients:
- 1 cup raw spinach
- 1 cup romaine lettuce
- ¼ medium cantaloupe
- ½ avocado
- ½ cup raw papaya
- 1 tbsp almond butter
- ½ cup coconut water

Instructions:

Put all ingredients in a blender and combine until smooth. Add more coconut water for a thinner smoothie.

Energizing Smoothie

This smoothie will help you perk up and keep going during these first trimester days when it may feel like your get-up-and-go got up and went. The coconut water and spirulina are revitalizing; the minerals in the greens will help your whole body function better; the fiber in the raspberries and flaxseed will keep you feeling full; and the natural sugar in the banana and date will give you access to slow-burning energy.

Ingredients:
- ½ cup water
- ½ cup coconut water
- 1 frozen ripe banana (I freeze mine— peeled—when they start to turn brown so I have plenty on hand for smoothies)
- 1 cup frozen raspberries
- ½ pitted date (cuts the taste of the spirulina)
- ½ cup spinach
- ¼ cup romaine (optional)
- ½ peeled cucumber (peel tastes bitter, so peel it)
- ½ lemon, juiced
- 1 tbsp organic spirulina powder
- 1 tbsp ground flax seed

Instructions:

Put all ingredients in a blender and combine until smooth. Add more coconut water for a thinner smoothie.

Other Nutrients That Are Important Now

- **Beta-carotene.** Vitamin A is essential for healthy organ development during the embryonic period (weeks three through eight). The only hitch is, if you get more vitamin A than you body needs, your body will store it in the liver. If it builds up too much in your liver, it can become toxic and has been linked to birth defects. To avoid this potential complication, focus on eating foods with plenty of beta-carotene, which is a water-soluble precursor to vitamin A; your body will use it to make the vitamin A it needs in just the right amount. Beta-carotene is found in brightly colored veggies like carrots, kale, squash, and sweet potatoes.

- **Vitamin B6.** Also called pyridoxine, this nutrient plays a role in your baby's brain and nervous system development. Proper levels of vitamin B6 during your first trimester may also help prevent the loss of your pregnancy. You should be able to get all the B6 you need for a healthy first trimester through diet alone. Good sources include bananas, chickpeas, eggs, salmon, carrots, and sweet potatoes. B6 may also help relieve pregnancy-related nausea.

- **Vitamin D3.** Technically a hormone, vitamin D3 is critical for healthy bones (for you and your baby) and teeth development (for the baby). A deficiency can lead to skeletal abnormalities and lowered growth. It can be found naturally in pastured egg yolks (also a good source of choline and omega-3s) and fatty fish like salmon, as well as fortified beverages, from milk to orange juice.

- **Phosphorus.** Like vitamin D, phosphorus aids in the development of your baby's teeth and bones. If you're eating a healthy, balanced diet, you should naturally be getting enough phosphorus. Foods particularly rich in this nutrient include meats, dairy products, fish, poultry, and eggs.

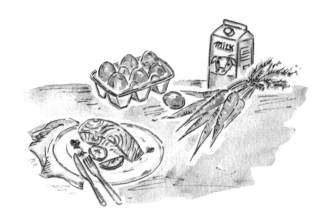

What If I Don't Feel Like Eating?

It's common to develop aversions to certain foods in the first trimester, or even to feel so nauseated that you don't want to eat much at all. But it's so important that you keep your nutrition up now. As Mari Mikel says, "In the first trimester you want to eat small amounts more frequently. It's getting an empty stomach that causes problems, because your blood sugar drops and it makes you feel nauseated and weak. You don't have to feel like eating; you just have to put the food in your mouth, chew it, and swallow it so that you keep your nutrient intake high." Make sure to check out the section on natural remedies for nausea in Chapter 7, as they can help prevent you from getting to that place where you've lost interest in food.

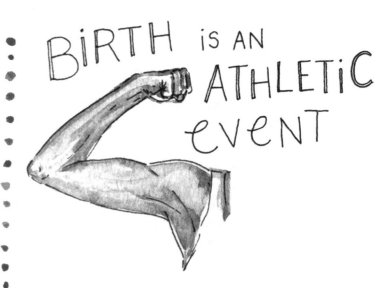

BIRTH is AN ATHLETIC event

Staying Active

I've talked to a lot of women, who once they get pregnant, seem to think it's an invitation to sit on the couch eating whatever they want with their feet up. Of course, I believe pregnant women should take great care of themselves by eating right and staying active.

I mean, yes, your body has an innate wisdom that is nothing short of magic—even if you did nothing but eat chips and drink soda the baby would likely still grow and still be born. But you have to go through some pretty significant transformations to make the magic of growing and delivering a baby happen. And make no mistake about it: Birth is an athletic event. One of the best ways to prepare for all the physiological changes to come, and for the event itself—and to handle them with strength and grace—is to exercise. What's more, exercise can help ease you through the mental and emotional shifts that often accompany the transition to motherhood.

If you've always exercised because it helps you maintain or lose weight, pregnancy is a great time to start to think about all the other things exercise does for you, some of which are listed below. Of course, exercising during pregnancy also helps you stay within a healthy weight range, which will help you recover from pregnancy and birth more efficiently.

- Helps lessen the aches and pains (chiefly back pain) that come with a changing body

- Strengthens your muscles, which naturally relax during pregnancy, and helps prepare you for all the pushing and physical exertion of labor

- Supports your joints and ligaments, which loosen as your body shifts and adapts to being pregnant

Should You Be Supplementing?

You should absolutely still be taking your prenatal vitamins (refer back to Chapter 2 for this information). Other than that, there are two nutrients that are extra important to both you and your baby now and that a lot of people are deficient in: omega-3 fatty acids and vitamin D. That's why it's a good idea to supplement these (after talking to your health care provider, of course).

Vitamin D3 dosage: 1,000–5,000 IUs a day

Omega-3 dosage: 1,000–3,000 mg a day in the form of a fish oil supplement; check the label to see what the total level of omega-3 is. It should be broken down into the two different types of omega-3 fatty acids, which are EPA (a potent anti-inflammatory) and DHA (important for brain development); your supplement needs to provide a minimum of 300 mg DHA. It should also be tested by a third party lab to assure that it's been purified, as many fish are contaminated with mercury and other heavy metals and toxins that could be harmful to your baby. This is one supplement it's really worth it to spend more on to ensure quality.

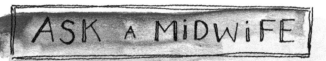

ASK A MIDWIFE

CAN I EVER HAVE A DRINK NOW THAT I'M PREGNANT?

(Mari Mikel shared her perspectives on drinking alcohol while you're trying to get pregnant in Chapter 2; if you missed it, go back and check out her wisdom on page 36, as it pertains to drinking while you're pregnant too.)

from MARI MIKEL:

"As I mentioned before, alcohol is a great stress-reliever, and really stress—and the hormones it creates—is just as dangerous for a baby, if not more so, than alcohol is. I tell the women in my care that it's OK to have one glass of wine a week to reduce tension, but that they have to think of it as medicine and not recreation. If you struggle to keep it to just one glass, you shouldn't have any. There are other things you can drink when you go out with friends [like a club soda with a splash of fruit juice and/or herbal bitters for a festive mocktail]—stick to those for your recreation and use your one drink a week to take the edge off of a really bad day, like the medicine that it is.

"While alcohol is stress-reducing, it's also a way to numb out, and you don't want to be numb now; your baby needs you to have your wits about you and to be present to all your feelings."

- Stabilizes blood sugar; it's normal for blood sugar levels to increase a bit during pregnancy—exercise helps your body better use the insulin it makes, which keeps your blood sugar levels in a safe, optimal range and helps you avoid developing gestational diabetes

- Boosts your energy; I know it might sound contradictory, but a little exertion can actually help you feel less tired and fatigued throughout your pregnancy

- Increases your circulation, which you want because your vascular system delivers oxygen and blood not just to all your cells, but to all the baby's cells too

- Improves your flexibility and balance, both of which will help you adjust to pregnancy effectively, with less pain, and safely (it's easier to lose your balance and fall as your center of gravity shifts as the baby grows)

- Helps you detox, both physically and emotionally, as sweat is purifying for your body and your mind

- Contributes to a good mood and positive self-image, even as the self you've known for years begins to look and feel much different than it ever has before

And that's just what it does for *you*. Science has shown that babies whose mothers exercised regularly have stronger hearts and more advanced motor development (able to grip and move) than babies whose moms didn't. Research also suggests that when you exercise during pregnancy, your child's brain may develop faster and they may even have a better chance of avoiding cardiovascular complications later in their life. Moving your body increases your blood flow, which delivers more oxygen and nutrients to the baby in addition to your own cells. Studies also show that women who are active and exercise in the first and second trimester have healthier placentas. If working out for yourself isn't enough motivation, think of what it can do for your child.

If you've been exercising regularly before pregnancy, it's generally considered safe, especially during the first trimester, to continue with relatively the same level of activity so long as it's moderate (walking, doing gentle yoga, light weights, etc.). I love an intense workout, so I know how important it can feel to break a sweat and push yourself, but pregnancy really isn't the time for that—you're already performing huge physical feats just by being pregnant. I'll talk a bit more below about the dos and don'ts of exercising while pregnant in the next pages, but honestly, for these first 8-12 weeks, you don't need to push yourself.

There are five main types of exercise that are perfect for pregnancy:

- **Walking.** Walking is great during your first trimester and beyond. It's low-impact yet can boost your aerobic capacity. And when you do it first thing in the morning, that early light exposure can lift your mood all day and help regulate your circadian rhythm, a hormonal orchestra that influences so many important things, like appetite and sleep. Even a 15-20 minute walk three to five times a week, preferably in the morning, is a great goal for this trimester. You can walk every day if you're feeling up to it.

   Mari Mikel suggests avoiding jogging or running during pregnancy—it's "too high impact," she says—as well as anything that has the potential for falling, like bicycling, skiing, rock climbing, etc. Your uterus is only held in place by ligaments and fascia, and it is increasing in size and weight daily at this point. When you run, you place significantly more strain on the ligaments than walking. If you miss the intensity of a run, go for a power walk and really swing your arms—that will get your heart rate up. The only caveat to walking is to watch your stride; shortening it will protect your hip joints.

- **Lagree Method.** This approach is similar to Pilates, and is what I used during pregnancy, in combination with Brooke's workouts and belly breathing, which I introduced in Chapter 1. As long as you only do pregnancy-safe core moves, Lagree is a great and very challenging workout. I'd only recommend doing this one if you already did it before pregnancy.

- **Yoga.** Stretching is an important part of any exercise routine, but especially a pregnancy exercise routine that helps you de-stress, maintain flexibility, and avoid some of the inevitable aches and pains. A prenatal yoga class will help you stretch all your major muscle groups. It also will compress and massage your organs and your muscles, which helps improve blood flow as well as the flow of lymphatic fluid, aka the trash collection service of the body.

   Mari Mikel believes that really focusing on the ligaments, tendons, and muscles of the pelvis saves you pushing time during labor. I believe it too. Stretching your pelvis helps make more space for the baby to come out—the squats, cobbler's pose, and pigeon poses that most prenatal yoga classes include will all help you prep your pelvis for birth.

Unless you're a very experienced yogi with a very well-trained teacher, stick to the prenatal classes even during the first trimester. Again, it might not be your sweatiest practice or your prettiest poses, but your goal now is to take care of your body and your baby, and prenatal yoga is great at helping you do both. Also, inversions except for downward dog are off limits—your hormones can make your ligaments loose and cause feelings of wooziness, and you don't want to do anything that presents a risk of falling.

> "WHEN YOU'RE PREGNANT, your BODY PRODUCES A HORMONE, APTLY CALLED **RELAXIN**, that MAKES your CARTILAGE and LIGAMENTS MORE FLEXIBLE."

An important note: When you're pregnant, your body produces a hormone, aptly called relaxin, that makes your cartilage and ligaments more flexible—it's how your belly is able to stretch to a size you may not have thought possible. This means you could overstretch your muscles if you aren't careful. Stretch gently and easily, never to the point of pain, and control your stretch every step of the way. Hold the stretches for about 30 seconds and avoid bouncing. And don't forget to breathe!

• **Swimming.** Swimming is a great form of cardio that strengthens the whole body, particularly the upper body where most women tend to be weak. (You'll need that upper body strength in spades once the baby is here!) A lot of women resist the idea of swimming for exercise, but it can feel so incredibly great when you're pregnant to be in a pool, where you're weightless, and swimming laps, where you can really tune into your body and your breathing. Wear a swim cap to protect your hair from the chemicals in the pool water. (It will also keep you warm if the water feels chilly at first—although swimming even a half a lap will warm you right up.)

Do the breaststroke to swim your laps—the frog kick is a great exercise for your pelvis, as it puts your hips through a broad range of motion, and the arm movement of the stroke will build your chest and back muscles. It's also an easier stroke with which to get your breathing right than the freestyle, where you have to turn your head to breathe. Mari Mikel even says that regularly swimming the breaststroke can help a breech baby decide to turn, as the movement will gently bump their head up against your ribcage and they will choose to go head-down.

If you're new to swimming, aim to stay moving in the water for 15-20 minutes. You can alternate a lap of swimming with a lap of using a kickboard and gradually work your way up to doing more laps without the use of a kickboard. Gradually work your way up to swimming a mile. I think you'll find that the weightless, quiet feeling can become addictive.

- **Strength-training.** I'm a big fan of light-to-moderate weightlifting throughout pregnancy. Toning your body with light weights will help with overall strength—which will come in real handy when you're carrying a baby and a diaper bag and a car seat everywhere you go. It will also improve your stability and reduce your risk of falls as you adjust to being a little top-heavy.

At this point, your body is pumping out the steroid hormones and human growth hormone that athletes cheat to get because they make building muscle so much easier—why not put them to work making you stronger?

I recommend using weight machines unless you're experienced at using free weights—you don't want to strain yourself trying to lift something that's too heavy, or without the right form, and the machines really make this harder to do. Aim to use a weight that's light enough that you can do 15 reps but heavy enough that it starts getting tiresome around rep 13.

- **Core-strengthening exercises.** Think about it: How will you be able to push a baby out of you without a strong core?! Unfortunately, the vast majority of us don't have a good relationship with our core. How we sit (a lot, and with not-great posture); how we breathe (typically shallowly, because we're often some level of stressed out); and how we move (because that not-great posture from sitting too much comes into play when we're active too) has impaired the function of the muscles that make up the canister that lines our abdomen.

Luckily, you don't have to do hundreds of crunches to get your core back online—in fact, please don't do them while you're pregnant.

Here's a circuit of exercises designed by Brooke Cates of the Bloom Method to help you keep strengthening both the muscles in your core and your connection to those muscles.

Core Circuit

Kneeling Belly Pumps

Duration: 45 seconds

Directions: Refer back to page 41 for a refresher on the belly bump. Then perform it kneeling, either with your booty off your heels for more of a challenge or resting on your heels for an easier option.

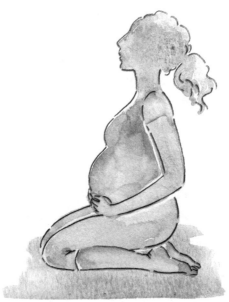

Bird Dog

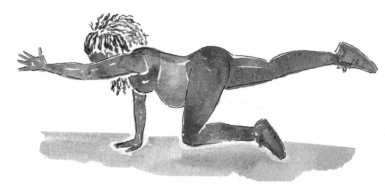

Duration: 1 minute

Directions: Start on all fours with wrists under shoulders and knees under hips. Exhale and engage the core and pelvic floor as you extend opposite arm and opposite leg out and away from the body. Inhale to lower back to starting and repeat on the other side. Continue to alternate lifting and extending with core activation as the guide and inhaling and relaxing through the core and pelvic floor to come back to all fours.

Side Plank on the Right Side

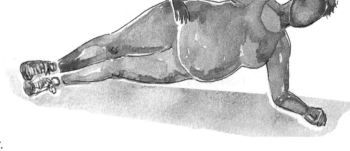

Duration: 45 seconds

Directions: Lying on your right side with your torso propped up on the right forearm, elbow directly beneath the shoulder, and with either legs straight or knees bent, exhale as in a belly pump, engaging the core and pelvic floor. Once they are engaged, lift the hips up, and go even deeper with your core and oblique engagement.

Modified Plank

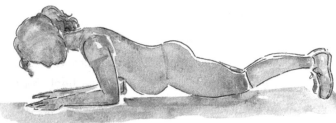

Duration: 1 minute

Directions: Coming onto forearms and knees, exhale and engage the core and pelvic floor as you angle the pelvis down towards the floor (while still keeping it elevated). Hold this position, taking sips of inhales into the chest while each exhale takes you deeper into core engagement. Don't lose your core engagement here! The breath is vital for helping you manage the pressure increase in your abdomen. If you see or feel a ridge or a bulge protruding out along the center line of your belly (in what's known as doming or coning), stop and come up to a more traditional all fours position, and then keep going with the breathing and the core activation.

Side Plank on the Left Side

Duration: 45 seconds

Directions: Setting up on the left forearm with either legs straight or knees bent, exhale as in a belly pump, engaging the core and pelvic floor. Once they are engaged, lift the hips up, and go even deeper with your core and oblique engagement.

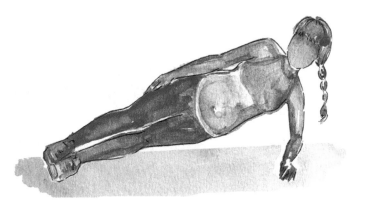

Supine Alternating Heel Taps

Duration: 1 minute

Directions: Lying on your back, exhale and engage your core as you lift one leg at a time up into a tabletop position. Exhale, engaging deeper as you slowly lower one heel down towards floor, then slowly return it to the starting position. Repeat with other leg. Move slowly and only go as far as you can with your core staying engaged (if your lower back pops up off the floor, you've gone too far).

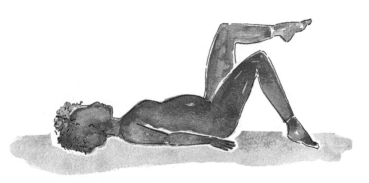

Overall, you really just want to embrace movement and give some thought to the fact that you want to be building muscle, getting your heart pumping, stretching your muscles, and strengthening your core. It might sound like a lot, but it doesn't have to be—especially now when your energy might be tanking. Whenever you can, get out for a morning walk (the light will perk up your mood all day), do a little stretching every day, and see if you can

Rest Is Part of Your Workout Now Too

Mari Mikel, says, "Your body is devoting a nuclear reactor's worth of energy to developing the baby and the placenta, taking the baby from two cells to a fully formed human being in only 12-14 weeks." If it's all you can do to get out of bed in the morning, it's OK to take a little time off from formal workouts now, and to take a gentle approach to the movement that you do get.

If you are feeling totally wiped out by pregnancy and don't feel you have the energy for anything that's not absolutely mandatory, honor that and rest as much as you need to. You should still stretch and do the belly pump and diaphragmatic breathing as close to every day as you can, and as you start to come out of the tired haze you can add in more walks, yoga classes, strength training, and/or whatever other form of exercise you truly love.

And even if your energy levels are pretty OK, or if you're type A about your workouts, know that resting now will help you get stronger later when your energy is back (for some women this happens as early as eight weeks; for others it takes 14 or 16 weeks—you've got to honor your body). Whatever you choose to do for movement now, it's not about burning calories, or setting a personal record. It's about improving health for you and your baby. And if you really love intense workouts, don't worry—you get to amp up your workouts in the second trimester.

find a gym nearby that has a pool, weight machines, and babysitting (you'll appreciate that option so much after the baby is born and you feel ready to get back out there with the exercise) and start getting there when you can to use the machines and swim in the pool. You can get in touch with your core at home, or really anywhere.

Of course, if you experience headaches, dizziness, chest pain, vaginal bleeding… stop exercising and consult your doctor immediately.

Pregnancy Exercise Dos and Don'ts

DOs

- Exercise as feels comfortable for you, regularly, at least three times per week

- Warm up and cool down

- Use proper posture: head up, shoulders relaxed, back straight, tailbone reaching down, and pubic bone reaching up (which will naturally engage and strengthen the core muscles)

- Hydrate, hydrate, hydrate

- Breathe, breathe, breathe

DONT's

- Exercise so intensely that you couldn't carry on a conversation while working out or to the point of exhaustion

- Bounce vigorously

- Engage in exercises that has you arch your back (such as the cow position in cat/cow pose)

- Hold your breath

- Do poses that cause your belly to push outward— like a plank (side and modified as shared on pages 116-117 are OK), or hanging from a bar, or a crunch; you want the muscles of the front of your stomach to stay together as the baby grows, and starting habits now that help that happen, even before you're showing, will help

- Exercise every day; your body needs a break

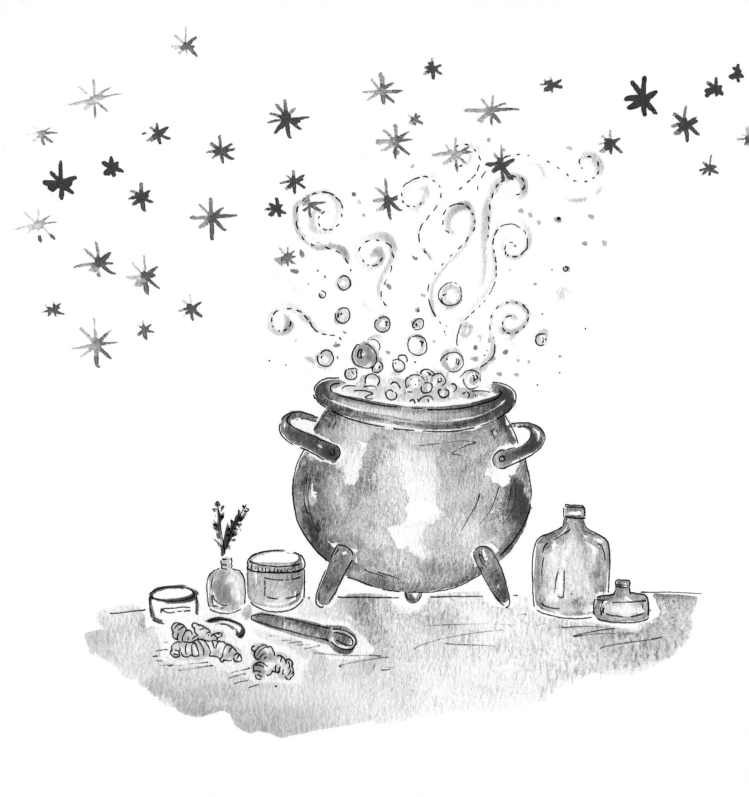

Chapter 7

NATURAL REMEDIES FOR FIRST TRIMESTER CHALLENGES

Now that you're growing a baby, there are a few different physical symptoms that can start to show up. Here are my best suggestions for the things that will help ease your symptoms and keep you feeling as good as you possibly can.

Some of these first-trimester challenges are really unpleasant—especially nausea. Just remember that typically, you'll feel a lot better in the second trimester.

Nausea

Nausea typically starts between weeks four and six and can worsen toward the end of the trimester, between weeks eight and twelve. Morning sickness is really a blood sugar problem—it tends to happen in the morning because that's when you've gone the longest without eating.

The best way to ward it off is to eat something approximately every three hours. That means eating right before you go to bed and then setting an alarm to wake up around 1:30 in the morning to eat something you've pre-prepared, such as half a sandwich, dinner leftovers, or a small baked sweet potato that you heat up in the microwave and have with a pat of butter. Choose something that has protein, complex carbs, and fat so it will stick with you. I know it's hard to sacrifice sleep, but you will ultimately sleep better and wake up feeling good instead of queasy.

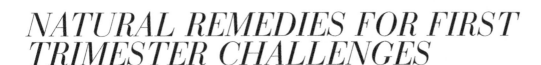

This also means you want to carry around food with you wherever you go so that you don't ever let your stomach get empty—always have nuts, apples, cheese and crackers, and low-sugar protein bars in your bag, your desk drawer, and your glove compartment.

Other remedies include:

- **Enjoy ginger,** whether that's by incorporating more fresh or powdered ginger into your meals, chewing on crystallized ginger, drinking ginger tea, or taking a ginger supplement (consult your doctor). Ginger is the only natural treatment for nausea recommended by the American College of Obstetrics and Gynecology, and countless studies prove that it works. It's thought to relieve nausea by stimulating the production of saliva and bile, thus promoting healthy digestion. You can try ginger ale as well; carbonated drinks may help quell nausea in general (find natural ginger ales that use actual ginger instead of artificial ginger flavor and less sugar than your standard soda).

- **Supplement with vitamin B6.** Take 25 mg three times a day to help keep nausea at bay. If you try it and at some point the B6 stops helping, keep taking it but skip it every fourth day.

- **Try acupuncture.** Acupuncture alleviates many of the symptoms of pregnancy, including nausea. It's also incredibly relaxing. If you've got the time and the budget, ask your mom friends for a recommendation for an acupuncturist who is well versed in pregnancy. (Acupuncture can also help you prepare for birth later in pregnancy by encouraging the downward energy of the body and loosening tight muscles and ligaments; it can even be useful in turning a breech baby.)

- **Get plenty of fresh air.** Sometimes various smells and odors can trigger your nausea—like the aromas released by food when it cooks or even things that you've never been able to detect before, like the odor of dirty clothes emanating from your hamper. Keeping a window cracked in the rooms where you spend the most time can help keep that queasy feeling away.

- **Avoid greasy and spicy foods.** Excessive amounts of oils and butter and fatty meats can upset your stomach, so be careful not to eat too much of foods such as fries, chips, bacon, pastries, croissants, and pie crusts—even if they sound appealing in the moment, they may contribute to queasiness later. Foods with lots of red pepper flakes, hot sauce, cayenne, chipotle, or other hot peppers may also promote stomach upset. It's best to keep meals kind of bland until your stomach rights itself.

An important note: If you haven't been able to keep anything down for 24 hours, contact your care provider. If pregnancy makes you consistently and violently ill, ask your doctor about Zofran, an anti-nausea medication used for hyperemesis.

Colds and Flu

The best way to avoid illness is to avoid people who are ill. If your partner comes down with something, sleep separately. If you have a co-worker who is sick, tell your boss, "Either they go home or I do."

Other than avoidance, stick to natural remedies, such as:

- Taking echinacea, oil of oregano, grapefruit seed extract, and/ or elderberry syrup, which are all supplements that boost the immune system and have antiviral and antibacterial properties. You can put the echinacea (one dropperful of tincture), oil of oregano (six drops), and grapefruit seed extract (10 drops) all in one shot glass of grapefruit or orange juice and toss it back so you don't taste it. Elderberry syrup (sold under the name Sambucol) tastes like grape juice already; follow the dosage directions on the package.

- Taking the homeopathic remedy oscillococcinum if you experience flu-like symptoms such as fever, chills, aches, and pains.

- Gargling with warm saltwater three or four times a day to kill the germs responsible for and relieve the pain of a sore throat.

- Using a neti pot with sea salt dissolved in it, or a saline nasal spray, to clean germs and mucous out of your nasal passages and sinuses.

- Drinking even more water when you're sick or fighting off something—a full gallon a day.

- Taking extra vitamin ester C, up to 3,000 mg a day; you can use effervescent ester C packets to make a drink (which will also help you meet your daily water needs), or take 500 mg every four hours.

- Giving yourself a steam treatment. When I was pregnant, I was prone to sinus infections, and the only thing that helped me breathe was to put a couple drops of organic lavender essential oil in the bottom of a large bowl then pour boiling water into the bowl and use a towel to make a tent over my head and inhale the steam. Amazon also sells facial steamers that make this process very simple.

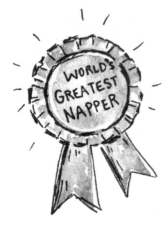

You'll also want to cut back on foods that are mucous producing, such as wheat and dairy, and on sugar, which causes a dip in immunity. Eat plenty of garlic, onions, greens, brightly colored vegetables, quinoa, and brown rice, as they are high in vitamins and minerals that will help your body fight the germs.

Rest is extra important when you're sick—resist the urge to push through and keep working. You need your energy to go toward the baby and to fighting off the virus right now, not to the laundry, the grocery store, or even your work.

Stomach Flu

Stomach flus are just miserable, and I pray you don't get one—they are bad enough anytime but just add insult to injury when you are pregnant. That being said, we all fall victim to them from time to time. If you get one, these guidelines should help you make them as manageable as possible:

- If you are vomiting, don't eat or drink anything (even water) until you haven't thrown up for two hours

- After you reach two hours, try having some very small ice chips

- Once you can keep ice chips down for two hours, take a dose of Pepto-Bismol

- Stick to clear liquids for the rest of the day, such as chicken or vegetable broth

- The next day, when you feel ready for solids, stick with things that are easy to digest such as applesauce, soups with well-cooked vegetables, quinoa, and rice cooked with plenty of water

- Call your doctor or midwife or have someone call for you so they can keep tabs on you.

Headaches

Most headaches are contributed to, if not downright caused, by dehydration. The next most common cause is not eating frequently enough. Remember, when you're pregnant you need at least 12 8-ounce glasses of water a day—that's a little less than one cup an hour for every hour you're awake. If you're getting frequent headaches now, the first thing you want to do is make sure you stay adequately hydrated. And then make sure you're eating throughout the day.

There's also an acupressure point in your hand called Joining the Union Valley that can help relieve headaches. To find it, extend all five fingers of your left hand with no spaces in between your fingers (bring your thumb right up next to your index finger). The point is located at the bottom of the crease that extends down from the inside of your thumb. Place your right thumb right on top of the bottom of that crease. Keep it there, then relax the fingers of your left hand and use the tip of your right index finger to press into your left palm just below where you right thumb is, and squeeze your right thumb and index finger toward each other. It should feel tender, but you don't need to apply so much

Stock Your Natural Medicine Cabinet

Keep these items on hand so that if you feel an illness coming on at any point in your pregnancy, you won't have to wait to start taking them until you or someone else can get to the store.

Arnica

Sold as a gel, cream, lotion, oil, and tablets, it helps relieve sore muscles and bruises

Astragalus

Supports the immune system and fights viruses

Cranberry extract

This supplement, sold in pill form, treats and prevents urinary tract infections. Look for one with D-mannose, a natural sugar that makes your bladder membrane less permeable to bacteria.

Echinacea

Classic immune booster that you can take regularly to ward off infection and/or at the first sign of illness (see page 126 for usage suggestion)

Elderberry syrup

Powerful immune booster often sold under the brand name Sambucol

Epsom salts

Reduces swelling and muscle soreness as well as constipation, as they promote relaxation and elimination. They are a form of magnesium, which is a relaxant for the nervous system and the smooth muscles of the body, including the digestive tract; pour a cup or more into a warm bath.

Grapefruit seed extract

Antibacterial, antiviral, and antifungal

Oscillococcinum

Homeopathic remedy that provides temporary relief of fever, chills, body aches, and pains

Pepto Bismol

Not 'natural' per se, but can really save the day should you catch a stomach virus pressure that it's uncomfortable. Keep applying pressure for one to two minutes while you breathe normally, then release and use your left thumb and index finger to press the same spot on your right hand. The earlier you do this when you first notice you have a headache, the more powerful it is. (You can also do this, gently, on kids to help them with their headaches.)

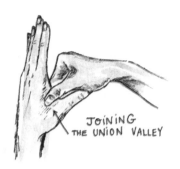

JOINING THE UNION VALLEY

   If you have a killer headache that doesn't respond to any of the other remedies suggested here, Mari Mikel says it's fine to take two ibuprofen; you don't want to take it every day, as there has been some research that suggests a link between taking non-steroidal anti-inflammatory drugs (NASIDs) such as ibuprofen and a higher risk of miscarriage and birth defects; this research is also highly refuted. If you were to take two ibuprofen every four hours for more than three days, it would likely have a negative effect on the clotting factor of your platelets. But if you're taking the occasional suggested dose of ibuprofen for a headache, it's OK. Talk to your doctor first; they may suggest you take acetaminophen instead, but ibuprofen is a better fever reducer than pain reliever, which is why Mari Mikel tells her patients to take a small amount of it for the occasional headache instead.

Breast Tenderness

Breast tenderness can be one of the first physical pregnancy symptoms you experience, and it can linger as your breasts grow along with the baby. The best way to counteract it is to keep your boobs well supported, even while sleeping. At night (or whenever you like), opt for a bra without underwire that will keep your breasts in place without cutting into your skin or impeding blood flow under your arms or anywhere the bra comes in contact with your skin.

Acne

Hormones do many amazing things… and some not-so exciting things. Like cause acne. From an external perspective, you want to keep the amount of bacteria on your skin as low as possible, so use a non-drying cleanser twice a day (because if your skin is too dry, it will only promote more oil production in an attempt to preserve moisture). Look for a nice cleansing milk or a cleansing oil.

As much as I love a great skincare product, clear skin is also an inside job. If you are breaking out you may be sensitive to wheat or dairy—cut back on both and see if it helps. When you replace those foods with fruits, vegetables, nuts, and seeds, you'll also get the benefit of adding a lot more vitamins and minerals to your diet, which benefit the whole body, including your skin.

Pelvic Pain

There are three basic sources of lower abdominal/pelvic pain. If you experience painful sensations in the middle of your lower abdomen, that is likely to be what's known as symphysis pubis dysfunction (SPD), which affects as many as one in five pregnant women. I had it—I experienced a strong burning sensation in the area of my pubic bone any time I had my feet wider than about shoulder-width apart. Everyone told me that it was round ligament pain, which is another possible source of pelvic pain. Round ligament pain is fairly common, and it's a sharp sensation on the sides of the low belly or groin caused by your round ligament, which attaches the uterus to the groin, stretching too quickly (also thanks to the relaxin). But I knew that this pain was in the region of my pubic bone, and not in the low belly, so I kept bringing it up with my doctor until finally I did enough research and reading online to self-diagnose the SPD. I watched videos of exercises that help alleviate symptoms and did them daily, and they brought a lot of relief.

Specifically, there's an exercise that resets the pelvis for about eight hours: You lie on your back with your knees bent and both feet on the floor, squeeze a yoga block between your knees for 30 seconds, and then remove the block and put your fist in between the knees and squeeze again for 30 seconds. You have to do it every day, sometimes even twice a day, but it makes the pain go away, at least temporarily, by bringing your pubic bones closer together. Wearing a Velcro belly band that you can adjust the fit of can also be helpful for some women, but didn't help me personally.

The belly pump exercise that Brooke shared in Chapter 2 also helps, as do glute bridges (lying on your back with your knees bent and feet on the floor, press into the soles of your feet, squeeze your glutes, and lift your hips up, holding for three to five breaths).

The third potential source of pelvic pain is a bladder infection; talk to your care provider if you suspect that might be the case.

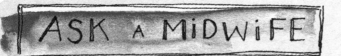

ASK A MIDWIFE

WHAT'S THE DEAL WITH FLU SHOTS?

from MARI MIKEL:

"I am a huge proponent of women who are trying to get pregnant and who are already pregnant getting a flu shot. Pregnancy can cause your immunity to dip, and the flu can be a very serious illness in pregnancy, even damaging to the baby. Pregnant women can be more at risk of severe respiratory symptoms due to viral illness, so minimizing your risk of getting the flu is a good move for you and your child.

"The only hitch is that I think you either want to get the shot before you're pregnant or in the second or third trimester. In the first trimester, your body is otherwise occupied by creating the baby, and your immune system is busy trying to identify whether the baby is an invader or not. Giving your body the extra challenge of launching an immune response to the flu shot really isn't the best use of your internal resources just now. Wait to get the flu shot until you are feeling better; it will be absorbed and acted upon by the body in a better way if you are feeling good."

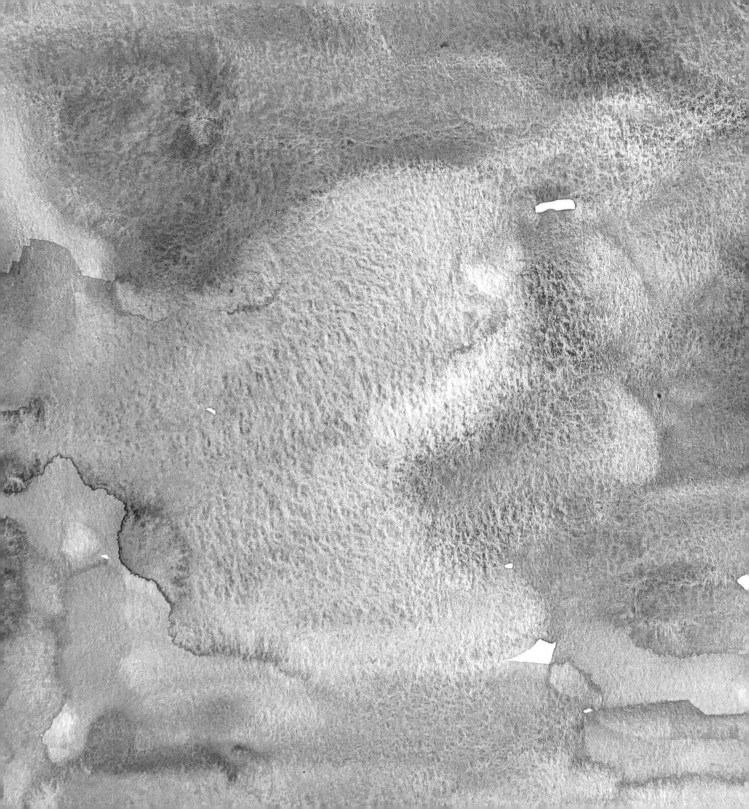

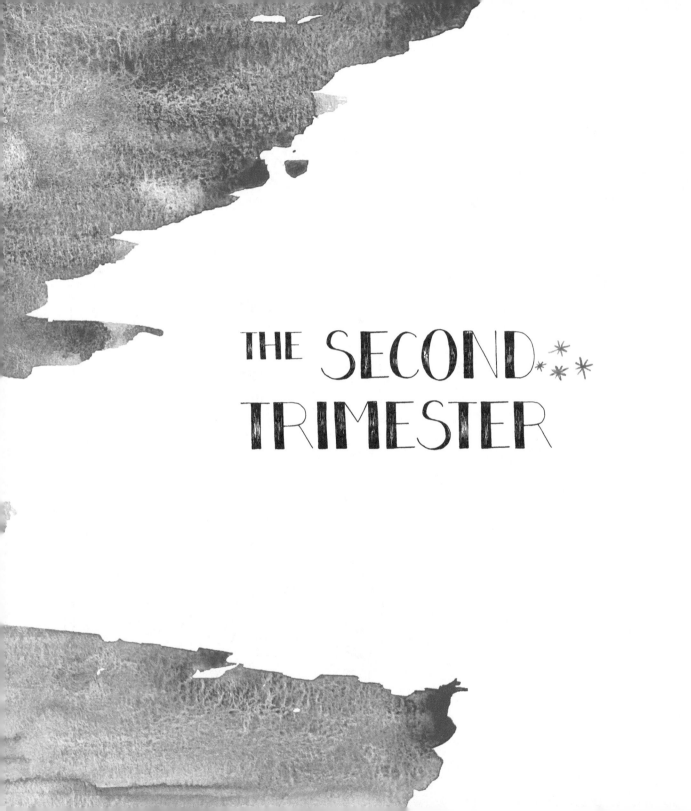

THE SECOND TRIMESTER

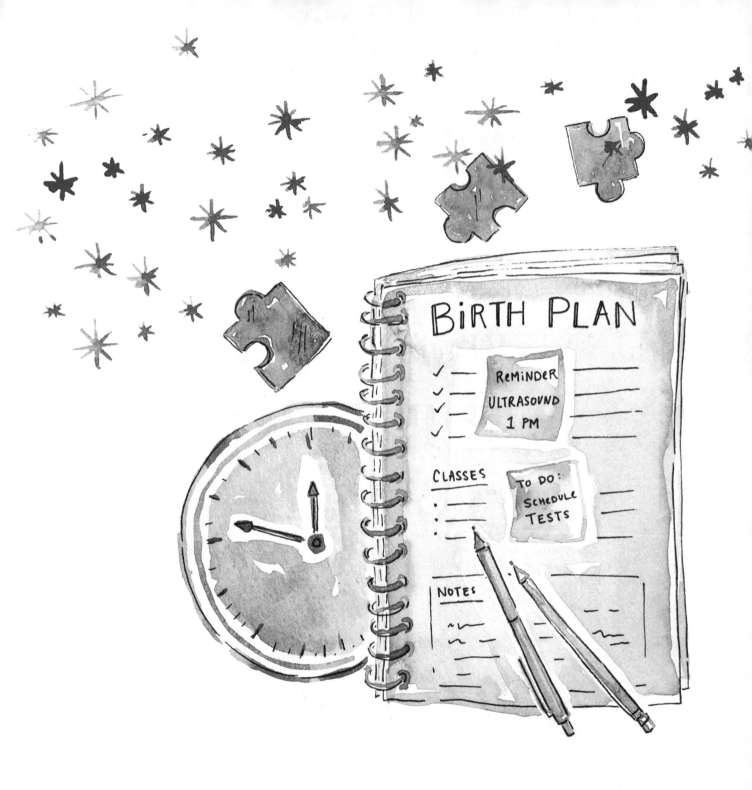

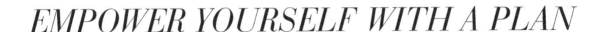

Chapter 8

EMPOWER YOURSELF WITH A PLAN

E ven though labor is still a long ways off, it's time to start thinking about the birth of your baby now—namely, the specifics of how you'd like it to go down. It's also a time when your care provider is likely going to start offering or suggesting a lot of different tests—most of them genetic screenings for any chromosomal anomalies. It's easy to get anxious about this phase, but if you know what to expect, and know what questions you need to think through, you'll emerge from this period of time feeling confident. It also helps so much to take a childbirth education class so that you can start to fill in the blanks of what you don't know about what's to come—I share some of my favorites later in this chapter so that you can get enrolled soon.

Remember, research, planning, and education are great antidotes for fear and worry. My hope is that this chapter will not only tell you what you need to be considering now, but also introduce you to some empowering viewpoints that can help you see just how many choices and how much agency you have over how your delivery will go.

Let's Talk Tests: What Are Your Options, and Which Are Right for You?

Fair warning: Now that you're in your second trimester, your health care practitioner is about to start asking if want to get a lot of tests now. I know it can be an intense time. After all, some of these tests could indicate that your baby has a genetic disorder. When your care provider starts asking you about procedures, screenings, and diagnostic tests, I want you to be ready with an answer—your answer. Whether or not a test is right for you is, well, up to you!

Ask your doctor or midwife to share the purpose of the test: Is it offered to all pregnant women? If not, why are they recommending it for you and your pregnancy specifically? Talk with them about how they will use the information the test provides and what that information will mean for you, so that you can make a decision you're comfortable with.

To help you do just that, here's a list of the tests that you are most likely to hear about, and as much information about each of them as I can provide in this space.

(Just keep in mind that it's not an exhaustive rundown of all the checks your doctor or midwife may want to perform. Throughout your pregnancy, they'll look to see if you have edema, or swelling in your ankles, legs, and feet. They'll measure your fundal height, or the distance from the top of your pelvic bone to the top of your uterus, which tells them how your baby is growing. They'll also monitor your blood pressure—on the lookout for high-blood pressure, which when you're pregnant is also known as pre-eclampsia or toxemia—and do basic blood work to look for any infections and issues like problems with blood clotting, which can lead to complications during your pregnancy and delivery. That's all completely normal—although you may not be used to how closely monitored your overall health will be, it's all for the sake of making sure that you and the baby are both doing well.)

Glucose Tolerance Test

I'm starting with this test for gestational diabetes, even though it's performed later in your second trimester than the others (usually between weeks 24 and 28), because it's recommended for all pregnant women. Although this condition often doesn't present with any apparent signs or symptoms, if not properly managed, it can lead to problems such as early birth, high birth weight (which can increase your odds of needing a Cesarean), and in very rare, unmonitored cases, even fetal death. What's more, babies born to mothers with gestational diabetes are more likely to develop type 2 diabetes as they get older.

Your doctor will likely start with a one-hour test, which has you drink a high-sugar solution (Glucola), wait one hour, and then have your blood drawn. If this test is abnormal, you'll need to repeat the test but this time waiting three hours between drinking the solution and having your blood drawn.

If you're working with a home-birth midwife, as I did, she'll likely have you have a breakfast with protein and complex carbs with a little bit of simple sugar, for example an omelet with toast and jelly, instead of drinking the Glucola.

Ultrasound

We talked a bit about ultrasonography, aka ultrasounds or sonography, in Chapter 5. One thing I didn't cover there is that ultrasounds don't produce ionizing radiation, or the potentially harmful type of radiation associated with X-rays and CT scans. And that the American College of Obstetricians and Gynecologists' (ACOG) Committee on Obstetric Practice believes ultrasounds are not associated with any health risks to a baby or pregnancy in general. However, ACOG notes that sonography should be used prudently and only to answer clinical questions or provide medical benefits. Meaning, the committee doesn't advise using ultrasounds to create keepsake videos, for example.

That said, they are a radiation-based tool, and you may wish to limit your baby's exposure to radiation in general and to limit the number of ultrasounds you receive throughout your pregnancy. They aren't mandatory. But if you want to at least do one ultrasound to get some, well, inside information about your pregnancy and how your baby is growing and developing, this is one to consider.

That's because it can further confirm what stage of pregnancy you're in, painting a more accurate picture of your due date within a week or so. And, it can check your baby's anatomy for chromosomal abnormalities. Note, however, not all anatomical issues are as easy to see as others, and it's not a perfect tool in this regard. It also locates the placenta (complications can arise if your placenta is too low, for example) and checks your amniotic fluid. It is usually given between 13 and 27 weeks, most often in week 20. This is also when you can find out the sex of your baby if you want to know.

Triple Screen Test

This blood test, also sometimes referred to as the second trimester screen or the multiple marker test, is used to detect chromosomal disorders (such as Down syndrome) and neural tube defects (like spina bifida). It is offered to all pregnant women, and is usually performed between 15 and 20 weeks; however, 16 to 18 weeks is said to be the magic window for this test. The multiple markers, hence the name, being evaluated are:

- AFP, a protein produced by the fetus

- hCG, a hormone produced by the placenta

- estriol, a hormone (you guessed it: a type of estrogen) produced by the fetus and placenta

Oftentimes, a fourth marker, inhibin-A, will be measured; if so, the entire screening may be called the quad screen. This marker can help the screen better detect Down syndrome.

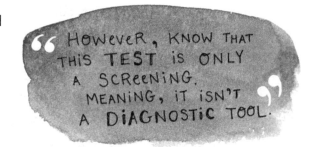

"However, know that this test is only a screening. Meaning, it isn't a diagnostic tool."

Again, abnormal levels of these markers may indicate a genetic disorder. However, know that this test is only a screening. Meaning, it isn't a diagnostic tool. It can't tell you for sure if your baby has a chromosomal disorder or neural tube defect, only indicate that more testing may be needed. The inhibin-A marker is said to detect about 75 percent of neural tube defects and between 75 and 90 percent of instances of Down syndrome. But, up to five percent or more of women will have an abnormal reading, yet their child won't be born with a genetic condition or neural tube defect. It is most accurate when combined with the results of the first trimester screen, which also checks for chromosomal abnormalities.

If you are at risk of having a baby with a chromosomal condition, this test may be a right choice for you. Likewise, if you have concerns and want to know as much information as possible about the health of your baby in a non-invasive way, this test might be the way to go: All that's involved is blood work. It can give you a baseline understanding and help you and your health care provider decide if the following additional tests are necessary.

Cell-Free Fetal DNA Test

Abbreviated cffDNA, this is a newer test that, like the triple screen, can evaluate your baby's risk of having a chromosomal disorder. It can be more accurate in this regard than the triple screen, but it does not check for neural tube defects. And, also like the triple screen, it is still just a screening tool and not a definitive diagnostic tool. It is usually offered to women who are at increased risk of having a baby with these abnormalities. Cell-free fetal DNA is genetic material that is created by the placenta and that can be detected in a mother's blood, and therefore is a low-risk screening method.

Amniocentesis

Amniocentesis is different from the triple screen and cffDNA in that it is a diagnostic test, meaning it can provide you and your doctor with a definite diagnosis of a chromosomal or genetic abnormality—remember, even ultrasound results may not be 100 percent accurate. A doctor performs an amniocentesis by inserting a needle into your amniotic sac through the skin of your abdomen; an ultrasound helps ensure the needle goes just where it needs to go. The needle removes a bit of your amniotic fluid, which the doctor can then check for abnormalities.

Clearly, it is an invasive procedure, and thus carries a small but real risk to you, the baby, and your pregnancy, including pregnancy loss. Thus, it's recommended when the benefits of the test outweigh its risks. For example, maybe the screens above indicate a high likelihood of a disorder that can't be confirmed by ultrasound. Ask yourself and talk with your partner: Do we want and need to know for sure? Will that change things for us, and if so, how? Will it make us more anxious to know?

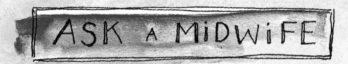

ASK A MIDWIFE

WHAT'S YOUR TAKE ON GENETIC TESTS?

from MARi MiKeL:

"There's nothing wrong with wanting to know as much as possible about your baby; it's perfectly natural to want your baby to be radiantly healthy. Yet I think that there is definitely a thing as too much information.

"I find that the genetic anomaly people are looking for with these tests is Down syndrome. And most people don't truly know much about the realities of parenting a child with Down. People with Down syndrome are very high functioning. Yes, they need a lot of stimulus to reach their full potential, but they are as limitless as any other human.

"In my practice, I have attended the births of over 3,000 babies. Out of all those, I have had only five Down syndrome babies in my practice: two were born to women in their 20s; two to women in their 30s; and one to a woman in her 40s. They were all surprises. And every single mom said, 'I am so glad I did not know, because if I had known, having known nothing about Down, I probably would have opted to terminate the pregnancy, and this child is the most wonderful person I've ever met and I'm incredibly glad that this person has come into my life.'

"When each one of these babies was born, I knew instantly, but the parents didn't, and I didn't tell them immediately. And each one of these parents was over the moon about their beautiful baby, they all nursed and bonded immediately. It wasn't until the next day that I said, 'You know, I think we should talk about something.' But by then they were already bonded and they didn't really care. You don't get that chance to bond with your baby while seeing it as a limitless creature if you get the news via a genetic test before the baby is born.

"I advise my clients to think about what they would do with the information. Half of them say, 'I would never have an abortion under any circumstances.' Then I say, 'You don't need to know.' What you need is to think of your baby as having unlimited potential, and you need to have a deep, abiding joy because the feel-good chemicals associated with joy will get imprinted on your baby's brain and benefit them immensely. And because of our culture's biases, if you discover that you're having a baby with a liva-with-able anomaly, you won't have that.

"There is a reason why you don't know what's going on with your baby when it's inside you—because you're not supposed to.

"On top of that, there are risks to some of the genetic testing procedures. I've had two cases where the baby died as a direct result of an amniocentesis procedure. As you can probably tell, I'm not a big fan of any kind of genetic testing unless you have a really great reason to do it, such as a genetic anomaly that is incompatible with life that runs in your family, or if you've already had a baby with a particular trisomy that is incompatible with life, then absolutely, find out. But start more low-tech, with an ultrasound, and then perhaps a blood test. Only do an invasive procedure if you have very good reason to think your baby may have a devastating anomaly. I know that 'devastating' might have different definitions for different people, so do your research, and search your heart, first."

The Birth Plan We Used When Our Twins Were Born

Understanding risks associated with twins, we prefer as little intervention as possible. Please discuss all procedure options with birther, spouse, and parents before the introduction of ANY medical procedure. We appreciate your time in doing so.

Thank you for respecting our wishes to the extent that is safely possible for the best outcome for all involved and for providing the evidence-based rationale when any of our preferences cannot be met. We are thankful you are here with us to support us all in this surrogacy journey!

DURING LABOR

Hypnosis birth	Food and fluids
Doula support	Natural water release
Free movement	No medications
Intermittent monitoring	Pitocin only in the case of emergency
Dim lights	No coached/forced pushing
Quiet/soft voices	No discomfort scale
Music	No vaginal exams unless requested
Hep lock	No episiotomy
Photography	No students
Access to shower	

OTHER SPECIAL REQUESTS DURING LABOR:

- Birth ball and peanut ball

- No epidural or discussion of it. I understand general anesthetic may be necessary if complication arises during birth of Baby B.

- No unnecessary pulling on baby or manipulating/stretching of vaginal area
- No forceps/vacuum unless emergency AND consent received

AFTER BIRTH

Immediate skin to skin with parents	No baths
Banking cord blood	Delay all exams, vaccines & eye ointments
Natural 3rd stage	Saving placentas
Do not wipe vernix	Delay cord clamp
Breastfeeding	Hope to cut cord
No pacifiers	

OTHER SPECIAL REQUESTS AFTER BIRTH:

- Prefer to wait for contractions to restart naturally for Baby B & breastfeed Baby A to restart contractions manually if necessary
- Babies to remain with their parents at all times unless special care required due to medical status

!!VERY IMPORTANT!!

Should parents not arrive in time for birth, twins are to stay in the care of surrogate/birther until parents arrive, unless there is a need for NICU or specialized care in which surrogate or surrogate's spouse will accompany twins at all times until parents arrive.

Writing Out Your Wishes: Crafting Your Birth Plan

I've come across quite a few fake, meant-to-be-funny birth plans on the internet. I've even watched a famous comedian do a, admittedly hilarious, spoof skit on her television show in which she and her girlfriends sit around and share seriously far-out-there birth wishes that poke fun at the desires of moms-to-be who want to do things as naturally as possible. If you watch or read one of these send-ups, definitely let yourself have a laugh. But don't laugh off the process of creating a plan. They are anything but frivolous, trust me. In fact, I think creating a birth plan is one of the most important moments in your entire pregnancy.

Here's why: They're the perfect tool for helping you, and your partner, get clear about the birth that you want—you, the woman responsible for delivering the baby and whose voice matters the most. And the second trimester is the perfect time to find that clarity. You may even find that as you develop a firm understanding of what you really want your labor and delivery experience to be like, you might have to change the decision you made during your first trimester about where you want to give birth. That's what happened to me! Thinking about my birth plan is when I opted to have my baby at home.

It may become apparent, for example, that because of its strict policies and produces, a hospital won't be able to accommodate your wishes. Or, that you want to have certain options you may not have at home or at a birthing center. In the same vein, you may also find that the health provider you've chosen won't honor some of your wishes for whatever reason, or that they aren't authorized to deliver your baby in the location you've chosen to give birth.

And that's another reason to make sure you have a birth plan—to share it with your provider and make sure that the things that you want are compatible with both the provider and the location where that provider is empowered to attend your delivery. You'll want to discuss your wishes in detail with your doctor and/or midwife well before your due date. If there are multiple parts of your birth plan that aren't allowed in the hospital where you're giving birth, or that your provider doesn't agree with, it may be significant enough that you want to consider changing providers and/or birth location. Better to know in advance than when you're in the throes of labor!

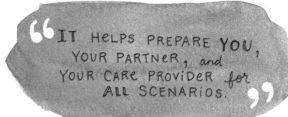
"IT HELPS PREPARE YOU, YOUR PARTNER, and YOUR CARE PROVIDER for ALL SCENARIOS."

Of course, there's a really, really, really good chance that your labor and delivery won't go exactly according to plan. For example, you may write a birth plan for a natural vaginal delivery but end up needing a Cesarean. That's okay. Your birth plan won't be a waste, because through the process of writing it, you'll also be prompted to think about what you want to happen if things do take an unexpected turn. It helps prepare you, your partner, and your care provider for all scenarios.

I've seen other pregnancy resources that advise thinking of the plan as more of a "philosophy," an opportunity to share your general preferences and ideas and then perhaps a more specific plan of the few things you are most adamant about. More importantly, to at least identify who will advocate for your philosophy on your behalf when you're swept up in the throes of delivery and to broadly share how you want decisions to be made in that moment, knowing that decisions may have to be made that are contrary to your wishes.

This said, your plan is *your* plan. You can make it as short and sweet or long and detailed as you want; I've included the birth plan my surrogate and I came up with on page 140 to help you see what it looks like once it's all put together.

Here are just a few of the MANY things to consider including in your birth plan. You'll also want to think about your feelings about common medical interventions—something I cover in depth in Chapter 15 (so skip ahead and read up on those, too, and make sure they're addressed in your birth plan):

Who will advocate on your behalf?

This can be your partner, a parent, a friend, your midwife, or doula. You need someone you can trust to represent your wishes. Of course, you have a voice and your voice matters the most. But the truth is, when you're having a baby, you're vulnerable. A choice that you've researched and know you don't really want to make unless there's no other option might start to sound really appealing when you're in transition (a distinct phase of labor that you'll learn more about in Chapter 19). You need someone who knows what you truly want, who can remind you of it, and who can confidently advocate for you.

What are your preferences for pain relief?

Do you want the option of having an epidural, and do you want one offered to you as soon as you are able to have one? Do you want to be able to control the dosage of the drugs yourself? Do you only want numbing agents or do you want narcotics? Do you want other pain interventions to be offered? Do you want as natural a birth as possible? Do you want to be able to explore a variety of different positions during labor in order to help alleviate pain?

What is to be done with your baby's cord blood and your placenta after you deliver?

If you're planning to either save or donate your baby's umbilical cord blood (see the box on page 150) or save your placenta for encapsulation (see page 146) these plans should be clearly spelled out so your doctor and/or midwife can make proper arrangements. Of course, you'll need to clear both with your birthing location before delivery.

What do you want to happen during labor and after delivery?

Your plan can contain as much or as little in the way of detail as you like. For example:

During labor and delivery:

- Do you want the freedom to move around? To use items like a birthing ball? Do you want to choose the position you're in when you deliver your baby?

- What kind of pain management are you comfortable with?

- What is your feeling on induction?

- What is your feeling on episiotomy?

- Who do you want in the room with you?

- What do you want to do to maintain an environment that's conducive to your being able to relax and focus?

- How much fetal monitoring do you want?

- How many internal checks of your cervix are your comfortable with?

- Do you want your membranes ruptured, or do you want them to break on their own?

- How do you want to handle the delivery of the placenta?

- Do you want to save the placenta, either for encapsulation or to bury it?

If you're having a Cesarean:

- Do you want to be awake?

- Do you want to be able to see the birth?

- Who do you want in the operating room with you?

- What type of incision and suturing do you prefer?

- Do you want your provider to swab your vagina and wipe it on the baby's skin to transfer some of the natural beneficial bacteria in your birth canal to the baby?

- Do you want to be able to hold and breastfeed the baby right away?

After delivery:

- Do you want to have skin-to-skin contact with your baby right away?

- Do you want your baby to stay with you at all times, unless there's a medical emergency requiring NICU care?

- Do you want to initiate breastfeeding immediately? How do you feel about bottles, formula, artificial nipples, and pacifiers? Is it OK for nurses to give these to your baby without asking you first?

- What is your feeling on newborn exams: Do you want them right away or want to delay them?
- What about newborn treatments, such as antibiotic eye drops, vitamin K shots, and the administration of the hepatitis B vaccine?
- Are you okay with your baby having a bath right away?
- If you're having a boy, do you want to circumcise him? (We'll cover this more in Chapter 15.)

Though you will have gone over your plan with your health care practitioner in advance, you will still want to take several copies with you in your hospital bag or home-birth kit when you deliver. And definitely make sure the person you have designated as your advocate has a copy and is up-to-date on any recent changes you may have made!

Your Magical Placenta

OK, listen, I'm about to talk about something that's probably going to make you squeamish. Prepare yourself mentally!

I want to talk to you about your placenta. This incredible organ—that you create out of nothing once you get pregnant, go, you!—does so many important things, including:

- Making estrogen and progesterone, which surge in pregnancy but then fall rapidly after delivery
- Seves as a repository for oxytocin, which floods the placenta during labor, and prolactin, which cues milk production
- Is a storehouse for nutrients, including vitamins, minerals, essential fats, and amino acids
- Contains stem cells, which are also magic (see the Should You Bank Your Baby's Cord Blood box on page 150).

For all these reasons, a growing number of women are doing something that women in traditional cultures have done for millenia: and that is, to eat their placenta. It's thought that ingesting your placenta will help replenish your hormone and nutrient levels after the hard work of growing and delivering a baby, which in turn is thought to promote milk production and ward off postpartum depression.

It's not like you have to eat it like steak. There's a process of storing, washing, steaming, dehydrating, and grinding the placenta so that it is small enough to place inside little capsules that you can then pop like vitamins. There are many small businesses who will do it for you; your midwife or doula may also provide this service, or be able to recommend someone who does. Just make sure that if you decide to go this route, your provider is certified and is happy to discuss her methods for sterilization and cleanliness with you. You'll want to do all this ahead of time, because you want the placenta to be as fresh as possible. If you wait until after birth, you've waited too long.

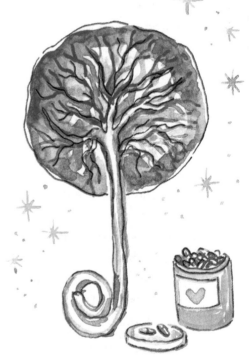

I had my placenta encapsulated with both of my first two babies. In each case, the placenta went right into my freezer and then my encapsulator came later that day. Since I've never not done it, I can't tell you the difference it makes. But I figured it couldn't hurt and could very likely be beneficial. If I could have had another baby, I would have done it again.

Finding the Right Childbirth Education Class

I've already shared that, as a planner, I read countless books and looked at even more websites with my first pregnancy. Did I take a childbirth education class, too? Of course! I wanted all the information I could get my hands on so that I could be as prepared as possible. I bet you do, too—you're reading this book after all. And while I consider it a robust resource, I still encourage you to attend a class as well.

Classes are dynamic, not static; that means childbirth educators are constantly keeping abreast of new developments and trends in birth and then they pass on all that latest info to you. What's more, taking a class can be an exciting way for your partner to take part in the learning process—and for you two to get even closer during a time when you're both going to need each other's love and support. And, you'll have access to a knowledgeable instructor to ask questions, as well as be able to add a great group of other moms-to-be and their partners to your network, and possibly even your group of close friends.

That said, you don't want the class to have too many couples enrolled; a smaller population allows for better discussions and individualized attention and instruction. It's nice for the group to be intimate enough that you feel free to talk about your fears as your due date inches closer and lessen any anxiety you're having about your baby's birthday (and the days that come after it!).

In general, classes cover the basics of medical interventions, potential complications that may arise, and your options for dealing with pain, as well as important elements of newborn care, like breastfeeding and diapering.

Even if you feel pretty well-versed in the ins and outs of childbirth, there might be one little piece of information that you learn in class that plays a clutch role in how your birth goes down.

It can be really surprising to learn how pushy some hospital policies can be—some may start suggesting that you give your baby formula right away even though you want to breastfeed if they think your milk isn't coming in fast enough. But if you've taken a class where you learn that a newborn's stomach is the size of a pea and that it's natural for babies to lose a tiny bit of weight after birth in the time that it takes for their mother's milk to come in, you'll be confident in saying that you don't need to supplement with formula.

You can attend an in-person class or take an online course, whichever you prefer. Know that hospitals offer in-person classes, but just keep in mind they aren't likely to be focused on natural births and also tend to spend a good bit of time going over specific hospital policies and practices. Classes taught outside of hospitals may be more in-depth and focus on natural birthing options and strategies.

Popular childbirth education classes include:

Lamaze. Perhaps the most well-known birthing class out there is offered by Lamaze International. While Lamaze classes are typically thought of as places to learn the trademarked breathing technique popularized by movies and the media, they also include a wealth of general information on labor, birth, and the early postpartum time, from pain-relieving techniques to breastfeeding tips. Lamaze incorporates these six Health Birth Practices into its philosophy:

- Labor works most smoothly when it is allowed to begin on its own
- Laboring women should be able to move around and change positions during delivery
- Laboring women do best when they have a loved one, friend, and/or or a doula for support
- Avoiding medically unnecessary interventions
- Avoiding giving birth on your back and honoring the body's natural urges to push
- Keeping mother and baby together to facilitate bonding, breastfeeding, and the health of them both (find more information at www.lamaze.org)

Bradley Method. This method of natural childbirth encourages you to tune into your own body to find the strength and resilience within and to nourish your body using nutrition, and exercise during pregnancy so that you feel confident in your own ability to give birth. It places a big emphasis on having your partner act as your coach during labor and teaches both of you how to work together. Bradley teaches plenty of breathing and relaxation techniques that are good both for calming you down and also providing a completely natural—and effective—source of pain management. (Find more information at www.bradleybirth.com.)

Do You Want to Bank (or Donate) Your Baby's Cord Blood?

The blood flowing through your baby, the umbilical cord, and the placenta contain cells known as hematopoietic stem cells, or stem cells for short. Unlike most cells in your body, which can only make copies of themselves, stem cells can mature in to a variety of different types of cells—brain cells, immune cells, nerve cells, etc. For this reason, stem cell transplants are a useful treatment for over 70 different types of diseases, including genetic diseases, neurological diseases, immune disorders, and some cancers, including leukemia and lymphoma. There's also promising research that suggests cord blood can be used to treat brain injury, spinal cord injury, and juvenile diabetes.

You can opt to capture some of the cord blood after baby is born and store it for future use as treatment for one of the 70 diseases stem cells are an effective treatment for. It's important to note, though, that stem cells are rarely used for the baby who donated them because they don't help treat that child's genetic disease or leukemia. The American College of Obstetricians and Gynecologists (ACOG) discourages the practice of banking cord blood as a "just in case" insurance plan should your child develop a disease that can be treated with stem cells later.

Cord blood is more typically used for either a family member who needs them or someone unrelated or unknown to the child.

In order to harvest the cord blood, you have to choose a cord blood bank where you will have the blood stored, order a kit (some but not all hospitals provide them; it's best to come to the hospital with your own), and the mother has to share a detailed genetic history and have her blood screened for genetic disorders and infections. This process takes up to six weeks, so now is the perfect time to get started if this is something you want to do.

There are two basic types of banks that store stem cells: public, and private. Public cord banks don't cost money as you are essentially donating the stem cells to anyone who needs them and who is a match, although some public banks allow you to make a 'directed donation,' where you can stipulate who you want the cord blood to go to (a family member with a neurological disease or leukemia, for example). Donating your baby's cord blood to a public bank is a generous thing to do all around, but especially if you're a member of an ethnic minority because there can be few matches in the cord blood banks. Donation of cord blood is encouraged by the ACOG.

Private cord banks charge for harvesting and storage (costing as much as $2000 up front) and the cord blood is typically only used for that child or someone to whom you choose to allow access. Not all private banks are created equally—there was a report in the *Wall Street Journal* in 2014 that found that many private banks at the time were going out of business, or had poor storage practices.

Cord blood banking can effect your birth plan because if you want to collect stem cells you want to cut and clamp the umbilical cord pretty soon after the baby is born. Some people prefer to wait until the cord has stopped pulsing to cut and clamp it (for reasons I cover on page 356). Whatever you decide about cord blood banking, make sure

to incorporate it and your wishes for cord clamping procedures in your birth plan. You'll also want to make sure that your hospital or other birthing location accepts cord blood donations, as not all do.

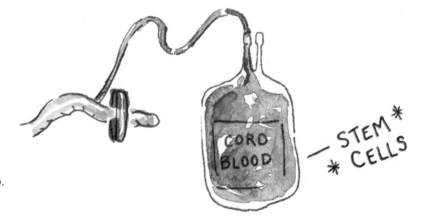

For more information on cord blood banking, visit www.parentshguidecordblood.org, and to find a hospital that collects cord blood, see the National Marrow Donor Program's website, www.bethematch.org.

HypnoBirthing®. Hypnobirthing is a philosophy and a mindset that aims to help moms-to-be hone and trust their instincts for giving birth; it also believes that the person giving birth has the most power in the birthing room and controls the pace of a delivery, not the care provider. Hypnobirthing is designed to help you get out of a fear response about birth and find your way to deep relaxation even during the delivery process. It's also a full childbirth education class that covers anatomy, nutrition, breastfeeding, and interventions as well as the mind-body techniques that help you find a tranquil mental zone and maintain it throughout delivery. (Find more information at www.hypnobirthing.com.)

Spinning Babies. This class teaches you how to work with your baby's positioning and your own anatomy to make pregnancy more comfortable and birth easier. It works with any birth plan. And yes, it can also help babies that are in breech (head up) or transverse (lying horizontally in your uterus instead of vertically) find their way to a more compact and comfortable head-down position (more comfortable for both of you), also reducing the need for interventions. Spinning Babies teaches you how to restore balance to the muscles and ligaments that support the pelvis and the uterus and find a better alignment. They provide a lot of free videos and content at spinningbabies.com; they also host single-day workshops around the country. (See www.spinningbabies.com for more.)

DONA International Birth Doula Training Workshop. One of the best pregnancy classes I took was the DONA Birth Doula Training Workshop, which is a three-day workshop all about birth. It's three full days that leaves you believing in your ability to give birth and feeling confident going into the process. Plus you'll be on your way to becoming a doula, should you decide later that you want to support other women through their transition to motherhood! (Find more information at www.dona.org/become-a-doula/birth-doula-certification/.)

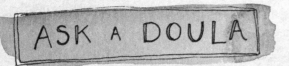

ASK A DOULA

WHAT'S THE DEAL WITH HYPNOBIRTHING?

My wonderful doula, Khristina Helmich, is also a certified HypnoBirthing instructor. I asked her to share a little bit more about it here.

from KHRISTINA

"HypnoBirthing really focuses on instinctive, gentle birthing. Your nervous system needs to feel safe in order for you to give birth gently, so HypnoBirthing talks about how to stimulate the parts of the brain that control the parasympathetic nervous system, which is what helps you feel relaxed and able to be comfortable with what your body already knows how to do.

"When I first got pregnant, I knew nothing about babies or birth. Everyone in my family was telling me I should just get a Cesarean. I don't like needles, and I certainly don't like scalpels. I wanted to be able to experience birth without all of that. So I Googled 'gentle birthing,' and HypnoBirthing came up. I had never done any kind of meditation before. I had no background in any relaxation techniques.

"I was hooked from the very first class. It gave me confidence that my body had the power to give birth. It helped me focus on what I needed to focus on—not what was happening in the room, but on allowing my body to birth my baby. As soon as it was over I wanted to help spread the word about it and eventually did my training in it.

"HypnoBirthing sounds like this hippie thing, but it's not. The average person hypnotizes themselves about seven times a day; say you're driving to the grocery store that you go to several times a week. You're not even fully aware of driving because you're in a deep relaxed state. The class teaches you how to purposefully put yourself into that state; you learn how to breathe, you receive scripts for guided relaxation that your partner can read to you, you practice visualizations—some that are self-guided, some that your partner can talk you through.

"We're taught to be afraid of birth; HypnoBirthing shows you that it can be a beautiful event, perhaps the most beautiful day of your life."

Writing Your Birth Plan

I think it's nice to think of your birth plan as more of a list of intentions and preferences. Again, I go into more of the details about the various interventions that you may be offered (or given without your consent, if you don't make your wishes known before hand), but it's good to start getting your thoughts down now and refine as you understand more. Here is a sample list to get you started.

While I understand the need to be flexibile for the sake of the baby's health and my health, I intend:

- To give birth at (location) in the care of (doctor or midwife)

- To have a natural, non-medicated, intervention-free childbirth

- To have my partner be an integral part of the birthing process

- To manage my pain with relaxation techniques, assistance from my partner and my doula, and use of a shower or tub

- To have/not have epidural anesthesia

- To labor at home for as long as possible and only come to the hospital when my contractions are 3 minutes apart and about 1 minute long

- To let my body dictate the pace of labor and to not be induced or have an externally-imposed time table for pushing

- To bond with my baby immediately after birth via skin-to-skin contact and breastfeeding

- To bank/donate/not bank the cord blood

- To circumcise/not circumcise my baby if it has a penis

- To breastfeed the baby; please do not offer the baby formula, pacifiers, artificial nipples, or sugar water without my prior consent

I prefer:

- To be able to walk, change positions, and have access to a birth ball, shower, or tub as I see fit

- To be able to try natural methods of stimulation of labor (pumping, sexual intercourse, nipple stimulation, etc.) before being induced with Pitocin

- To only have an IV if medically necessary, and if it is required, to use a saline lock so that I can move around

- To have as much privacy as possible in the delivery room; please have a nurse screen any new visitors or medical personnel (unless it is an urgent, emergency situation)

- To be able to eat and drink as desired throughout labor

- To have intermittent external fetal monitoring; only continuous and/or internal fetal monitoring if medically necessary

- To not to be offered pain medication unless I request it

- To adjust the lighting in the room and bring battery-operated candles with me to create a more tranquil environment

- To NOT have my membranes ruptured

- To minimize routine internal examinations once the membranes rupture

- To have my partner cut the umbilical cord after it stops pulsing

- To avoid an episiotomy with counterpressure, warm compresses, perineal massage, and slow crowning unless the risk for a major tear is significant

- To delay the routine post-birth procedures until after I have had a chance to bond and breastfeed the baby (bath, vitamin K, weighing, etc.)

- To have/not have the Hep B injection administered to my baby

- To have/decline the anitbiotic eye drops

If a Cesarean is medically necessary, I prefer:

- To have my partner and doula present during the procedure

- To remain awake

- To be able to see/to not be able to see my baby being born

- To have my baby placed in my arms immediately after birth

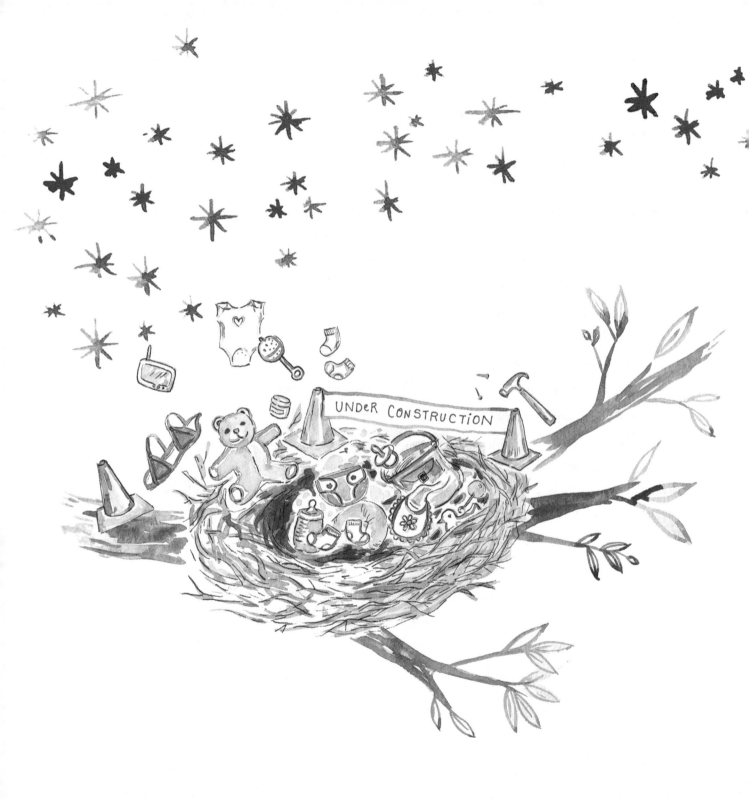

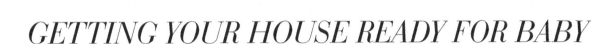

Chapter 9

GETTING YOUR HOUSE READY FOR BABY

Now it's time to talk about the fun part of pregnancy: shopping for baby things! All those tiny onesies, soft blankets, and adorable toys are so fun to shop for, especially for your first child, or your first child of a different gender if you already have a child. That drive to stock up on supplies is *real,* and can even spill over into an urgent need to re-do parts of your home, or perhaps even move. Before I take you through the lists of things you definitely want to have an hand (and a few nice-to-haves, too) for the baby, I want to talk about that urge to re-do your whole house, which I completely identify with, so trust me, there is no judgment here.

When I was pregnant with our first child, I added a second washer and dryer to our laundry room—I just knew how much more laundry was in our future and I wanted to be prepared. But I didn't stop there. I ended up wallpapering or re-painting every room in the house, changing up the furniture in our living room (twice!), and turning a set of cabinets into a pantry in the kitchen. I also added three new rooms to our house and caused a huge headache of construction that went well past when I ended up giving birth. I drove a lot of people crazy because there was no place in our house that wasn't in transition. If you had told me at the time that it was the hormones talking, I would have waved you off. But looking back I can see that I was completely in the grip of hormones.

Oxytocin and estrogen, which are coursing through your body right now, both have roles to play in your drive to spruce up the house—they are the same hormones that drive expecting mama birds to feather their nest. It's nature's way of making sure that infants are protected from predators and the elements. It's completely natural to feel like your home needs improving. But there's something else at play that can contribute to your taking on projects that are way bigger scale than you perhaps you need or is good for your mental health (being surrounded by moving boxes or construction materials can definitely add a whole other layer of stress to your pregnancy). And that is a desire for control and an outlet for anxiety.

As your body seems to take on more and more of a mind of its own and you get less and less say in how you feel and what plans you can make in the months ahead, it feels extra good to have some say in your life—and you've got a lot more control over the color of the nursery walls and the shelving in your closets than you over when the baby will be born or what pregnancy symptom will pop up in the next few weeks.

As you look around the house and imagine the projects you could do, just check in with yourself before you pull the trigger by asking, *Is this significantly going to add to my family's quality of life? Or am I just looking for a project to keep me from freaking out?* Because there are plenty of things to buy and decisions to make now—enough to keep you sufficiently busy without turning your whole house upside down.

In this chapter, I walk you through the things you need, as well as the things it's OK to borrow or to skip, so that you can have plenty of fun—and, OK, control—feathering your nest and making a nice, functional space for your growing family.

Getting Your Home Ready for Your New Life

If you haven't already, it's time to switch to nontoxic cleaners. (I talked about this in Chapter 2.) There are so many good ones out there, why take the risk of exposing

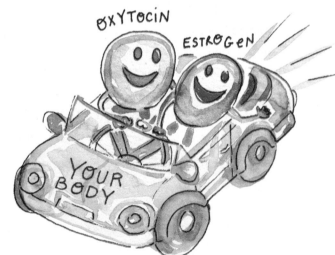

your baby to chemicals when you don't need to? That includes a non-toxic, allergen-free detergent to wash everything that fits in a washing machine before you use it on the baby—such as clothes, sheets, blankets, towels.

Now is also a great time to start babyproofing the house. Even though the baby won't be mobile for several months, you've got the hormones behind you at this point; it can't hurt to start thinking about any items you want to move, sell, or donate because they don't really fit the lifestyle of having young kids. Maybe it's a white upholstered couch (because there will be spills), or a glass coffee table that just screams "breakable."

I recommend getting outlet plugs and cabinet locks so that the baby can't get their fingers somewhere they could get hurt. Also consider those foam corner guards for your coffee table—although I ended up switching out our coffee tables for soft, square ottomans and used trays on top of them for drinks. (I told you, I had a project going in every room of the house.)

Something else you may want to consider: having a lock installed on the inside of your bathroom so that you can shower in peace. As much as you love that child, it's nice to know you can get alone time now and again—just remember that your kids will soon be old enough to figure out how to use it too.

When it comes to the nursery, think about what the baby will gladly live with (and will last) until they are seven or eight—wall color, dresser, even wallpaper if you want to go bold. You can keep the soft furnishings—the bedding, the pillows, the art on the walls— more baby-centric because it's easier to switch out as your child (and your child's bed) gets bigger. And of course, I advocate using non-toxic or organic everything: paint, sheets, changing pad covers, towels.

With my first child, I didn't find out the gender, so I decorated the nursery in grays and clear Lucite. Same with my second—I stuck to gray and minimal touches of light blue— still very gender neutral. With the twins, because I knew they were girls, I went all-out with the pink. It was pink *everywhere*.

What to Buy, What to Borrow, What to Skip

The first time you walk into a baby supply store, prepare to be overwhelmed. There are so many options for everything (15 different types of bottles, 50 different pacifiers, a dozen different diaper brands), and gadgets you've never even heard of. You might want to walk right back out! The following lists can help you head in with a plan—or go right to buying the perfect thing online.

What to buy

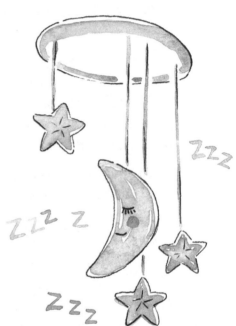

Sleeping

- Crib (I've used several kinds, including the Nurseryworks Vetro crib, one from Restoration Hardware, and one I got on Amazon that was less than $100 but still modern and stylish)

- Mattress (should be firm, to minimize risk of suffocation, and non-toxic)

- 2 waterproof mattress protectors (one to use while the other's in the wash)

- 2 fitted sheets

- Co-sleeper (if you're interested in having the baby in your bed for a while, there are many products designed to help you do that safely—our kids slept like champs in the Dockatot)

- Swaddlers (I'm a swaddling pro and prefer using muslin or organic cotton large thin blankets, but if you are not a swaddling pro, buy the SwaddleMe; it makes swaddling so easy)

- Sleeping sacks (for when the baby is a little older and can sleep swaddle-free, but still too young to have covers because they can pose a suffocation risk, especially to babies who can't yet roll over)

- Diapers, in a range of sizes (but just one or two packs of the newborn size—they outgrow these quickly)

- Wipes

- Diaper cream (preferably without minerals and petroleum products, although I admit, I love Triple Paste but I'm busy making one that's all natural now)

- Changing pads (one or two for home and one or two for travel)

- Changing pad covers

- Diaper pail

- Baskets (I keep one in every room full of everything I need for a diaper change)

- Burp cloths (get more than you think you'd ever need so you can keep some in every room—my favorite are made by Burt's Bees)

- Maty's and California Baby (for shampoos, diaper creams, moisturizers, and other personal care products for the baby that are all-natural and petroleum-free)

- NoseFrida (aka "The Snotsucker," really helpful for unclogging stuffed noses)

- Gripe water for upset tummies

- Washcloths

- Towels

- Bath tub or two (a tiny one for newborn, and a bigger one for later—or buy a sling to hold your newborn in a bigger tub)

- Inflatable bath tub (for travel)

- Baby-wearing shirts, one for you and one for

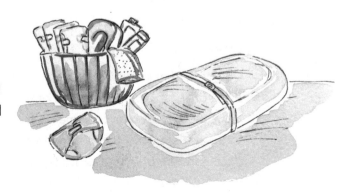

your partner (these T-shirts have a compartment for you to put the baby right on your bare chest for skin-to-skin contact, but they allow you to be covered up; my husband and I both loved the ones from NüRoo)

- Little Remedies gas drops and saline drops for stuffy noses

Feeding

- Bottles (since 2012 all baby bottles have been required to be BPA (a hormone-disrupting chemical)-free; I used plastic bottles so I didn't have to worry about dropping a heavy glass bottle on the baby) I prefer Dr. Brown's.

- Several different sizes and styles of nipples (you just don't know what style will work with your baby, and as they grow they need a larger opening)

- Formula (even if you're breastfeeding it's good to have at least some formula on hand in case your milk runs low or you're away from the baby—it's also great for helping your partner or baby nurse handle a night-time feeding)

- Bottle warmer (if you're using formula, I loved the Baby Brezza, which looks like an espresso machine and lets you choose how many of formula you'd like prepared and the temperature you'd like it warmed to; if you're breastfeeding and pumping a bottle warmer is good because it doesn't heat the milk too quickly or too warm so that it preserves the vitamins in the breastmilk)

- Bottle brush

- Drying rack

- Pacifiers if you use them

- Baby food maker (OK, you don't need one of these as a blender works well too, but the BÉABA babycook makes it so easy—it steams, purees, and maintains the temperature of whatever fruits, vegetables,

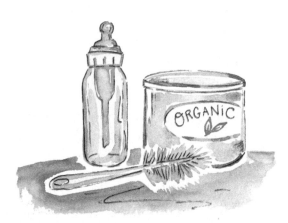

meats, or grains you put in there, with only one button to press; and dishwasher safe, too! You won't need this until the baby starts solids, but it's something worth registering for.)

- High chair (you'll need this eventually; I used one from Joovy and one from Stokke, which is earth friendly, easy to clean, convertible into a chair for when your baby is older)

- Clip-on chair (for travel or eating out once the baby is old enough to sit upright)

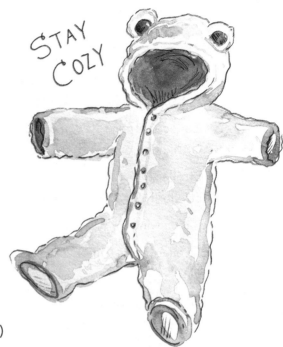

Clothing

- Going home outfit (if you're planning a hospital birth)

- 2-4 newborn hats (newborns can't regulate their own body temperature so these lightweight cotton hats help keep them warm; Etsy has cute ones, much cuter and softer than the ones at the hospital)

- 8-10 footie pajamas in a variety of sizes—0-3 months, 6 months, and 12 months (I loved KicKees, Aden + Anais, Primary, and Burt's Bees; some use magnets instead of snaps, which makes middle-of-the-night changes so much easier)

- 3-5 plain white short-sleeved onesies (great for layering)

- 3-5 long-sleeved onesies (depending on climate where you live and season baby is born)

- 3-5 elastic waist pants in a variety of sizes

- 3-5 pairs of socks (I love the socks from Primary)

- Small hangers, clips, and hooks for hanging tiny clothes

- Props for newborn photos (again, look on Etsy; I got a snap pea mat with two beanies so my girls literally looked like two peas in a pod)

- Car seat (I love the Doona car seat; a car seat that has wheels and a handle that pops out so that you don't also need the next item on this list)

- Car seat stroller (if you prefer a regular stroller that doesn't accommodate a car seat, you'll need one that reclines fully until the baby is 6 months old)

- Stroller (I love the Babyzen YOYO for its incredible collapsibility and the double stroller from Joovy—although it's not good until the baby is about 6 months)

- Baby swing for when you want to put your baby down to get some actual you time

- Stroller hooks (I'm obsessed)

- Baby-wearing device (for babies past 20 pounds, the Ergo or Baby Bjorn carriers are great; for younger babies I prefer the baby K'tan—a soft sling-type carrier that's very simple; for twins the Weego is life changing)

- A stroller sack (keeps the baby warm and lasts longer than a newborn coat)

- 2 fleece hats (if you live in a cold climate)

- 2-3 pairs of mittens (again, if you live in a cold climate; look for those that can flip open in case your baby is a thumbsucker)

- 2 fleece blankets (to tuck in around the baby—and over the car seat or stroller straps—for warmth; you don't want anything puffy, such as a blanket or winter coat, between the baby and the car seat or stroller harness because it can leave too much space underneath the straps in an accident; also, once the car warms up you want to be able to remove the cold weather gear so the baby doesn't overheat)

What to borrow

Unless you're planning on having more than one kid, there are a lot of things that you'll only need for a couple of months—these are the perfect thing to get as hand-me-downs or borrow from a friend who hasn't cleared out how baby stuff yet.

- Activity mats
- Bouncy seats
- Baby chairs (like a Bumbo)
- Bassinet

What to skip

Some baby items you just flat-out don't need; a couple are actually great things to have, but also very popular presents so you don't need to buy more.

- Baby shoes (my boys used grippy socks that I bought on Amazon—if someone gifts you a cute pair, great, you just don't need to buy them)
- Crib bumpers (they pose a risk of suffocation and the American Academy of Pediatricians advises against them)
- Baby blankets (baby blankets are great; it's just that you will likely receive several as baby gifts)
- Newborn clothes (you probably won't need these, as they're designed only for babies up to 7 pounds—you'll probably get a couple newborn outfits at your shower; those are plenty)

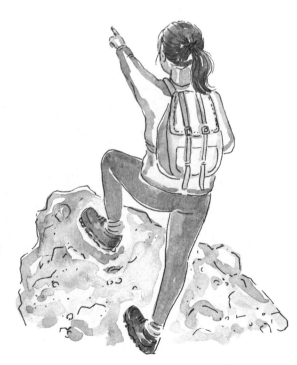

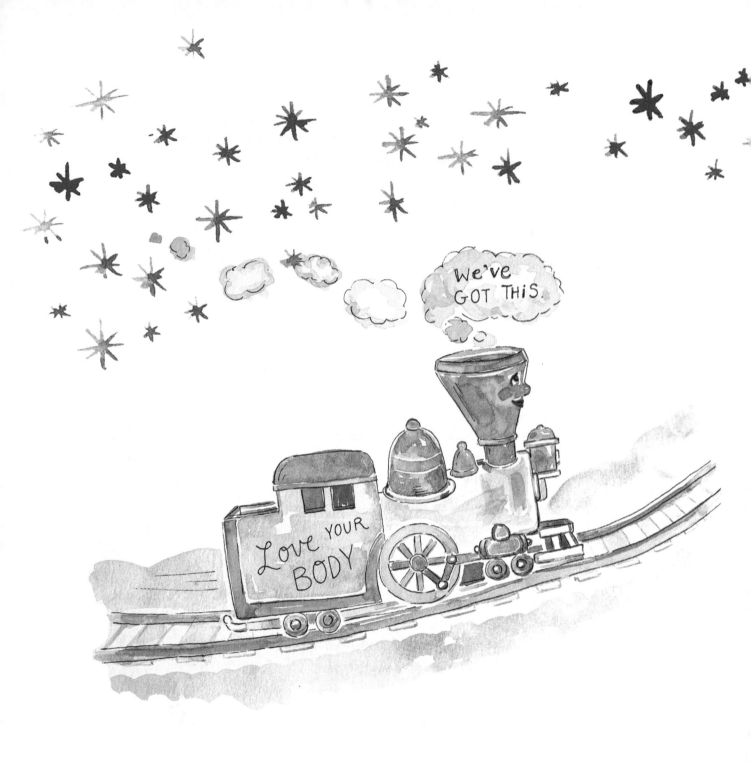

Chapter 10

HAVE A BODY-POSITIVE PREGNANCY

One day, after your baby is here, and you can gaze at the beautiful creature you created and give birth to, it will be clear to you just how miraculous your body is and how powerful you are. But a lot of times, that appreciation for your body isn't easily accessible when you're actually pregnant. I get it—your body is changing right before your eyes, both in how it looks and how it feels. It can be easy to get hung up on the changes that are happening on the surface.

For me, learning about how my body was working behind the scenes, all on its own, to do exactly what was needed to grow a baby helped my confidence grow, both in my ability to give birth and in my appreciation for my body.

Learning about each of the hormones that rise and fall in perfect synchronicity made me completely in awe of my physiology in a way I never had been before. It also made the idea of giving birth much less scary because I could see how my body was supporting me. Even on days when I felt tired, or nervous, or overwhelmed, it just kept chugging along and that knowledge helped ease my mind. I hope it will do the same thing for you.

Holy Hormones: Pregnancy's Magical Chemicals

In its innate wisdom, your body will produce each and every chemical needed to help your baby grow, to allow you to safely carry and birth your child, and then to nourish them once they're born. Not only that, but your body will produce these chemicals all on its own (barring any medical issues), at just the right times and in just the right amounts. It's like, well, magic!

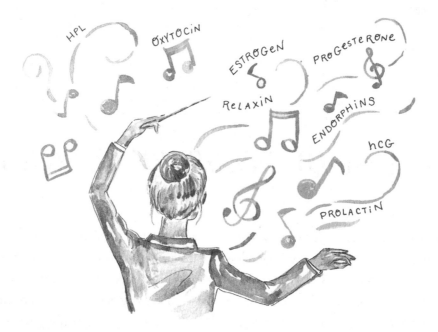

(Generally speaking, the more natural your delivery, the more labor hormones will come into play then and do the work they were designed to do.)

Here are some of the main players involved:

- **Human chorionic gonadotropin (hCG)**: hCG is only produced during pregnancy, and it kicks off the whole entire process*—it's thanks to hCG that you and your doctor can find out, almost ASAP, that you're pregnant. That's because it's excreted in your urine and can be detected by urine analysis, at your physician's office and at home with a store-bought pregnancy test; a high concentration confirms you've got a baby on the way. hCG can also be detected by a blood test. The hormone can first be identified by either method about a week and a half to two weeks after conception.

  hCG is produced by cells that eventually form your placenta. It's a chemical messenger, telling your body to begin readying itself for a new life. It signals a ramp up in production of the equally important hormones progesterone and estrogen (more on the coming pages), and even suppresses your immune system so that your body can focus on your growing baby. Levels are highest in the first trimester; during the first 10 weeks, hCG levels double approximately every two to three days, or every 48 to 72 hours. Circulating hCG will reach its peak sometime between 60 and 90 days after ovulation, or roughly weeks eight to 11 of your pregnancy. After that, levels decline and eventually level off for the rest of the nine months. It's no coincidence that morning sickness often occurs during the first 12 weeks, as it's possible rising hCG is a cause. Women with higher levels of this hormone might experience worse nausea than women with lower amounts.

*We're talking major players here, but know that **follicle stimulating hormone** and **luteinizing hormone**, while not present during pregnancy, could be said to really jump-start everything. Together, they stimulate ovulation, or the release of a mature egg from the ovary.*

- **Progesterone:** Like hCG, progesterone is key in early pregnancy. In fact, it prepares your uterus for pregnancy by thickening its lining, or endometrium, so that it's an ideal environment for an embryo, or fertilized egg. Progesterone levels actually peak after the embryo implants in your uterine wall. If you're undergoing IVF, you'll likely get supplemental progesterone in order to encourage the embryo to attach successfully.

  Levels remain high during your pregnancy, though the initial surge in progesterone begins to plateau after your first trimester. Remember, the rise is triggered by hCG, and is eventually produced by the placenta. Once the embryo has attached, progesterone focuses on other jobs, from nourishing the fetus and aiding in development to loosening and softening your joints and ligaments to prepare you for labor. It also helps spur the growth of breast tissue, helps your body's immune system tolerate and not fight against the fetus (which could be seen as foreign to your system), and expands your uterus to make room for your baby as they grow, as well as relaxes uterine muscles so they don't contract until labor. Because it has a relaxing effect on the body, it can also relax your blood vessels, which may cause your blood pressure to drop and may explain the occasional dizziness that often occurs with pregnancy. It may also be responsible for pregnancy symptoms such as heartburn and constipation, as well as contribute to excess hair growth.

- **Estrogen:** In general, estrogen helps you have a healthy pregnancy. Your body produces more estrogen during one pregnancy than it does throughout your whole life. Along with progesterone, it plays an important role in fetal growth, triggering the development of your baby's organs, including their lungs, kidneys, and liver. Estrogen also serves as the conductor of the hormone symphony playing in your body over these nine months: It helps maintain and regulate the production of other vital pregnancy hormones. In particular, it helps the body utilize oxytocin (which I'll cover in just a bit). Although, that's not all: Estrogen also enlarges milk ducts for breastfeeding during the second trimester. A rapid increase in estrogen in the first trimester may, along with rapidly rising hCG, trigger morning sickness. It may also contribute to early pregnancy fatigue, as well as what some people call a pregnancy "glow."

- **Relaxin:** This hormone's name gives you a good idea of its main job: relaxing your ligaments, joints, muscles, and bones later in your pregnancy to prepare your body for the big job of labor—to make room for the growing baby and to allow for delivery through the birth canal. It is produced throughout your pregnancy. Unfortunately, soft and loose joints can sometimes lead to pain, particularly experienced in the pelvic area and sometimes in the back, as well as throw off your balance. Relaxin may also contribute to constipation.

- **Oxytocin:** This hormone is made in the hypothalamus—the brain's "master gland"— and is secreted by the posterior pituitary gland. When the time has come to deliver your baby, it's oxytocin that stimulates the contractions to get labor going, to dilate your cervix and move the baby down and ultimately out of the birth canal. (Because it helps the uterus contract, it also helps protect against hemorrhage.) Oxytocin levels appear to surge with labor; receptors that make your body more responsive to it also increase right at the end of your pregnancy. Which, clearly, is a good thing! Not only does it encourage contractions, oxytocin also stimulates milk release during breastfeeding.

But there's more at play with oxytocin. Called the "love hormone" or "cuddle hormone," it's regularly released when you're hugging and snuggling up with someone you love or having an orgasm. (I've seen it described as being released in "pulses.") In fact, that's why you may have heard that it's a good idea to have sex, to the point of orgasm, in order to help bring on labor. It's also possible that oxytocin is responsible for the urge to "nest" before delivery, just as it's responsible for helping you bond with your newborn baby and cement a strong mother–baby connection as you hold them (preferably skin-to-skin contact, which enhances oxytocin release) after birth—your baby even produces oxytocin during the labor and delivery process! During pregnancy, oxytocin also helps your body better absorb nutrients, handle stress, and conserve the energy you need for labor.

It's possible you can actually help your body release oxytocin during labor and delivery by stimulating your nipples (you can even get out the breast pump even though your milk hasn't come in yet), or having your partner stimulate your nipples (which is more fun, if you ask me)! Staying as calm as possible may also help. Breastfeeding shortly after birth stimulates oxytocin's release to make the bond with your baby even more concrete.

• **Endorphins:** Your body regularly produces pain-relieving hormones called endorphins to help you cope with painful or stressful situations. It makes sense, then, that it would produce higher levels of endorphins near the end of your pregnancy and during labor and delivery. In fact, if you don't opt for pain medication (it interferes with this production), your body will pump out more and more endorphins to get you through the birth of your baby. You may even feel euphoric!

One endorphin responsible for producing an "altered-state" during this time is beta-endorphin. It's a naturally occurring opiate, really, as it has been shown to work on the same brain receptors as opioid drugs like morphine. High levels of it are also present, like oxytocin, during sex. And, it helps facilitate the release of the hormone prolactin (see below) and consequently plays a role in breastfeeding.

Not only do endorphins serve as analgesics, they also help strengthen your bond with your baby, inducing bringing on feelings of joy and dependency. If levels drop early postpartum, postpartum depression could result.

- **Human placental lactogen (HPL) and prolactin:** Both of these hormones play a role in breastfeeding. Produced by the placenta, HPL is thought to prepare your breasts for breastfeeding, primarily by stimulating milk glands. It also helps feed your growing baby inside the womb by breaking down the fats you consume and desensitizing your body to insulin, which frees up more glucose in your bloodstream that can then be used as nourishing fuel for you baby. (For this reason, in some women it may be the cause of gestational diabetes.) Levels rise during pregnancy and then drop after pregnancy. HPL is said to have prolactin-like properties.

  The hormone prolactin, released by the pituitary gland, is responsible for the growth of your breasts and for telling the body that it's time to produce breast milk. It also helps activate your desire to put your baby's needs before your own; i.e., their need to be fed and nourished. It makes sense, then, that only low levels can be found in the body when you're not pregnant.

  The next time you start to worry about anything pregnancy or delivery related, just remind yourself: *My hormones have got things covered.*

Feeling Sexy and Confident as Your Body Changes

Some women feel like a glowing goddess when they are pregnant. While it is entirely possible that you will too, it's not necessarily a given. It can feel like your body has a mind of its own, especially as the weeks progress and your breasts get bigger, your nipples darken, your ankles swell, and perhaps even your face starts to look different either because of melasma (the natural darkening of pigment that can accompany pregnancy), retaining fluids, or gaining weight.

 # BODY-POSITIVE AFFIRMATIONS

MY BODY is A SAFE and PLEASURABLE PLACE for MY BABY.

MY BODY and THE BABY are NATURALLY DOING JUST WHAT THEY SHOULD.

I LOVINGLY ACCEPT my CHANGING BODY.

I TRUST my BODY'S WISDOM and KNOWLEDGE.

I AM CONNECTED to MY BABY; MY BABY KNOWS MY HEART BEAT, MY BREATHING, MY VOICE, the feeling of MY LOVE.

MY BODY WAS MADE for THIS.   I TRUST MY BODY.

I LISTEN to MY BODY.   I LOVE MY BODY.

MY BODY is AMAZING.   I AM AN AMAZING WOMAN.

In addition to educating yourself about just how incredible your body is with its orchestration of all the hormones (which you just did, so...go, you), it's also so important that you exercise regularly now. Not only are you in training for birth, as I discuss in Chapter 14, but you also stand to benefit so much from producing endorphins and doing things that get you into a state of appreciating what your body is capable of, whether that's salsa dancing, walking to run your errands, or lifting weights. It will help you embrace yourself as you are, now. Remember, it's temporary.

You might not love how your thighs look during pregnancy but you need all that extra weight to assure that you'll have the calories on hand that you need for breastfeeding; and you need the extra muscle mass to carry your additional body weight. It's all happening for a reason.

Please resist the urge to talk badly about yourself. I know we all fall prey to it now and again, but please, talk nicely to yourself! The affirmations in the box on page 173 will help you do just that.

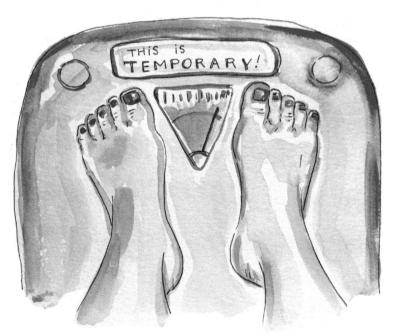

Pregnancy Weight: Adding Up the Pounds

I know it can be both a beautiful and difficult experience to look in the mirror and see your body changing—i.e., to see your waistline expanding… and expanding… and expanding. You know the extra pounds are there to benefit your baby, yet you may still have to fight against seeing yourself as "fat," and even the urge to call yourself the F word to your partner or friends. I hope you'll flip to this page and this box any time you start to feel this way, to see the magic of your pregnancy body laid out in detail and to remind yourself just how needed each pound is.

Remember, there's no one-size-fits-all approach to weight gain during pregnancy. You may gain anywhere from 25 to 55 pounds, depending on your pre-pregnancy weight and BMI and if you're carrying twins or multiples. On average, most women will gain around one to four pounds in the first few months and then about a pound a week until delivery, for a total that is typically between 25 and 35 pounds. Of those:

- 7-8 pounds is your baby

- 1.5-3 pounds is your placenta

- 2-3 pounds is your amniotic fluid

- 3-4 pounds is increased blood supply

- 2-4 pounds is increased fluid volume in general

- 1-3 pounds is your larger breasts and maternal breast tissue

- 5-9 pounds is stored fat and other nutrients for your baby and for breastfeeding

- 2-5 pounds is your enlarged uterus

You don't want to "lose" blood, or the materials you need for breastfeeding, or parts of your uterus, do you? Of course not. So I hope that this knowledge can help steer your thoughts away from losing your pregnancy weight. The vast majority of these pounds will fall away naturally after the baby is born and your body comes back to a non-pregnant state.

My Best Tip for Looking—and Feeling—Great

With a changing body and a limited maternity wardrobe, it's not always possible to feel like a million bucks based on what you're wearing when you're pregnant. Lean in close while I share my best advice on how to feel glamorous, no matter what. You ready? Here it is: Get your hair blown out. Regularly.

You can hit the Dry Bar once a week; after all, your pregnancy hormones are giving you the glossiest, thickest head of hair you've ever had. Rock it! You can be in a pair of sweats and your partner's T-shirt, but if your hair's on point, you're good to go. I still did color my hair using balyage, but only the ends, not the roots. It's important to minimize the chemicals you're exposed to, including in your nail polish and hair color. Look for the most non-toxic versions you can find and save the pedicures for special occasions.

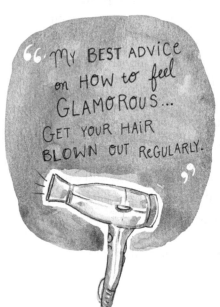

My second best tip is to get eyelash extensions; just be sure that the glue the salon uses doesn't contain formaldehyde, which can cause allergic reactions. Even a half-set of lashes can help you feel bright-eyed from the moment you wake up for a month or more.

Finding Your Maternity Style

Anyone can pull on a pair of yoga pants, and why not? Comfort is more important than ever when you're pregnant. However, if you have an office to go to, you don't really have that option, and we all need to present ourselves in a put together way from time to time.

My overall strategy for dressing myself while pregnant was to put off donning maternity clothes as long as I could. I didn't buy new things until I absolutely had to—I used a rubber band that I looped around the button of pants to make the waistband bigger. I admit, though, that when I finally bought maternity jeans, I wondered why I didn't buy them sooner.

In general, I bought normal clothes in bigger sizes so that I could keep wearing them after I had the baby. I also recommend buying three pairs of maternity pants: one blue denim, one black denim, and one gray dress pant. For any times I didn't need to look respectable, I wore high-waisted workout pants that came up and over my belly, just sized up from my regular size. They felt great to wear because they helped support my belly. I also became a huge fan of dusters, so I could wear a fitted shirt or tight camisole and show off my belly but still be adequately covered.

If I had to dress up, I bought a regular dress in a larger size in a jersey or stretchy material. I wore the same coat the entire time, although by the end my belly was definitely sticking out (luckily, pregnancy makes you run hot, so I rarely felt cold).

When your breasts grow enough that you need new bras, I suggest going ahead and buying nursing bras so that you can wear them longer and start getting used to how they open and close. I tried to find pretty bras, but I ended up going with comfort—more of a spandex material with no underwire. You've simply got to be comfortable!

In general, I say to show off your bump and celebrate your big belly. It's adorable, and so are you. Wear the fitted things. You certainly don't have to hide it—and as your pregnancy progresses, you won't be able to hide it anyway, unless you wear a poncho or a tent, so why try?

It's All About the Self-Care

People often go out of their way to be nice to pregnant women, and now that you're showing, perhaps you've experienced a stranger giving up their seat on the subway for you, or holding the door long past the time they'd hold it for someone else. But you cannot depend on the kindness of strangers, or even your partner, to get the extra care you need and deserve right now. People learn how to treat you by how you treat yourself, so give them a great example to follow by taking exquisite care of yourself now. You will need these self-care muscles to be strong after the baby is here and all your instincts will be take care of the baby first and forget about giving yourself what you need.

Self-care doesn't have to be extravagant to count. I got really in to tea, in particular a rooibos tea with dark chocolate and mint called Better Than Sex by Tay Tea in the Catskill region of New York State. It's hard to describe the taste but it is delicious and smells just as good. Taking that time to sit and enjoy a hot beverage is really nourishing. You won't feel like you're missing out on anything (like caffeine or sugar) when you're drinking this tea—or whatever variety is your favorite.

Taking baths also becomes a next-level act of self-care when you use bath salts and essential oils. It feels great to be weightless and I like to think that floating in the tub helps you imagine what your baby is experiencing in your belly.

I also indulged in prenatal massage; it's amazing how much a massage can help your body reset. Ideally you'd get a prenatal massage from someone certified in it, at least once a month. Toward the end of my pregnancies I got them every week. A gift certificate for a series of prenatal massage is an excellent thing to put on your baby registry; it's an incredible gift.

Real Talk about Pregnancy Symptoms and Fears

Unfortunately sometimes we can start to feel bad about things that haven't even happened yet. Here's some insight on some of the side effects of pregnancy and birth that I hear my girlfriends worrying about the most:

Skin changes

Something else that happens as a result of your hormones surging during pregnancy is that your melanin (the substance responsible for skin pigmentation) glands get stimulated. As a result, you may notice certain parts of your body getting darker, including:

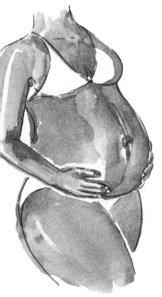

• **Parts of your face.** Known as the "mask of pregnancy," and officially called "melasma," you may experience areas of the skin on your face darkening.

• **A straight line between your belly button and your pubic bone.** This is called the *linea negra* ("black line") and Mari Mikel tells me that it happens at the exact spot where you once folded in two when you were still an embryo. So this line growing darker is just a reminder of the process you took on your journey to being born. Try to at least appreciate the intricacies of your body, if not downright marvel at what's happening in your body without your conscious effort.

• **Your nipples.** These get darker too. Some people say it's to help the baby, whose eyesight is severely limited at birth, see your nipple better thanks to the higher contrast, some say it's just a hormonal fluke. Either way, it won't last. None of these pigmentation changes will. By the time you have breastfed your baby you hardly remember what your nipples used to look like. They might go back, they might not. Before you have kids, you think everything's big and the end of the world, but after you become a mother, trust me, your tolerance will be so high and you'll have so many other things to worry about that you won't remember what your nipples used to look like.

Stretch marks

The best way I know to combat stretch marks is to give your skin the conditions it needs to stretch; and that is to keep is hydrated. The two most important ways to do that are:

• First, use a glycerine-based soap, not a traditional soap, on your skin, because traditional soap is very drying, and dry skin lacks elasticity. You want to maintain as many of your own natural oils as possible, and harsh soaps strip them away.

• And second, be religious about using a thick cream on your skin, so thick that even if you just showered you can still feel the cream on your skin. Not something that feels greasy, but that doesn't fully absorb or get fully washed away. Avoid petroleum-based moisturizers—most of the ones on the shelves at the drugstore are. Instead, buy pure shea butter or cocoa butter, they're hard at room temperature you have to warm them in your hands before they become spreadable, but they're thick enough to stay on. My company, MUTHA also makes a Body Butter that is loaded with shea, cocoa, and mango butters, as well as aloe, rosehip oil, avocado oil, beeswax, and grapeseed oil that I specifically formulated to nurture the skin of pregnant mamas—no filler, all stretchmark killer.

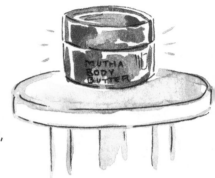

Also, doing the belly pump breath regularly (refer back to page 41 for instructions) helps condition the skin to expand and contract, which helps to minimize the risk of stretch marks. It's the opposite of trying to hold your belly in all day long—something so many of us have internalized—which then keeps your skin taut and thus, less likely to be able to stretch along with your belly without developing stretch marks.

Different physique

I'm betting you know at least one woman—or a lot of women—who say, "I just never lost the baby weight." It can definitely happen that your body is different after having children, but it's not necessarily because you carried a baby. The good news is your body has an incredible ability to bounce back, and you're reading this book, where I've gathered a dream team of experts to guide you through how to take care of your body as it recovers.

Honestly, being a mom for the rest of your life is more of a challenge to your future physique than pregnancy and birth, which only take up nine months of your life. When you're a mom, it's easy to stop taking care of yourself; to get the exercise that makes you feel great and keeps you strong, and to eat the food that helps you look and feel your best. It can be awfully easy to start eating for convenience instead of health, or to tell yourself you're too tired or too busy to move your body. All the more reason to take great care of yourself now, while you're pregnant, so that once the baby's here you've got the memory of how to do it—and how good it makes you feel—in your bones.

It's definitely possible to have great abs post-baby, especially when you follow Brooke Cates' guidance on how to strengthen and stay connected to your core that are sprinkled throughout the book. She certainly helped me feel great both while I was pregnant and after the baby was here.

I'm not trying to delude you. Yes, having babies and being a mom can have a very real effect on your body. But it's not a definite. And, even if your body does take on a new reality, kids are worth it.

Different vagina

I know it's crazy to think about a baby coming out of your vagina—how could that not have an effect? Well, of course, your vagina is different after the baby comes out, but that effect is temporary, particularly when you follow the fitness guidelines in this book that help you keep your core strong and your pelvic floor healthy.

An important way to help your vagina and pelvic floor heal well is to recline as much as possible in those first days after birth. Why? Right after the baby comes, your vagina is going to be softer than it ever will be again. At the same time, your uterus is still really big; it weighs as much as five pounds, when it typically weighs four to eight ounces when you're not pregnant. You don't have the support structures in place to support those five pounds. Mari Mikel says that if you're up and on your feet a lot right after birth, your uterus will be hanging down lower than it should and then it will heal that way. She advises that you try to stay lying down as much as possible for the first week post-birth, with just four or five times a day when you get up for 10 minutes or so—no cooking, no cleaning, no taking care of kids. The second week, you can have five or six of those 10-minute periods. Brooke has breathing exercises you can do while you're reclined that will help your core and pelvic floor come back together (that's coming in Chapter 26). So whenever you start worrying that you'll pee your pants when you sneeze or have a stretched-out vagina forevermore, start thinking about how you can get the support you need that will make it possible for you to rest as much as possible those first two weeks after birth. You don't need the worry—you need a plan.

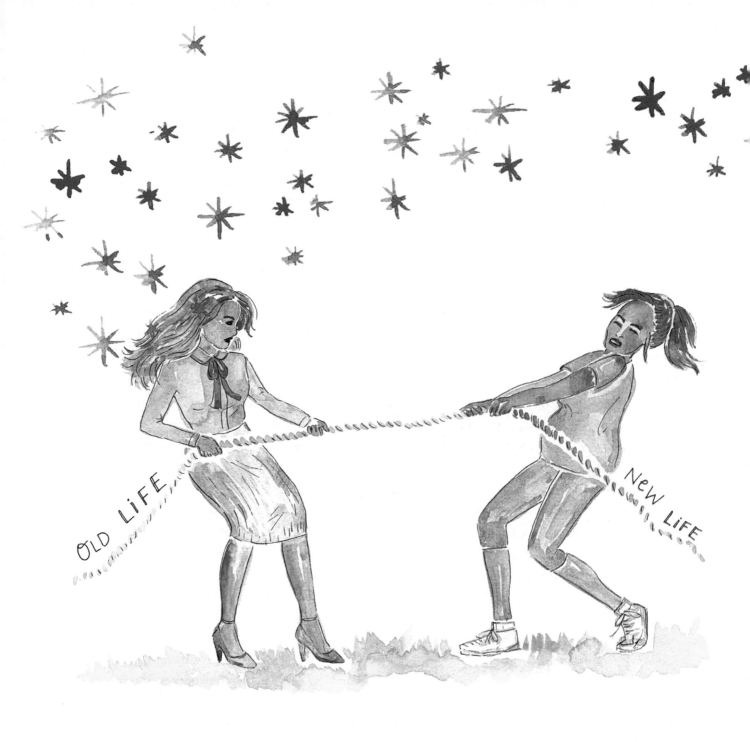

Chapter 11

NAVIGATE CHANGING RELATIONSHIPS

W hen I was pregnant, and in my second trimester (so that I was showing), I remember a woman coming up to me in a store, grabbing me by the arm, and saying, "Your whole life is about to change." I knew her intentions were good but it also made me bristle. What did she know about my life? And why do strangers feel they can say anything to you, at any time, simply because you're pregnant?

Here's the thing: she was right. And I'm about to tell you the same thing, so try not to hate me. You already know that your life is changing in so many ways—adding another human to the planet and to your family, and one that you are responsible for keeping alive, healthy, and happy. You get it. But you may not be considering how your relationships to other people are going to shift, too. And that's why I wanted to include this chapter—to give you a little heads up so that it doesn't catch you by surprise. It's been said it takes a village to have a baby. If you can be prepared to for the changes that are coming to your relationships, your village will be as supportive and strong as it can be. Let's start with the person who is most important to your health and happiness: you.

How You See Yourself

You might be surprised to see the relationship you have with yourself covered in this chapter about changing relationships, but how you think of, talk to, and stay connected to yourself is changing now too. You are becoming a mother. That is a huge deal.

In all honesty, I resisted my new identity as a mom, and I was in denial about what my life would be like after I had kids. To be clear, I love each of my kids like crazy and wanted to spend as much time with them as I could, because I knew that their babyhood would fly by. But I also struggled with accepting that my life revolved around them. I wanted to have my kids and my old life—getting dressed, going to events, being social. It was so confusing to know that all my friends were going out to a restaurant and feeling in one way like I should be there, and in another that I wanted to spend every single second possible with my babies. On the rare occasions when I did go out and join my friends, I felt guilty about it and like I should be home with the kids. I think a lot of moms can relate to that feeling of not feeling 100 percent good about where you are no matter where you are.

"Let's start with the person who is most important to your health and happiness: YOU."

It's true that the day your baby is born, your identity as a mother is born too. But I took some time to accept mine. I wanted to be thought of as cool enough to stay out all night. It would have been a lot easier if I had let that go.

It's important to remember that you can be the kind of mother you want to be; society will heap expectations on you and there will be some days you'll feel like you couldn't be a 'good mother' even if you did everything absolutely perfectly (which, let's face, isn't even possible anyway). While your kids will definitely have their own ideas about what they need from you that you'll have to adapt to once they're here, when you decide what kind of a mom you want to be, it makes it easier to fully embrace your new identity. Give this idea some thought—do you want to be a mom who has a life outside of her kids? Or the mom who really goes in 100 percent to being a mom? Or somewhere in between? You're not setting anything in stone at this point, but think about what version of motherhood inspires you, and then let that be your guide as you make decisions in the coming weeks and months. You may come to realize, like I did, that the identity you want for yourself is in conflict with your reality, and that's OK. It's perfectly acceptable, even expected, to keep re-calibrating your identity as a mother. But the first step in being able to do that is always to recognize what you're currently doing so that you can understand how you want to modify it.

Your Ties to Friends

Nobody gets through this life without friends. Before I had kids, I said I would never be friends with someone just because we both had kids the same age—it was another way I didn't want my life to be defined by motherhood. Well, I was wrong! It's just so true that you can relate to someone who is also worried about how much their baby is eating, and who is also not sleeping, than a friend who is still on the dating apps and going out most nights. It's not that I stopped being friends with my old friends, but we had a lot less in common. You've got to have a really strong bond to stay close over the long-term. Just logistically, it can be hard to find a time to get together or even talk on the phone. I absolutely still love my old friends and love seeing them when I can, but it is different.

Be open to making new "mom" friends; whether you meet them at your childbirth education class or your doula connects you or you strike up a conversation in the pediatrician's office. It's really helpful to have friends who are in the trenches with you. As for your old friends, just be as honest and open with them as you can about each of your expectations for how your relationship may change once the baby's here. The ones who are in it for the long haul will stick with you, even if there are periods of time when your connection isn't as frequent or as close as it once was.

Your Relationship with Your Parents (and Your Partner's Parents)

If you got married, or if you've been in a long-term relationship, you probably felt things shift within your own family of origin as you essentially started your own new family unit. That feeling will likely only intensify as you now become a mother yourself. And if you're having your baby on your own or with someone you haven't been with for very long, prepare for a lot of change in your family dynamic. Having a child may be the first time your parent or parents truly see you as an adult. That's a big deal.

An interesting shift happens with your partner's family, too; a lot of times, before you have kids, you're the new kid on the block. Maybe even seen as an interloper. But once

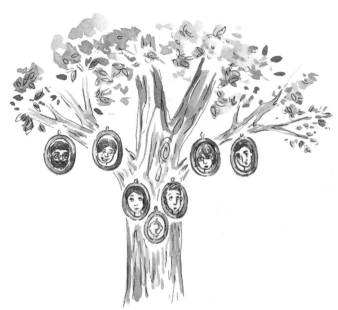

you give birth to a grandchild, you are family. Where before you were the wife or the girlfriend, now you're a family member's mother. It's like you really become blood. And you are very likely to be in a lot closer contact than before, sending pictures, getting advice, and hearing more stories about when your partner was a baby.

Things definitely change within your own family, too. Within the first year of my being a mother, my relationship with my mom got approximately one thousand times better than it was before. (We were not close when I was between the ages of 12 and 25.) I realized how hard it must have been for her to raise four kids as a single mother. I grew a different level of respect for her, and it made all the difference between us. (Sorry, Mom, that it took as long as it did!)

That being said, it's not a given that your relationship to your parent or parents will get better. It may get more difficult, especially if you feel that they are projecting their expectations on what kind of a parent you are. Or you may feel sort of forgotten if they go hog wild over your baby and don't think to check in on you. It's all within the realm of possibility and I will only say that you are entitled to all of your feelings. Sometimes it takes a really big event like having a baby for unhealthy dynamics to come to light. Stay true to yourself and communicate with everyone as openly as you are able and trust that you will get through to the other side.

Also, it's really important that you talk to your family members about each of your expectations for how much they will be involved in your child's life. A lot of new moms have fantasies about their mothers being a regular caregiver to their child. And a lot of grandmas don't share that vision.

It's so tempting to envision your mom or your mother-in-law being your own personal Mary Poppins, but it's definitely not a given. A lot of how involved your parents will be in your baby's life depends on their age, employment status, relationship status, and energy level. My mom had me when she was 16, so as I write this, she's only 52 and happy to hold babies, carry babies, and get down on the floor with kids. Whereas my mother-in-law recently turned 80—she's legitimately past the point of caring for babies.

I hit the timing jackpot with my mom. When my sister had her kids—10 years before I had mine—my mom was still working as a nurse. My sister had hoped that my mom would stay over some nights and help her care for my niece, but mom, who was still working a lot of nights, really didn't have the bandwidth for that. I actually have a little guilt because my mom is very involved with our kids, and primarily because of timing. Just expect that your family relationships will go through an adjustment period; again, talking about expectations and feelings openly goes a very long way. Because there is probably a gap between what your expectations are and what theirs are. And if you don't talk about those expectations, your relationship is likely to fall into that gap.

If you do end up having a family member take care of your kids regularly, think about paying them at least something for their time (if you can swing it). Even a small amount of payment helps keep things out in the open. Your family member knows you value their efforts because you're paying them. You feel more empowered to ask them (or tell them) how you want them to take care of your baby, because you're paying them. Trust me, if you don't pay them—and I know that it's not possible for everyone and this tip may not be all that relatable—it's very easy for resentment to build on both sides. It helps maintain the power dynamic, that you're the parent. Grandparents are great, but they do tend to spoil kids more than a parent would, and if your kid is spending a lot of time with its grandparents, it can start to get problematic.

With Your Partner

Your relationship with your partner goes through a huge change after the baby comes. You have probably already started to feel the tectonic plates of your relationship shifting even before the baby is here.

I think it's very easy for the partner to feel like a third wheel. You and the baby are in a circle, and the other parent can feel outside the circle. It's important to give thought to how you're going to keep the circle big enough for the three of you. When our girls were born, I bought my husband one of the Nu Roo baby-wearing shirts I talked about on page 162; it made it so easy for him to wear the babies on his chest and bond with them.

It can be really hard to let other people—even your partner!—do things for the baby, especially in those early days when your hormones are making you break out into a sweat and start leaking breast milk every time the baby cries, but try to find duties that can be your partner's domain. For example, I always hand our girls to my husband to burp. Some dads claim diaper changes as their territory. And some take over one of the night-

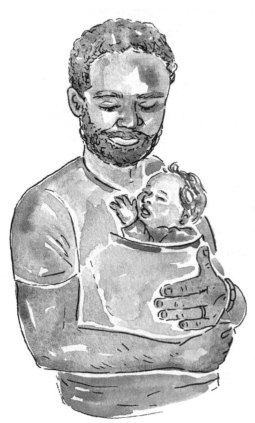

time feedings—so you'll want to be sure to pump enough for a feeding if you're breastfeeding, trust me it makes a huge difference if you can get that extra sleep and you don't feel like the only sleepless one in the relationship!

Until the baby is here, just try to enjoy these last few weeks or months of the two of you being able to go out to dinner or even away for the weekend or a true vacation on your own schedule. Taking a 'babymoon'—a relaxing vacation before the baby comes—is a really great idea so that you can enjoy each other's company, undisturbed.

Once your baby is here, it will depend on you for everything. Your schedule won't be your own for a long time. Even with my Mom helping out and a nanny and a baby nurse, it is really challenging for my husband and I to find time to go to dinner, much less spend the night away from home. I know it's hard to hear, but just try to appreciate the freedom you have now. Go on dates. Go places. Enjoy it.

Speaking of Babymoons, When Is it OK to Travel?

The American College of Obstetrics and Gynecology (ACOG) suggests you can safely travel up until 36 weeks when pregnant with a singleton, and that the best time to travel is now, in the second trimester, because your energy is highest and your risk of complications lowest. If you are flying internationally, make sure your return ticket is before you are at 36 weeks. Some airlines restrict international travel for pregnant women starting at 28 weeks—check the fine print of your ticket before you purchase. ACOG also recommends you avoid traveling to places that have a risk of exposure to malaria or the Zika virus, as both pose risks to pregnant women and their babies (you can visit www.cdc.gov/travel/ notices for the latest travel advisories, including those for pregnant women, from the Center for Disease Control and Prevention.)

For your own comfort, and to reduce the risk of deep vein thrombosis (DVT), which is when a blood clot forms in your leg or other extremity due to long periods of sitting and then travels to your lungs once you are up and moving again, take shorter plane trips (or divide a longer flight into two legs) and break up longer car drives with plenty of breaks—every two hours or so—for getting out of the car and walking around. The risk of DVT is elevated in pregnant women, and this may be your last trip for a while when you can travel at your own pace, so why not take your time and take care of yourself along the way?

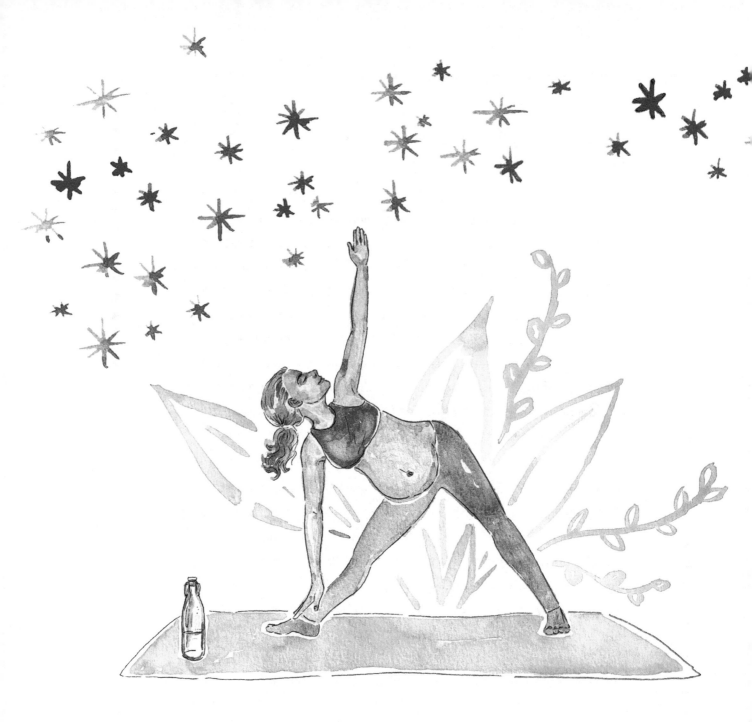

Chapter 12

TAKE CARE OF YOUR BODY NOW

I hope that by now you're over any nausea or fatigue and that your appetite and energy are back. Just because you're feeling good doesn't mean you don't have to take great care of yourself, however. You are in training for an athletic event (aka birth) and a new reality; your nutrition and exercise choices now can go so far toward setting you up for success. Don't just check out and eat all your favorite junk food and let yourself be sedentary because you're already gaining weight, so why not? The better you treat yourself now, the stronger and more prepared you'll be later.

Plus, now is a perfect time to develop a greater appreciation for your body and what it's capable of. Realizing that you are growing a new human can really empower you to respect your body more. I felt it: When I was pregnant, it was a like a door opened in my mind, and I realized I needed to take great care of myself. All I can say is, go with it. The more you get into nutrition and exercise now, the deeper the roots of these healthy habits will grow and the less likely you'll be to let them all go once the baby is here and it seems like you've got a great (and adorable) excuse to.

Foods and Nutrients to Prioritize Now

Do you still need to focus your diet on all the nutrients—and their corresponding foods—I discussed in Chapter 6? Absolutely! After all, your baby's tissues, major systems, and vital organs are continuing to develop rapidly, and each of those nutrients plays an important role in making that growth happen. In addition, there are some different

" NOW iT'S REALLY TiME to START EATING for TWO. "

nutrients that you need to prioritize at this stage. Mainly, it's time to concentrate again on iron, which I last discussed in Chapter 2, and to take in some extra protein.

And, now it's really time to start eating for two. While guidelines can vary, the general recommendation is to consume an extra 340 calories per day during your second trimester from clean, healthy foods. Ideally, they'll include the following nutrients, which are more important now than ever.

Iron. Iron helps your body produce hemoglobin, found in your red blood cells, which transports oxygen around your body to other cells. When you're pregnant, it's iron that gets all-important oxygen to your baby. And it's more important now because your blood volume increases a lot in your second trimester, by up to 60 percent, so you need more iron to keep up with that boost. If your diet is deficient in iron, you could become anemic. If your diet is deficient in vitamin C, it increases the risk, because your body requires vitamin C to absorb iron. Anemia increases the risk of complications with your pregnancy, including premature birth. In fact, your health care practitioner will likely test you for anemia around the very end of your second trimester.

I shared a few foods rich in iron in Chapter 2, which I'll include again here along with some additional options to consider adding to your plate now:

- Beans
- Beets (and their greens) & beet powder
- Blackstrap molasses
- Butternut squash
- Chicken
- Dark chocolate (a little is okay!)
- Dried fruits (apricots, peaches, raisins)
- Egg yolks
- Green leafy vegetables (broccoli, kale, spinach, sea vegetables/seaweeds)
- Legumes
- Nuts and seeds (especially pumpkin seeds)
- Oysters
- Quinoa
- Turkey
- Whole grains

Remember, you can also cook with cast iron pots and pans, which can increase the iron content in the foods you're cooking by as much as 50 percent.

A note about calcium: Adequate calcium intake is very important in your second trimester, as well as in the first, because it helps build your baby's bones and teeth; it's also vital in healthy muscle and nerve functioning. That said, try to avoid eating calcium-rich foods (yogurt, leafy greens, nuts and seeds, some fish) with iron-rich foods in the same meal, because calcium can reduce iron absorption. On the flip side, vitamin C-containing foods can increase iron absorption, so consider including those foods in your iron-rich meals: oranges, red bell peppers, broccoli, etc.

In general, the body absorbs iron from animal foods (heme iron) way more efficiently than from plant foods. While I talked in Chapter 2 about eating less animal protein, a little is certainly okay, and important now. Especially because your iron and protein needs increase during your second trimester, you can confidently incorporate some animal foods at this stage to ensure adequate intake. It's still a good idea, though, to opt for leaner cuts and to select organic, pasture-raised, hormone-free meats whenever possible.

Protein. I'm guessing you've heard protein referred to as the building block of the body. So you can understand why it's important to pile on the protein in your second trimester. Your baby is growing and developing quickly; their brain and tissues need all the building blocks they can get. Your placenta is growing, too, and your blood and amniotic fluid are increasing. What's more, your breasts and uterus are growing. Protein may also keep swelling down in your body, as it helps balance the amount of fluid in your tissues.

In this stage of your pregnancy, protein should comprise the bulk of your meal. And you should be eating a serving of protein at least three times a day. General guidelines typically recommend at least 75 grams a day or 0.8 grams per kilogram of bodyweight. But a recent study, which focused specifically on the protein needs of pregnant women, found the needs may be higher. It showed protein needs to be 39 percent higher in early pregnancy and 73 percent higher in late pregnancy than that 0.8-gram recommendation. (We'll talk about protein again in your third trimester too.) That means 1.22 grams in early pregnancy and 1.52 grams in later months. So, if you weigh 130 pounds, you multiply that by .45 to get the number of kilograms. That gets you roughly 59 kilograms. Then multiply that by 1.22 or 1.52 depending on which trimester you're in. That means 72 grams of protein a day (or about 24 grams per meal) if you're in your first or early second trimester, and 90 grams (about 30 grams per meal) if you're in the second half of your pregnancy.

Good sources of protein include:

- Beans, peas, and lentils
- Bone broth
- Dairy (full-fat)
- Eggs
- Fish (see page 196 for more information about safe seafood)
- Lean meats
- Nuts and seeds
- Nutritional yeast
- Poultry
- Tempeh

You may want to consider a daily protein drink to help you meet your needs. You can blend almond milk or juice with ice, fruit, and protein powder to make a delicious smoothie. Here's my favorite protein-rich smoothie recipe:

How to Know How Many Grams of Protein You're Eating

While you can always check the label, it's also helpful to use an online database to see how much protein is in the foods you eat. I like the one at nutritiondata.self.com.

Organic Superfood Smoothie

Ingredients

- 1 organic banana
- 1½ cups frozen berries
- 1 generous handful organic spinach
- 2 tablespoons organic virgin coconut oil
- 2 tablespoons ground organic flaxseeds

- 2 tablespoons organic hemp seeds
- 8 ounces unsweetened vanilla flavored almond milk
- 1 scoop your favorite flavored protein powder
- 1 tablespoon açai powder

Instructions

1. Blend all ingredients until smooth and enjoy.

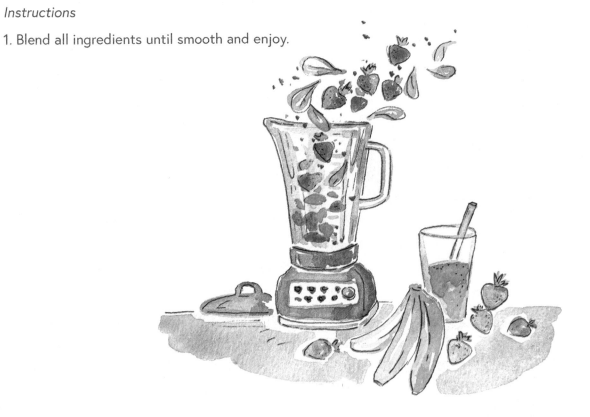

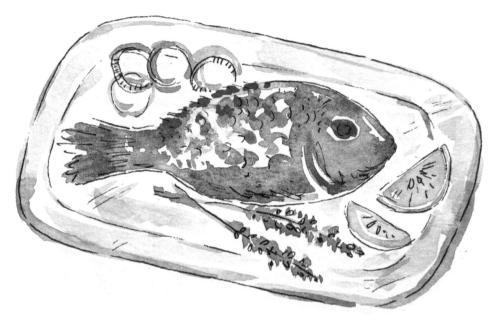

Safe Seafood

While it's always prudent to choose
safe seafood, it's absolutely critical when you're pregnant. Again, you want
the important nutrients fish and seafood provide for your health and that
of your baby—but without any mercury that can cause serious damage
to a developing fetus. Here's a guide to help you make the right selection
when shopping at your local store or market. The information comes from
data provided by the FDA and EPA and compiled by the Natural Resources
Defense Council. For more about safe seafood, visit www.nrdc.org and
www.ewg.org seafood.

LEAST MERCURY	MODERATE MERCURY	HIGH MERCURY	HIGHEST MERCURY
Anchovies	Bass *(Saltwater, Striped, Black)*	Croaker *(White Pacific)*	Bluefish
Butterfish	Buffalofish	Halibut *(Atlantic, Pacific)*	Grouper
Catfish	Carp		Mackerel *(King)*
Clam	Cod *(Alaskan)*	Mackerel *(Spanish, Gulf)*	Marlin
Crab *(Domestic)*	Lobster		Orange Roughy
Crawfish/Crayfish	Mahi Mahi	Perch *(Ocean)*	Shark
Croaker *(Atlantic)*	Monkfish	Sablefish	Swordfish
Flounder	Perch *(Freshwater)*	Sea Bass *(Chilean)*	Tuna *(Bigeye, Ahi)*
Haddock *(Atlantic)*	Sheepshead	Tuna *(Albacore, Yellowfin)*	
Hake	Skate		
Herring	Snapper		
Jacksmelt *(Silverside)*	Tilefish *(Atlantic)*		
Mackerel *(N. Atlantic, Chub)*	Tuna *(Canned chunk light, Skipjack)*		
Mullet			
Oyster			
Plaice			
Pollock			
Salmon *(Canned)*			
Salmon *(Fresh)*			
Sardine			
Scallop			
Shrimp			
Sole *(Pacific)*			
Squid *(Calamari)*			
Tilapia			
Trout *(Freshwater)*			
Whitefish			
Whiting			

Speaking of Protein, Can I Really Eat Fish?

Yes! And you should—but it's all about moderation and selecting the right type (more in a minute). Not only is fish a great source of lean protein, oily fish are also extremely rich in omega-3 fatty acids. And remember, omega-3s are crucial in the development of your baby's brain, eyes, immune system, and nervous system. Adequate intake also reduces your risk of developing preeclampsia.

Yet, it's true that fish can be contaminated with unhealthy toxins like mercury, which can negatively affect your baby's nervous system (not to mention your own) and brain development. That's where selection and moderation come in. Aim to eat no more than 12 ounces of low-mercury fish weekly. Keep consumption of higher-mercury fish much lower: no more than three six-ounce servings a month. And always avoid consuming species of fish that are highest in mercury concentration, including shark, swordfish, tilefish, and king mackerel. For more about mercury and which fish to put on your plate during pregnancy, see the box on pages 195-196.

Dietary Don'ts

Here are some important don'ts to remember this trimester, when you're trying to meet your increased calcium, protein, and other nutrient needs. **Don't:**

- Eat any raw or undercooked meat, fish or shellfish, or eggs (including those in salad dressing and mayonnaise).

- Enjoy deli lunch meats or hotdogs (even if the label says precooked) *unless* they've been heated until hot. They could carry the harmful bacteria *listeria*, which is killed by high heat. Deli salads are prone to it too. If you're worried, skip these foods altogether. I know it can be tempting to grab a turkey sandwich from the deli, but don't do it. It's not worth the risk. *Listeria* is dangerous enough for adults; for fetuses, it is life-threatening.

- Consume high-mercury fish (see page 197).
- Eat soft/cultured cheeses like feta and Brie unless they're cooked, and cooked thoroughly; they can also harbor *listeria*.

Supplements to Consider

In addition to your prenatal vitamins, there are a couple of supplements you might want to add to your repertoire (although, of course, check with your health care provider first). They are:

Magnesium. If your leg cramps are severe, you may want to consider taking supplemental magnesium. If you're experiencing ligament pain, consider a magnesium orotate supplement, which is magnesium with the addition of orotic acid.

Vitamin E. Vitamin E helps your skin remain elastic, and thus can possibly help prevent stretch marks from the inside out (and reduce varicose veins and hemorrhoids)! Importantly, it also aids in the development of your baby's reproductive system and placental attachment—and detachment. One thing to be cautious of, though, is that if your doctor has recommended you supplement with iron, the two should not be taken together.

Evening primrose oil. Because preeclampsia becomes a concern in the second and third trimesters, you may also want to consider taking evening primrose oil, which can help combat hypertension, if your blood pressure is elevated.

Vitamin D. This fundamental vitamin will help your baby grow strong bones and teeth. Because many Americans are deficient, and because it's not naturally present in many foods, if you didn't start taking a vitamin D supplement in your first trimester, this is a good time to begin.

FITNESS: YOU'RE PREGNANT, NOT DEAD

From BROOKe CaTeS *of the Bloom Method:*

"We're often led to believe that pregnancy robs us of strength, forcing expecting moms to dial back on their exercise. I don't buy it, and you shouldn't either. It is possible to tap into a deeper connection to and appreciation of your body—including your core strength—DURING pregnancy than you had prepregnancy. Pregnancy and motherhood can transform you into a stronger version of yourself. Anytime you doubt whether you're strong enough to give birth, remind yourself: I'm stronger now than I've ever been.

"In this trimester, you want to start focusing on strengthening and lengthening the pelvic floor, because it's a valuable player in both overall core strength and in preparing for and healing from birth. You may not have given much thought to your pelvic floor before, but it plays a key role in your posture, your breath, and how you move throughout your day. The muscles of the pelvic floor are commonly tight because of all the sitting we do—and the squatting and kneeling and other traditional movements we don't do—and a tight muscle is a weak muscle. You want to be able to contract and lengthen these muscles as needed; it's something that should happen naturally, but if you haven't given this group of muscles much thought, you are likely more in contraction mode, even baring down on them more than is necessary. Getting your pelvic floor online will better prepare you for birth, prevent future pelvic floor dysfunction (such as incontinence—urine leaking—and uterine or bladder prolapse), and lead you to your strongest core now and after you're pregnant."

Pelvic Floor Circuit

Here are the four exercises Brooke recommends you do during the second trimester to start to prepare and connect to your pelvic floor, so that it is both stronger and more pliable for your delivery—and beyond. Brooke says: "Throughout this circuit, the pelvic floor muscles should lengthen or feel like they are opening towards your vagina on the inhale, and engage and contract (much like a Kegel) on the exhale. You may notice that in one of the positions, it is easier to feel the lengthening phase, while in the other it's easier to feel the contraction phase. Aim to reach a point where you can feel the lengthening and the contraction phases equally, regardless of the position."

Child's Pose with Diaphragmatic Breath   *Duration:* 1 minute

Description: Come into a child's pose (knees wide, big toes kissing, chest and forearms relaxed on the mat beneath you) and find your diaphragmatic breath. Observe the subtle (not forced) sensations that come with each inhale and exhale: On the inhale, feel the ribcage, abdomen, and pelvic floor lengthen and expand. As you exhale, feel the rebound of this sensation first in the pelvic floor, then the abdomen, and lastly the ribcage—think of the subtleness of a flower opening and closing.

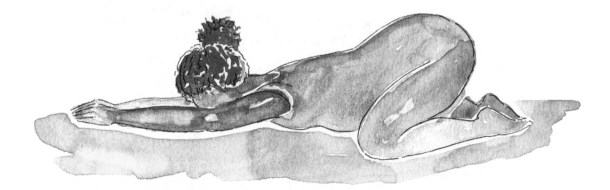

Child's Pose with Belly Pump

Duration: 1 minute

Description: Staying in your child's pose, it's time to increase your core awareness by shifting into the belly pump technique. On the inhale, continue feeling into the natural expansion from ribcage to abdomen, down into the pelvic floor musculature. (Remember not to force it; you should not feel as though you are pushing outwards against your abdominal wall or baring down on the pelvic floor.) As you exhale, contract the pelvic floor in either a Kegel exercise or go deeper by imagining all four sides of the vagina coming together like a claw crane and moving upward. At the end of your exhale, contract your deep core and hug your baby. Keep going, noticing what you feel in the pelvic floor and the difference between the sensations of the belly pump versus diaphragmatic breathing.

All Fours with Diaphragmatic Breath

Duration: 1 minute

Description: Come onto all fours, stacking your shoulders over your wrists and your knees directly under your hips, and find your diaphragmatic breath. Remember, the sensations should feel subtle and not forced. You're not trying to contract anything; rather, you're focusing on the subtle movements in the pelvic floor as you breathe.

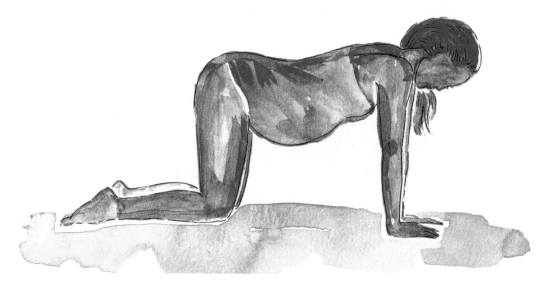

All Fours with Belly Pump   *Duration:* 1 minute

Description: Remaining on all fours, shift into the belly pump breathing pattern, noticing what you feel in the pelvic floor and the difference between the sensations of the belly pump versus diaphragmatic breathing.

Once you've performed all four exercises, do one more round, starting again with Child's Pose with Diaphragmatic Breath.

Take Care of Your Core to Prevent Diastasis Recti

You may have heard of diastasis recti, a condition that can occur after pregnancy where the connective tissue that runs down the front of your abdomen and connects the two sides of your rectus abdominis (the six-pack muscle) separates.

It's important to know that a natural and healthy level of abdominal separation occurs in almost all expecting women, and it is very possible to avoid an injury level of separation by learning how to properly recruit your inner core system during exercise and your daily life. The most important way to do that is to avoid what's known as doming or coning, which is when your baby moves into the very front of your abdomen and your belly takes on a dome or even a triangular shape. This typically can happen when you're lifting something heavy, sitting up from lying down, holding a plank position, or reclining in a chair. That doming is a sign of pressure being placed on the connective tissue, weakening it, and increasing the risk of injury.

You can prevent doming with a few simple strategies:

1. Doing the belly pump breathing on page 41 and in the Pelvic Floor Circuit in this chapter will help you strengthen your core muscles and connect to your ability to engage and lengthen them—you need both lengthening and contracting to be strong.

2. Apply optimal core connection—which is the same action as on the exhale portion of

the belly pump—both during your day and your workouts to ensure that you're minimizing the pressure within your abdomen and continuing to challenge the core muscles as your belly grows.

3. Minimize doming. Chances are it will happen at least a handful of times, but catching yourself and creating the necessary core engagement will limit any lasting effects.

When you're aware of how to protect your core, and you've done your diaphragmatic breathing and belly pumps, you're taking important steps to protect yourself from the trashed abs and leaky bladder that you may have heard other moms lamenting or joking about. Those things are not a given; remember, your body is magic, and perfectly designed to both carry and birth babies and recover from those efforts. Practicing your breathing exercises is how you support your body in doing its incredible work.

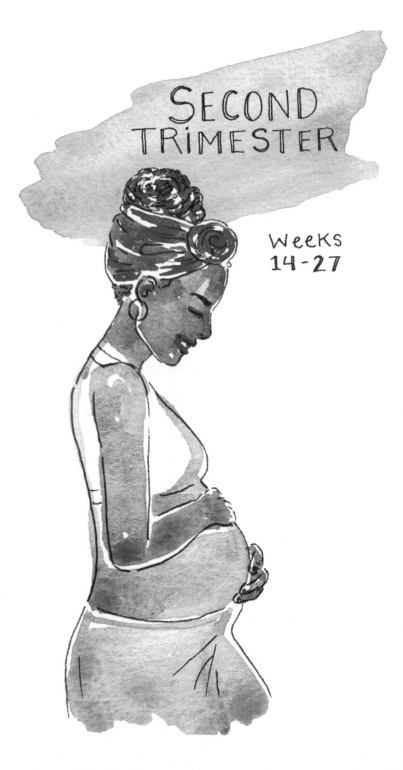

SECOND TRIMESTER

WeeKS 14-27

What's Happening Now: Second Trimester (Weeks 14-27)

Now that you're in your second trimester, you should be feeling more energetic and less nauseated. But while this time may feel like more of a "vacation" for you than the first trimester, your body isn't taking any time off when it comes to your fetus's development, so you may still experience some less-than-pleasant symptoms that go along with those shifts. You may also feel a little increasingly anxious about your approaching labor and all that's to come as a new mom. Just remember, you are one in a line of billions of women who have given birth and become mothers; you were born to do this. You've got this.

With Baby

At 20 weeks, you've reached the midpoint of your pregnancy, and things are getting pretty far along in terms of your baby's development. In fact, a baby born prematurely after 23 weeks may survive—with intensive care, of course.

By the end of the second trimester, your baby will weigh around two pounds; they really pack on the lbs during this stage. But that's not all that happens:

- **Senses are coming online.** Your baby is starting to see, hear, smell, and even taste. Their eyes are beginning to open and move, albeit slowly at first. They can recognize and even respond to your voice. And because their digestive system was fully formed in the first trimester, they can even start to taste the foods you eat via the amniotic fluid now. They are also urinating and releasing it into the amniotic sac. Since they can swallow and suck at this stage, they may also begin sucking their thumb.

- **Sleep cycles are happening.** Your baby has begun developing a sleep/wake cycle. They spend most of their time either in active or REM (rapid eye movement) sleep. They can even yawn at this stage—and baby yawns are one of the cutest things in nature.

- **Things are getting a little hairy.** Your baby's scalp hair pattern is beginning to form, and they also now have eyebrows and eyelashes. Around 19 weeks, they're covered with what some people call a "fur coat," technically known as lanugo. These fine, downy hairs will help keep them warm, because they don't have much body fat yet. Also around this time, their skin forms vernix caseosa, a greasy or creamy white layer that provides them protection from the amniotic fluid, which is quite acidic. On a hair- and skin-related note, they also develop tiny fingernails and toenails now, and their fingerprints (and toeprints!) form. (OK, maybe baby toes are the cutest thing in nature.)

- **You may be feeling movement.** You may start to notice the baby's delicate movements as a fluttering feeling in your belly that's referred to as quickening. (Some of the baby's new jerking movements could be caused by hiccups.) Brain developments are allowing for control over their motor function, although much more brain development takes place in the final trimester.

With You

As I mentioned above, you should start feeling more energetic and more like yourself this trimester. That's why it's a good time to think about your birth plan (see Chapter 8) and get your home ready for your new arrival (see Chapter 9). Your body is still working hard to make a new human, however, so you'll likely feel some effects of that effort; although, they shouldn't derail you the way morning sickness and fatigue did in the first trimester. Also, now you'll start to get a legitimate baby bump! As your belly develops, your breasts will grow too.

- **Back pain is a possibility now.** As you gain a little extra weight, your back may feel a bit more achy. I found that sleeping on my side with a pillow between my knees helped relieve the pressure. It's also a good time to treat yourself to a prenatal massage or an appointment with a chiropractor who specializes in pregnancy. Backache can also be a symptom of urinary tract infections, which are more common during pregnancy.

- **You may be more stuffed up.** All those hormones can irritate the mucous membranes in your nose. You may find that you're more congested during your second trimester, and even that you experience nosebleeds. Using a saline spray or humidifier can help, and both are entirely natural solutions.

- **The appearance of a whole new kind of cramps.** Just because you're not getting your period doesn't mean you won't have any cramps… leg cramps, that is. Leg cramps are common in the second trimester and often continue into the third. Be sure to stretch before bed, and to stay active and hydrate, hydrate, hydrate. Supplements can also help; see page 199. It's common to begin to experience a slight swelling of your ankles and feet later in these months too. Again, this swelling can last through the rest of your pregnancy. Staying active helps reduce this puffiness, as does drinking enough water and limiting your salt consumption.

- **Your oral health may take a hit.** It's common now to experience sensitive gums; they may even bleed a little. That's normal. But definitely take good care of your teeth and be sure to see your dentist at least once during your pregnancy.

- **You've got to protect your skin.** All those pregnancy hormones can affect your skin—specifically, your skin's pigment. For example, you might notice brown patches on your face or a dark line that runs down your abdomen. Your skin is also more sensitive to sunlight in the second trimester, and sun exposure can worsen pigmentation changes. Be sure to use a natural sunscreen and to limit your time outdoors when the sun is at its afternoon peak in the sky.

- **Things to watch out for.** Hopefully it's relatively smooth sailing for you during this time, with only mild discomfort from the symptoms above. Of course, if you have intense vaginal bleeding, severe belly pain, or a high fever, you should contact your health care provider right away. Keep an eye out for symptoms of gestational diabetes, which often begins around your 24th week, as well as preeclampsia: These include excessive urination and extreme thirst, as well as serious swelling in the hands and face, among others.

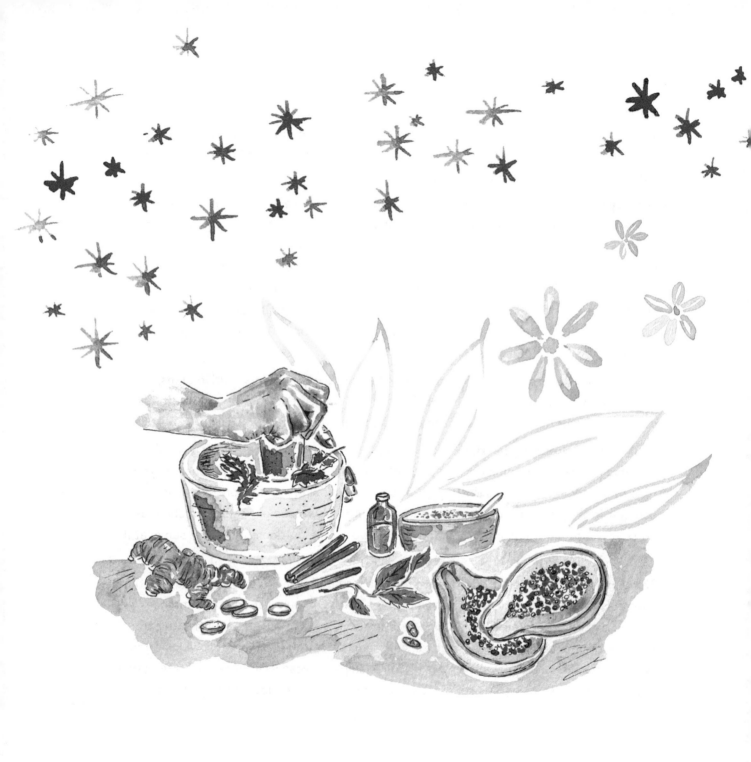

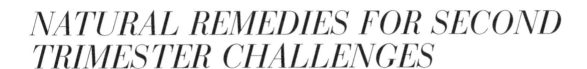

Chapter 13

NATURAL REMEDIES FOR SECOND TRIMESTER CHALLENGES

Now that your baby and belly are growing, you'll probably start experiencing a new set of symptoms—many due to the fact that the baby is taking up more space in your torso, which can impact your lower back, your digestion, and even your sleep.

These natural remedies can help you feel your best. Just remember to consult with your health care provider before starting any new supplements or herbal remedies. Even though you are the ultimate authority on your experience, you want them to know about everything that's happening with you and the baby.

Heartburn

There's an old wives' tale that says if you experience heartburn as a pregnancy symptom, your baby will be born with a full head of hair. I don't know about that—what I do know is that heartburn in pregnancy can be caused by the same hormone, relaxin, that loosens your tendons, ligaments, and muscles, because it can also cause the flap between your esophagus and your stomach to get lazy, allowing stomach acid to flow back upward. You've also got a growing baby that can exert pressure on your stomach from the bottom up, and perhaps indigestion or constipation to boot.

Some of the same remedies for other pregnancy symptoms help with heartburn, including ginger (which also helps with nausea; you can either add to your food or steep for tea), apple cider vinegar (which also helps with constipation, see below for instructions on how to take it), and exercise (even a little walk around the block after eating will help your food pass out of your stomach more quickly so that there's less upward pressure). You can also try taking digestive enzymes derived from papaya or pineapple 30 minutes before eating (check with your health care provider first) as they help you break down food more efficiently.

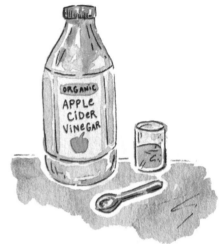

Also, if your heartburn just won't seem to go away no matter what you do, try limiting the wheat, meat, dairy, and sugar in your diet as these are hard on digestion. I know it's hard to avoid all four, but if you try it and find that it does make a big difference in how you feel, it won't feel like a sacrifice—it will feel like you've figured out a secret to feeling good.

Constipation

Constipation is common during pregnancy, especially during the second trimester. That's because changing hormone levels can slow things down—not only that, when you do go, you might find things painful.

I got constipated during both my pregnancies—I found that a one- to two-ounce shot of apple cider vinegar first thing in the morning really helped keep me regular. It's definitely intense, but you get used to it. I actually started to crave it. Look for apple cider vinegar that has "the mother"—that means the vinegar was naturally fermented and delivers gut-friendly bacteria.

It's also important that you make sure you've getting plenty of fiber—at least 20 grams per day, and as much as 35 grams—which will help food move through your digestive tract. You can easily get that amount by eating plenty of fresh fruits and vegetables; nuts and seeds; beans and legumes; and whole grains. That also means you should cut down on the processed wheat, meat, dairy, and sugar, all of which are low in fiber and take a long time to move through the GI tract; sugar and most dairy (especially if it's sweetened, such as flavored yogurt) also feed your unfriendly gut bacteria, which takes a toll on your digestive health.

In addition, Mari Mikel believes that up to 90 percent of constipation is due to not drinking enough water. Make sure you are drinking plenty of water—more than you think you need.

Finally, exercise helps. If you're not moving, neither are your bowels. Get up and do something to move your body.

If you need more support, try a magnesium supplement. Magnesium relaxes your smooth muscle tissue, which is what lines your digestive tract. To gauge how much magnesium to take each day, start by taking 50 -100 milligrams a day (depending on the dosage of your supplement—powder is best if you can find it because it is more easily absorbed than a capsule or tablet), increasing by 50 - 100 milligrams a day until your stools become loose, and then to back off by 50 - 100 milligrams.

One thing you should not do is take laxatives, including castor oil, or use an enema. The same nerves that enervate the uterus also enervate the intestines (that's why you may have gotten loose stools when you've started your period in the past—and why you may again when you go into labor), and by activating the gut you might also activate labor. (I'll talk more about castor oil as a means to get labor—its plusses and its perils—in Chapter 18.)

Backache

As the baby grows and your center of gravity is pulled more and more forward, your posture can get whacked out and take a toll on the muscles of your lower back, resulting in back pain. The tendency is to lock your knees in an effort to stabilize yourself and lean the upper torso back to counteract the weight of the belly, which contracts the muscles of the low back. You want to stand so that your eyes, shoulders, hips, and ankles are all in one line so that no set of muscles has to work overtime to hold you up—you'll probably have to look at yourself from the side in a mirror to see when you've got it.

Also, some kind of support around your belly (like the high-waisted exercise pants I loved to wear that come up over your belly) makes a big difference in preventing your belly from just falling forward and pulling on the muscles of the low back.

And I'm probably starting to sound like a broken record by now, but working out and making sure you're both moving and strengthening your core and back muscles really helps—as do the breathing exercises I shared in Chapter 12.

If it's really bad, try chiropractic care, prenatal massage, or acupuncture—just make sure the practitioner is well versed in pregnancy.

Fatigue

Make sure your prenatal vitamin is up to snuff—in particular, all the B vitamins make a huge difference when it comes to fatigue. Also, file this under "obvious advice," but make sure you're sleeping enough. You really need a minimum of seven hours a night and preferably eight or nine. Make sure you're not staying up too late watching shows or online shopping or catching up on work. I know that you may feel like late nights are the only times you get to yourself (particularly if you are already a mom), but making a baby takes a nuclear reactor's worth of energy—you need the sleep now. The work you're doing is harder and takes more of a toll than you think it should.

This is another place where being adequately hydrated makes a big difference. Drinking 25 percent more water provides 75 percent more energy; so if you're feeling wiped out, start drinking two to four more glasses of water a day. And here's yet another reason to get plenty of exercise! Walking to your car doesn't count. Inactivity breeds fatigue.

Trouble sleeping

Another reason pregnant women are often tired is that it's not easy to sleep when you're uncomfortable. I highly recommend investing in a big body pillow to throw your top leg and arm over when sleeping on your side, and/or a foam wedge to place under your belly so it's not pulling on your back muscles as you sleep. It's worth some trial and error to find the pillow situation that will help you get your rest. I used a wedge under my belly for support and couldn't image sleeping without one.

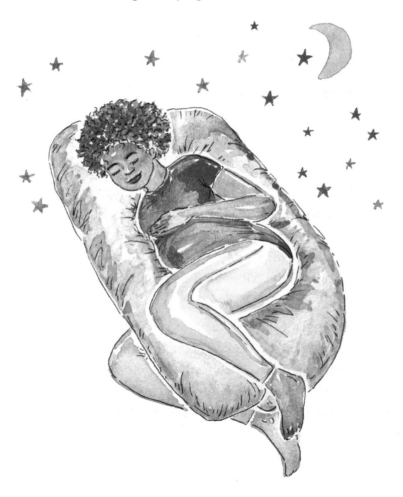

Leg cramps

Leg cramps are such a pain, particularly when they also interrupt your sleep. Most of the time, leg cramps are about a lack of ample minerals. Even if you're eating a super healthy diet filled with lots of dark leafy greens (which are a strong source of minerals), you may not be getting enough because our soils have become depleted of minerals and as a result, even organic veggies don't contain as many minerals as they once did. I recommend taking Ultra-Mins by Nature's Way, which provides calcium, magnesium, manganese, zinc, chromium, potassium, iron, phosphorus, iodine, and selenium. Mari Mikel has her clients take three tablets a day.

Varicose or spider veins

You may notice new varicose or spider veins sprouting now that you're pregnant—definitely discuss this with your health care provider as they indicate that your capillaries (the tiny blood vessels that carry a majority of your blood supply) might need some shoring up.

The herbal remedy white oak bark helps to support your capillaries and can keep the problem from getting worse—Mari Mikel suggests one or two capsules every morning and evening; one capsule twice a day if your veins aren't that bad, and two capsules twice a day if they are painful. Vitamins E and C also support the circulatory system—both yours and your baby's.

On a practical level, you can wear compression socks. I know it takes dedication, but they really help, and varicose veins can be painful and can get inflamed and perhaps even contribute to forming a blood clot, which you definitely don't want—compression socks are a more desirable choice! You want to put them on before you get out of bed in the morning because that's when you'll have the least amount of blood in the vessels of your feet and legs.

If you are prone to varicose veins you may want to avoid taking evening primrose oil because it helps tissues soften (which is why it's good for softening the cervix—something I'll discuss in Chapter 18). Also, gluten seems to be a really big factor. Cut way back on gluten-containing foods and see if it makes a difference for you.

Anemia

The second trimester is when you might experience low levels of iron, otherwise known as anemia. That's because the baby starts to store all the iron they are going to need until they eat solids, as there is no iron in breastmilk. And nature always prioritizes the health of the baby, so the baby will get the iron it needs but you might be left depleted.

Common symptoms of anemia are fatigue, dizziness, shortness of breath, insomnia, leg cramps, rapid heart beat, and difficulty concentration (it almost reads like a description of pregnancy, doesn't it?). Your health care provider can diagnose you with a blood test, but there are natural ways to support your iron levels too.

Red meat and greens are the best sources of iron, but you need plenty of vitamin C to convert that iron into a usable form and then to absorb it, so be sure to take at least 1000 mg of vitamin C a day.

You can also take yellow dock, an herb that boosts your body's ability to absorb iron. Look for a tincture at your health food store and discuss dosage and suitability with your health care provider.

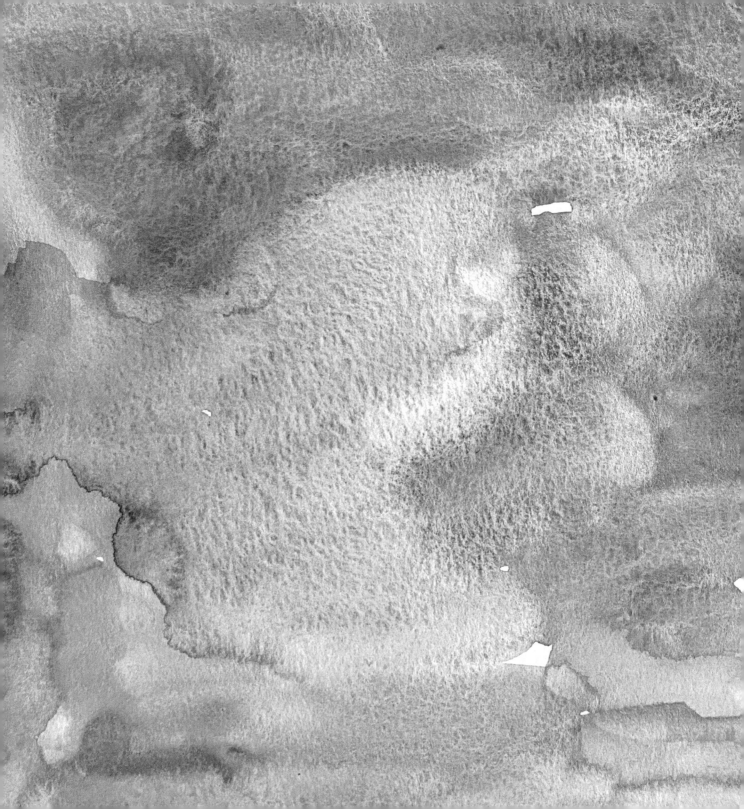

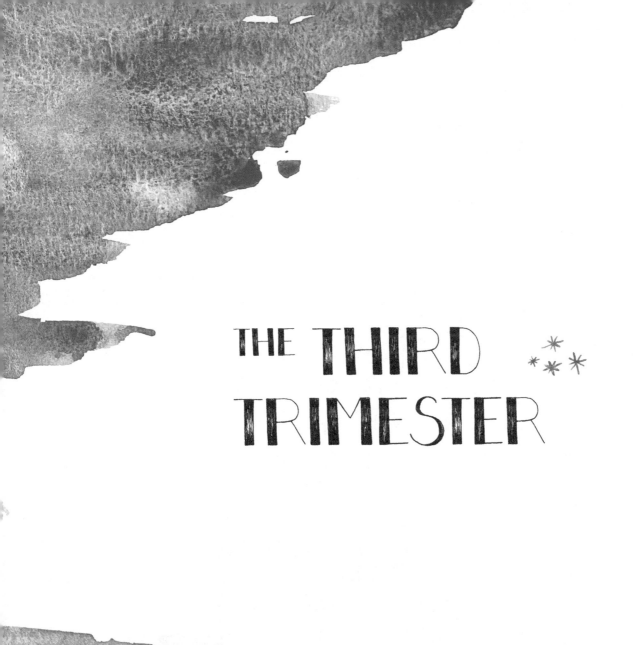

THE THIRD
TRIMESTER

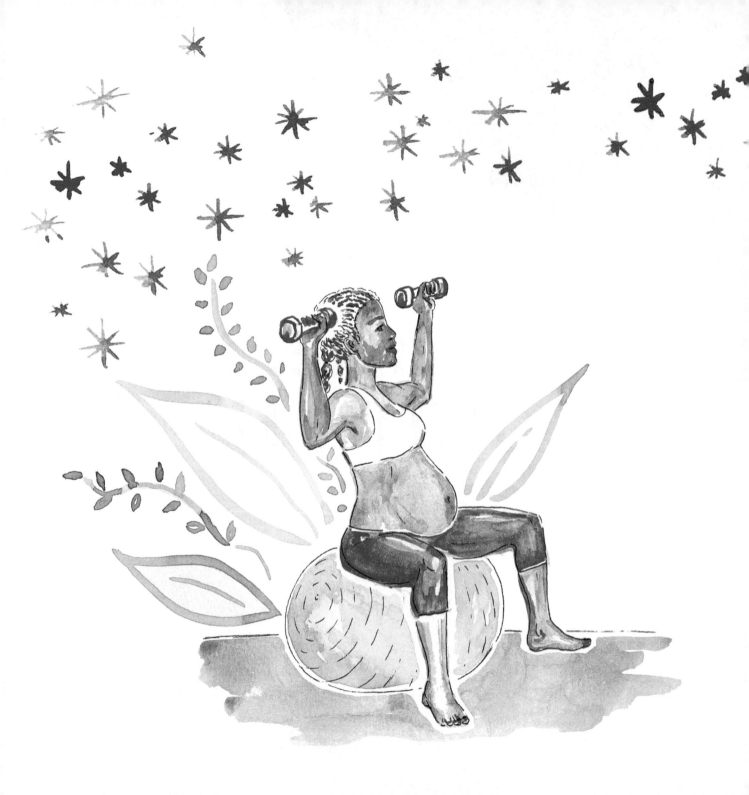

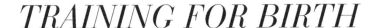

Chapter 14

TRAINING FOR BIRTH

Y ou've rounded the final curve in your pregnancy lap and are on the straightaway toward birth. Now is the time to make sure you're at your best physically and emotionally—and that's what this chapter will help you do.

Keep Training Your Body

If you haven't started exercising regularly yet, by all means, NOW is the time. (Refer back to Chapter 6 for general information about fitness.) And if you have, now's the time to a) keep going and b) fine-tune your efforts so that you're really focused on building strength in the muscles you'll need during birth and on boosting overall stamina. You don't want to "hit the wall" before the baby is out, do you? Nor do you want to be so wiped out from the birth that you can't really be present or engaged in bonding with your baby once they are in your arms.

You are an athlete in training at this stage: It's like you're going to be competing in the Olympics in two to three months. Trust me, you'll appreciate every second of physical prep you've done once labor starts. Just imagine that every squat you do or mile you walk takes one minute off your pushing time. That ought to get you motivated!

Brooke, the creator of The Bloom Method who has contributed a circuit of exercises in these pages for every phase of your pregnancy, says, "A birthing mom expels three times the amount of oxygen during birth than an avid runner

"A BIRTHING mom EXPELS THREE TIMES the AMOUNT of OXYGEN DURING BIRTH than AN AVID RUNNER DOES DURING A MARATHON."

does during a marathon. Meaning, you need to train both mentally and physically so that you arrive at birth prepared to ride the waves of intensity while feeling more in control of your birth experience." Brooke's BirthPREP circuit, below, can make you feel more empowered before, during, and after labor.

That being said, it is an intense workout. Chances are you'll need to focus and dig deep to get through it—which is also great training for birth. "The mental body is often ready to quit before the physical body needs a break. Using verbal cues can help you push through each exercise while training the mental body for the challenge. When you get to your edge, breathe and dive deeper—this is where you get stronger," Brooke says.

The Bloom Method's BirthPREP Circuit

In this circuit, you'll do each of the exercises first with the right leg doing the majority of the work, and then repeat the exercises using the left leg as the primary leg. If you need it, take a 15-second rest between exercises and a 45-second rest between each circuit, working up to being able to perform them without any rests in between.

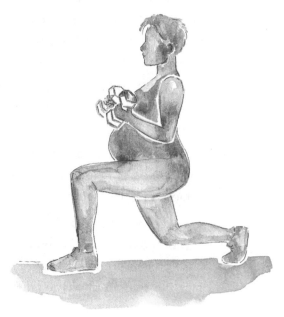

Single Leg Lunge with Bicep Curl

Duration: 2 minutes

Directions: Holding a set of dumbbells in each hand, hands hanging down by your sides, step right leg forward into a single leg lunge, with front knee stacked on top of the ankle and the back knee underneath the hip and the majority of your weight on your right leg.

As you inhale diaphragmatically, bend right knee to lower down into full lunge. At the bottom of your lunge, contract your pelvic floor and deep core, and as you exhale, drive through the heel of your right leg to rise up, performing a bicep curl as you do. Keep going for two minutes. For an extra challenge, when the two minutes are up, come into your lowest lunge and perform little pulses, using your belly pump or diaphragmatic breathing, for an additional 30 seconds.

Single Leg Static Squat with Alternate Leg Tap Outs with Tricep Extensions

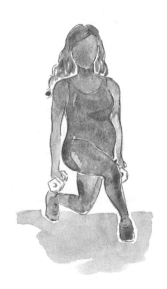

Duration: 1 minute 30 seconds

Directions: Holding a set of dumbbells in each hand, step your feet a little wider than shoulder-width. Transfer your weight onto your right leg, and lift your left foot onto the toes. Bring your elbows to 90 degrees with palms facing in.

As you exhale, engage your core and pelvic floor and extend your left leg and arms back behind you into a tricep extension. As you inhale, return the arms and left leg to the starting position. Continue for 90 seconds, focusing on driving through the right heel to fire up your glutes.

Single Leg Curtsy Lunge

Duration: 1 minute 30 seconds

Directions: Holding a set of dumbbells in each hand, stand with your feet hip-width apart. Take a big step back with your left leg, crossing it behind your right leg. Inhale and bend your knees and lower your hips until your right thigh is nearly parallel to the floor.

Exhale and contract your deep core and pelvic floor muscles as you drive through your heel and rise up to the starting position, taking care not to lock your right knee at the top. Continue for 90 seconds. As you move, keep your torso upright and your hips and shoulders as square as possible.

Glute Bridge with Chest Fly

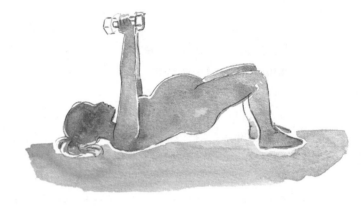

Duration: 2 minutes total

Directions: Lie on your back with your knees bent and your arms out to the sides, holding a dumbbell in each hand. (If you get light-headed on your back, place 1 or 2 pillows under your shoulders to lift you up slightly.) Exhale and squeeze your glutes as you lift your hips off the mat and bring the dumbbells up and together with your palms facing each other.

Inhale diaphragmatically as you lower your arms and hips back to the starting position. Continue for 90 seconds. On your last rep, hold the lifted position with your glutes squeezing as much as possible before lowering back down.

Single Leg Kneeling Get Up (with Double Pulse at the Top)

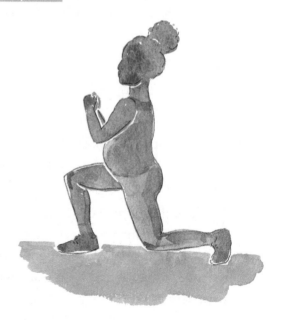

Duration: 2 minutes total

Directions: Begin in a kneeling position (with your backside lifted up off your heels). Exhale and step forward with right leg, driving through your heel to rise up into a low squat position. Do a double pulse (lifting and lowering your body by slightly straightening and bending your right knee, twice) before inhaling and lowering back down to kneeling position. Continue for 2 minutes.

Repeat this circuit on the left leg.

Stick With Your Breathing Exercises, Too

Aim for at least five minutes a day of diaphragmatic breathing (bonus points for extra minutes of the belly pump). Refer back to page 40 for detailed instructions.

from BROOKE Cates

"When you breathe slowly, deeply, and diaphragmatically, you create the space for your body to stimulate the parasympathetic nervous system, which sends calming, restoring, and de-stressing signals to every cell in your body. Even better, your baby experiences this same reaction.

"The more you practice these now, the easier it will be for you to use these breaths during labor, which will turn on your body's natural pain-relieving response system and help you stay calm through the intensity of birth. The breaths also allow your labor to progress without the presence of adrenaline, which is often present when women labor in a more amped-up, stressed-out sympathetic nervous system state and can slow your progression, because the body has to feel safe in order to give birth.

"Physically, your diaphragmatic breath also prepares the pelvic floor for the pushing phase with its ability to soften the muscles of the pelvic floor, perineum, and even the jaw. The more relaxed your mind and body are, the more likely you are able to surrender to the full experience while minimizing the core and pelvic floor injuries that can occur during birth.

"Next time you're feeling stressed or anxious, shift your breathing to slow, diaphragmatic breaths. Notice how quickly this shift helps you move out of stress and anxiety. Its power is GOLD!"

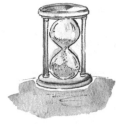

Countdown to Labor

Throughout this trimester, and especially in the two weeks leading up to your due date, make it your priority to do the following things to head into birth as strong and vital as possible.

Eat exquisitely. Minimize wheat, meat, dairy, and sugar in your diet; load up on high-fiber, colorful veggies, clean protein, healthy fats, and unrefined grains (such as brown rice and quinoa). You want to fuel up on nutritious foods—resist the urge to indulge in processed junk foods "because you can." You really can't afford to be feeling sluggish because you ate too much crappy food now, and you don't want to gain too much weight at this stage because your baby will gain it too, and then you'll have a large baby to birth.

Stay hydrated. Keep drinking water. Every day.

Stick with supplements. Don't neglect your vitamins; they're refilling the stores that the baby is taking, and that you'll need for breastfeeding.

Continue (or start) drinking red raspberry leaf tea or a tea blend designed specifically for pregnancy. It will help strengthen your uterus—and it's the muscles of the uterus contracting that squeezes the baby out. I drank it throughout my pregnancy.

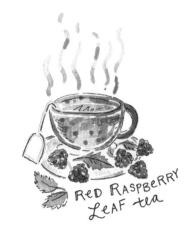

RED RASPBERRY LEAF tea

Keep working out. Not only will exercise help your strength and stamina, it will release endorphins, which are needed to create adequate contractions once labor starts. It will also help clear your mind of any worries about birth, becoming a mother, or anything else.

Start doing perineal massage. You can do it yourself, but it's hard to learn how to relax while your perineum is getting stretched, so I think it's better to have your partner do it. (See box at on page 234 for instructions.) The more familiar you can get with feeling a strong sensation and pressure in your perineum, and learn how to relax the muscle while feeling this pressure, the more comfortable you'll be during labor.

Have sex. Sex got you pregnant (unless you had IUI or IVF), and sex can help you come to the end of pregnancy (by giving birth), too. You'll learn in Chapter 18 all about how sex can help kickstart labor—in the meantime, just know it's relaxing. (And if this is your first child, these will be some of the last times you won't have to worry about your kids walking in on you!)

Practice your diaphragmatic breathing and belly pump breaths. They'll calm you and prepare your pelvic floor and core for birth.

Stop sitting with crossed legs. Keeping both feet on the floor while you sit will help ensure that your pelvis and low back don't get pulled out of alignment as the baby gets heavier and heavier.

Say your affirmations. They keep your mind in a positive place. Also spend time visualizing your birth going smoothly. (Read more on this in Chapter 15.)

Do fun things. Resist the urge to work like crazy either at your job or around the house (or both) before the baby comes; doing things you love will help you and the baby be in a good place before, during, and after birth. As Mari Mikel says, "Anything that makes you relax and have a good time will help you have an easier and happier childbirth."

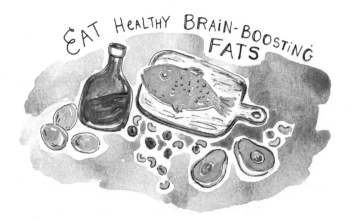

EAT HEALTHY BRAIN-BOOSTING FATS

Nutrition for Your Third Trimester

The third trimester may be the time to eat even more —anywhere from 300 to 500 extra calories per day, based on your particular needs. Some women gain weight very easily at this stage, and too much weight gain will make the baby bigger. So if that's you, you may not want to increase your overall caloric intake. Regardless of how many calories you're taking in, it's a good idea to bump up how frequently you eat so that the nutrients available to the baby remain high at all times; you want your baby to be as nourished and strong as they can be for birth.

This doesn't mean you should forget the healthy eating habits you've adopted in the first and second trimesters and just pig out on chips and other junk food, tempting though it may be. In fact, the science says that what you eat now, during these final three months, is extremely important and can affect your baby's health long after they're born.

The baby is growing up to a pound a week in the final weeks of pregnancy. You may feel ravenous because your body is fueling that growth. To get the calories you need without overdoing it, weight-wise, and without overtaxing your digestive system—which is really cramped and will have trouble accommodating large meals—it's best to graze on healthy foods (vegetables, salads, beans, clean animal protein, fruit, quinoa, etc.) pretty much all day. Save the mac and cheese with a side of bread for later.

In one animal study, researchers found that mice offspring born to mothers who ate a high-fat diet during the lactation phase (which is equivalent to the third trimester in human pregnancy) were more likely to be overweight throughout their lives than mice whose mothers consumed a normal, balanced diet during lactation. In addition to being prone to obesity, they were predisposed to impaired glucose function as well. Turns out, the fatty diet caused changes in the offsprings' brains, specifically in a region that regulates metabolism. Interestingly, those changes occurred even if the offspring were born to thin mothers who ate a high-fat diet. Meaning, nutrition really matters, regardless of weight.[22]

It makes sense: Your baby's brain is developing rapidly in the third trimester, which includes developing the neural connections that are associated with metabolism. That's why you want to be focused on eating more healthy fats, which provide brain-boosting nutrients and won't contribute to metabolic dysfunction; they also help your body prepare to breastfeed. In general, healthy fats come from whole foods (and not processed foods). Think nuts, seeds, fish, eggs, avocados, yogurt, and olive oil, as examples.

Some other eating principles you want to follow now are:

Double Down on DHA

I've already mentioned omega-3s in earlier pages, because adequate intake is important for your baby's growth at every stage. Omega-3 fatty acids aid in the development of their immune and nervous systems, their eyes, and, why it gets a big mention again here, their brain. Remember, their brain development is all systems go at this point. Now's a good time to focus on the omega-3 docosahexaenoic acid, or DHA, in particular. Foods high in DHA include:

- Salmon*
- Anchovies*
- Trout*
- Mackerel*
- DHA-fortified eggs
- Algae, like seaweed

*Note that, thankfully, these fish are all low-mercury options and thus safe to eat in moderation during pregnancy (refer back to page 196). While vegetarian foods like walnuts and flax seeds are high in omega-3s, they're rich in the omega-3 ALA. The body can convert ALA into DHA, although not very efficiently. So it's a good idea to up your intake of animal sources of this essential fatty acid now as well as vegetarian, plant-based sources.

Consuming enough DHA in your third trimester may also help prevent preeclampsia, a cause of early preterm birth. One analysis of two large randomized controlled trials found that getting 600-800 mg of DHA a day during pregnancy could reduce women's risk of preterm birth anywhere from 40 to 64%.[23] And, DHA may help lower your odds of developing symptoms of postpartum depression, too.

Eating eight ounces of DHA-rich fish a week would get you to these levels. If you're not a big fish fan, you might consider supplementation. Just know that not all prenatals contain DHA. If you take a specific omega-3 supplement, check to see that it provides both DHA and EPA.

Don't Count Out Calcium

I've shared that calcium is important in both your first and second trimesters, but it remains important in your third trimester, too, as well as during lactation (it fortifies your breast milk). Calcium is vital for bones, and your baby's skeleton is developing with superspeed now. You don't want them leaching calcium from your bones, so extra intake is crucial. Although, the body is, as I keep saying, magical: Knowing your baby needs more calcium, it amps up production of vitamin D now, which helps you better absorb calcium from your food. Calcium may also help prevent preeclampsia. If you're concerned you're not getting enough from your diet—it is predominantly found in dairy products, although greens are also good choices—talk with your healthcare practitioner about supplements. You just don't want to overdo it.

Keep Prioritizing Protein

Your baby is going through their last growth spurt now (at least, their final growth spurt in the womb). To help them pack on the pounds they need, protein is key. Protein also positively influences brain development at this stage. Indeed, protein is required for all aspects of prenatal development, and as I've stressed many times here already, their growth is on the fast track in these later months. Experts recommend around 75 to 100 grams of protein per day. The fish mentioned as being high in omega-3s are great sources of protein, as are poultry, lean meats, eggs, beans and legumes, nuts, and soy options like tofu. If you prefer vegetarian protein sources, just know that you'll need to eat more, quantity-wise, than you would animal sources to meet your increased requirements.

Fit in More Fiber

Things may feel a little out of whack in your tummy now, and you may experience the worst constipation yet of your pregnancy. Luckily, you can address constipation simply by eating more fiber. It helps bulk up your stool so it can pass through your digestive system—which, again, is operating under really cramped conditions at this point—much easier. What's more, fiber can help keep your blood pressure low, thus reducing your risk of preeclampsia, as well as regulate your blood sugar, helping to ward off gestational diabetes. Of course, the foods richest in fiber also contain a bevy of other important vitamins and minerals to be eating now. Plus, they're good sources of carbohydrates that will keep you energized at a time when you might be feeling sluggish and fatigued. Try enjoying more fruits, vegetables, whole grains, and legumes. Some of the best fiber-rich choices in these categories are:

- Acorn squash
- Sweet potatoes
- Green peas
- Kidney beans
- Lentils

- Quinoa
- Avocados
- Dried figs
- Raspberries
- Pearled barley

Consider adding more kale to your plate this trimester. It's rich in all the nutrients your baby is storing up now before birth—nutrients they'll use in the first few months of their life. Not to mention, greens are a great way to round out a meal of omega-3- and protein-packed fish plus fiber-rich beans and grains. It's a third-trimester recipe for a healthy you and a healthy baby.

Kale and Strawberry Salad | Serves 1

This salad is a great way to get your greens. The tang of the lemon and the sweetness of the agave are an exciting flavor combination for your taste buds, and the strawberries, almonds, and coconut add fiber, protein, and healthy fats, making it a healthy (and filling) meal.

For the salad:

1 cup organic strawberries, sliced

3 cups kale, chopped

½ cup slivered almonds, toasted

¼ cup coconut flakes

For the dressing:

¼ cup plus ½ teaspoon canola oil, divided

½ to 1 tablespoon agave nectar

2-3 tablespoons lemon juice, to taste

Salt, to taste

Pepper, to taste

In a medium salad bowl, add ½ teaspoon canola oil to chopped kale and gently massage with your hands until kale softens. Add strawberries, almonds, and coconut flakes.

In a glass jar, stir together agave nectar and two tablespoons lemon juice. Add a few drops of canola oil at first and completely stir in before adding the rest of the canola oil a bit at a time, mixing each batch in completely before adding more. Taste the dressing and adjust the amounts of agave, lemon juice, salt, and pepper little by little until you love it. Then add to the salad bowl and toss salad before serving.

Should I Be Supplementing with Iron?

Iron remains an important nutrient throughout your pregnancy. I haven't mentioned iron supplementation yet, though, because it's generally not considered a wise choice in early trimesters (refer back to pages 192 and 193 for good dietary sources and cooking tips to increase iron). But it could be right for you during your third trimester, because levels decrease toward the end of your pregnancy. And, because your baby is pulling the vitamins and minerals they need from the foods you eat now, and from your body, in order to create the nutrient stores that will fuel them after they're born.

Your care provider will likely test you for anemia in your third trimester and can thus advise if supplementation is needed, as well as the best way to take supplemental iron for absorption and to avoid unwanted side effects.

Getting Extra Sleep

Sleep is just as important as exercise when it comes to preparing for labor, birth, and early parenthood, so make it your goal to get as much shuteye as possible in the last weeks and days before birth. Naps are great; if you can't fully fall asleep, just allow yourself to rest and relax.

In fact, sleep can actually impact your labor and delivery. Lack of sleep has been linked to preeclampsia and preterm births. And studies show that women who get less than six hours of sleep nightly are more likely to have Cesarean births and experience longer labor than women who get seven hours or more. So, again, it's important to rest up. Not to mention, you'll just feel like doing so: Any energy that returned in your second trimester is likely waning now and you're back to feeling fatigued.

Unfortunately, it may be harder to get quality sleep in your third trimester.

Here are some helpful tips...

Try eating smaller, more frequent meals to help with digestion and heartburn, which can keep you tossing and turning at night. Also avoid spicy and rich, fatty foods like fried foods, especially later in the evening. You may also want to have a snack right at bedtime or even wake up to have a snack in the middle of the night: The baby can't go for long periods without eating and will give off hunger signals, whether movement or hormonal changes, that will wake you up in an attempt to get you to take in more calories.

Just make sure the snack isn't something sweet, but rather something savory and nourishing, like leftovers from dinner or a bowl of really hearty soup or a half a sandwich. I know this may sound like a crazy idea, to willingly sacrifice sleep, but if you have the food ready to go before you get in bed and just have to wake up and eat it without having to think about or prepare it, you won't wake all the way up and will be able to fall back asleep—and sleep well—once you go back to bed. The routine will also prepare you for having to get up in the middle of the night to feed your baby after they're born.

Drink fewer fluids at night. Cut back on the amount of liquid you drink leading up to bedtime, so you don't have to wake up and get up to go. This means you need to drink more water earlier in the day, because you still need plenty of fluids to stay adequately hydrated.

Find a comfortable position:

- The best position is on your left side, which might help improve blood flow and the flow of nutrients to your baby, as well as improve blood flow to your kidneys, uterus, and heart.

- You can try using pillows between your knees and a wedge under your belly for support and increased comfort.

- Stay off your back, especially during this trimester. Because your uterus is so heavy now, in this position it can press on nerves in your spine and the inferior vena cava, which is a major vein that carries blood from your heart to your lower body. You don't want to cut off blood flow to you and your baby!

Pick your pajamas wisely. Get comfy options, and avoid tight waistbands.

Start Thinking About Your Exit Strategy

I know that if you work the temptation is to work as much as you can right up until the baby is born, so that you can enjoy more downtime once the baby is here. But think about how much more ready for and relaxed about birth you'll be if you give yourself a buffer of one or two weeks. If you can at all swing it, I really, really, REALLY want you to think about how you can slow down on the "get stuff done" front at this time. Mari Mikel shares that in her practice, she notices that a large percentage of women who have complications are the ones who worked up until the bitter end. Being stressed, tired, and frazzled is not a great way to head into one of the most physically challenging events of your life! (Refer to page 269 for more of Mari Mikel's thoughts on the subject.)

How to Do Perineal Massage

Your perineum is the area of your genitals between the vagina and the anus. And it is the part of your body that can get stretched to the point of tearing during birth. I know that sounds like a very scary thing, but the good news is that you can help this area become more relaxed, more elastic, and less prone to tearing by massaging it—ideally daily—in these last weeks of your pregnancy. Think of it as birth canal widening. Studies show that it works: A 2013 review found that women who practiced perineal massage for their first vaginal birth were significantly less likely to get an episiotomy and less likely to experience pelvic floor pain three months postpartum.[24]

Starting about six weeks out from your due date, with the okay of your health care provider, have your partner do the following routine as close to daily as possible. If you don't have a partner, you can do it yourself; you may not be used to being this hands-on with your body, but you can do it. You do want to make sure your hands, or the hands of whomever is doing the massage for you, are clean because you don't want to introduce bacteria or viruses to this area, particularly at this point in your pregnancy.

Perineal Massage Steps:

1. Lie on the bed propped up on pillows with your knees bent and feet on the bed.

2. Have your partner lube up their index fingers with almond, jojoba, or vitamin E oil; if you're performing this on yourself, use your thumbs. Wearing gloves can make things slippier, which is good—you want to apply pressure, but not friction.

3. First, have your partner insert one finger about an inch or inch and a half into the vagina, then press gently down toward your rectum until you feel the tissues relax (your partner should be able to provide you feedback about that).

4. Once you've relaxed after this first step, they can insert the other index finger and again apply pressure downward until you feel a change in the tension of the muscles and tissues. If it's ever painful, stop.

Then your partner should repeat, applying gentle downward pressure and holding for a few moments to different spots along the bottom half of the vaginal opening.

In addition to prepping the tissues of the area for delivery, perineal massage also helps relax the muscles of the pelvic floor, which, paradoxically, strengthens them—because tight muscles are weak. What's more, your mind will appreciate knowing that your body is well-prepped for birth.

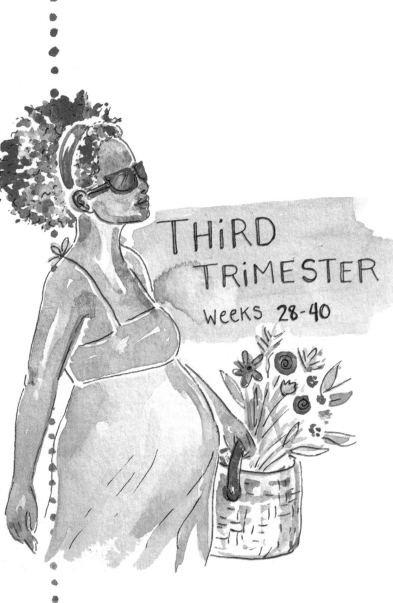

THIRD TRIMESTER
weeks 28-40

What's happening now: Third Trimester (Weeks 28-40)

As your due date nears, you may begin to feel a bit more uncomfortable. After all, your body is doing a lot, making its final preparations for labor and delivery. And, your baby is continuing to grow and mature, doing their own getting ready for the big day.

Around week 34, most babies—except those who stubbornly stay breech—start to move themselves into a head-down position and settle there until it's time to greet the world. Interestingly, when their head engages into your pelvic area, it's called lightening.

With Baby

This final trimester is primarily about growth. Your baby keeps packing on the pounds; they will typically weigh between six and nine pounds by your due date.

- **Fattening up.** One reason your baby gains weight now is that they're accumulating more fat, which is a good thing, as it helps keep them nice and warm now and once they're outside your body. That means there's no more need for lanugo, which almost completely disappears before delivery. It also means their skin is no longer translucent and is instead opaque.

- **Finishing touch.** Your baby's touch receptors fully develop in this trimester, meaning they now experience all five senses. They're really opening their eyes now, too, and even blinking.

- **Boning up.** Adequate calcium intake becomes especially important now (see page 228) because your baby's cartilage hardens into bone at this stage, all except for the skull, which remains soft and pliable so it can pass through the birth canal more easily.

- **A little brainiac.** Your baby's brain began its most important phase of growth back around month five, and things really kick into high gear now—by the time they're born, they'll have around 100 billion brain cells. The brain is now beginning to regulate your baby's body temperature, and is even causing them to dream.

- **Take a breath.** Your baby's lungs are continuing to develop into the third trimester, only fully maturing between weeks 38 and 40, or basically all the way through delivery. At this point, your baby is able to practice breathing through rhythmic breathing movements; they breathe six to nine times per minute throughout the day.

With You

You're very obviously pregnant now and, as a result, perhaps a bit clumsier. Many of the same symptoms from your first and second trimesters—particularly leg cramps, swelling, skin changes, varicose veins, heartburn, back aches, and the frequent need to urinate—may continue. While some women don't experience increased discomfort, many do, including:

- **Tiny contractions.** You may begin experiencing practice contractions now, as your uterus builds the might it will need to get the baby out. (Some women have these contractions earlier, in their second trimester.) They're irregular, infrequent mild contractions in your abdomen, which often occur after physical activity (that includes sex) and can also occur as a result of dehydration. They may become stronger as your due date inches closer. It's your body's way of preparing for labor; however, because they go away and don't intensify, these contractions aren't the same as true labor contractions. They should be mostly just uncomfortable and not painful. To relieve the discomfort, try drinking water or some herbal tea, or changing positions.

- **Ready for feeding.** It's normal for your breasts to begin to leak colostrum, the earliest form of breast milk; they're just getting ready for the important job of feeding your newborn. It's a good idea to start toughening up your nipples by spending more time braless and using a washcloth on them in the shower so that they get used to contact.

- **Possible secretions.** You may notice mucousy vaginal discharge toward the end of your pregnancy; it may even have a little blood in it (if it does, it's very likely normal, but tell your care provider anyway). Also notify your provider if there is an excessive amount of discharge or blood, if you suspect that your amniotic fluid is leaking, or if the discharge is a color other than white or clear and has any kind of unpleasant odor.

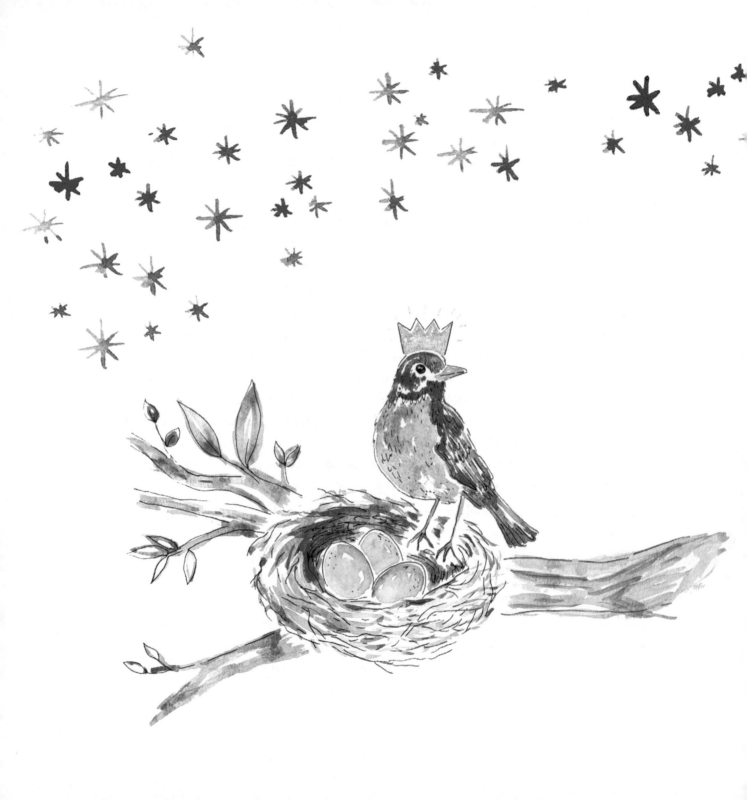

Chapter 15

THINK LIKE A MOTHER

As important as it is to take care of your body in preparation for birth, it's every bit as vital that you tend to your mind, emotions, and spirit now, too. You are a whole person and you'll want your whole self feeling its best as you head into birth and the transition to motherhood.

In this chapter, we'll talk about how to address your fears so that you can get your mind and spirit in a good place, and how to use that clarity to start making decisions on behalf of your baby—beginning with the various newborn tests and procedures that are typically done very soon after birth. You really want to think these through ahead of time, because after the birth you'll a) be tired and b) want to use all your available energy on bonding with your baby and recuperating.

Name and Research Your Fears

If worry and anxiety about childbirth is creeping in as your due date gets closer, know that it's totally normal. If you're a first-time mom, it's especially normal. After all, the labor and delivery experience is a total unknown to you, and there's so much to think about, so many things that could go differently than you've planned and than you desire. I know for me, deep down, I wasn't entirely sure that the process would actually result in a baby, or that the baby would truly be able to come out through my vagina. It's hard to imagine something as miraculous as birth happening via your own body. (I hope that reading this book is helping to convince you of just how powerful you—and your body—are.)

Even if you've already given birth, fear can still set in. Maybe things didn't happen the way you wished they had the last time around. Or maybe it's not the birth itself that's got you nervous, but rather it's all the ways your life is going to change once you have another child. Or something else entirely.

Whatever is making you nervous, it's OK. You are entitled to your feelings. Just remember that feelings aren't always based on facts. They will pass. But you do want to give yourself the space to feel and process them now, before it's time to deliver your baby. Fear and anxiety can cause you to resist the changes in your body, your mind, and your life that giving birth requires, and that resistance can make labor and delivery more difficult and uncomfortable.

So how can you move through and get past your fear? One potent way—and the one that calmed me down when I was pregnant—is to name your fears and do your research.

You're already reading this book, so you're already educating yourself about all things labor and delivery. You've thought through or are thinking through a birth plan, and you've likely attended a childbirth education class, which are great steps. The more you know about what will and can happen with your body and your baby, the less there is to be afraid of.

When I was pregnant, I found it very helpful to ask my friends, family members, and doula about their children's births. I asked them how long their labors took, if there were any complications, what they felt like physically and mentally during the process, and so many more questions.

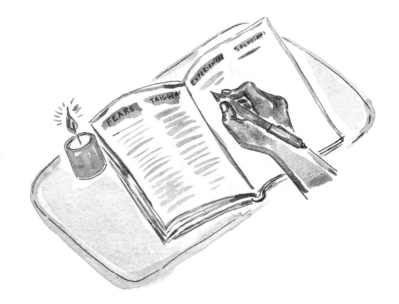

Of course, to research your fears, you have to know them. That means you have to look for them—you can't just ignore them and hope for the best. Dig deep and identify what you're most worried about. Journal about them or challenge yourself to make a list of them, and see what comes up. Maybe you're most worried about pain, or getting to the hospital on time, or specific interventions, or having a Cesarean. Once you know what is triggering for you, you can pay careful attention to that information shared here and do additional research beyond these pages. Knowledge really is power.

Addressing the Subconscious

Often a big piece of what's behind fears about birth is a subconscious response to things you've experienced in the past. Pregnancy can actually be a very healing time, because it brings you face to face with some of your deepest held beliefs about life, which can trigger big emotions, maybe even past traumas. That may sound like a bad thing, but it's actually a great opportunity, because you can only heal and release what you are aware of. It's when you're unaware of the fears and thoughts that are in your subconscious that you get mad, sad, or irritated on a daily basis without understanding why. I hope you can take some time now to process anything that might be coming up for you, whether in your journal, with a friend or partner you absolutely trust to help you see the big picture, or with a therapist.

You have a powerful opening now for healing anything that may be lingering in your subconscious. Your baby's birth is one of the most important events of your life, and the story of bringing your baby into the world will be with you forever. You want to go into it as emotionally healthy as you can. Don't try to stuff those intense feelings down; they're coming up because they're ready to be seen, healed, and released. Addressing them, and taking great care of your emotional health, now will only help you go into birth more attuned to your needs and your strengths. It will help you write a better birth story and be a better mother.

Something I encountered when I was pregnant was a subconscious fear of "messing my kids up" once they were born. I became uber-aware of the parenting I received as a child, remembering situations that had occurred and getting upset about them. I am lucky that my mom and I are close and I could talk to her about these things. (Thanks, Mom, for being receptive and open with me.) With many fears, I felt better as soon as I gave voice to them. I also went to therapy after I had my son, so that I could learn more about who I am and become better equipped to not repeat negative past patterns. I loved the experience and found it super helpful. If some part of you is thinking that maybe talking with a therapist is a good idea, I encourage you to do so.

AFFIRMATIONS to PREPARE YOU FOR BIRTH

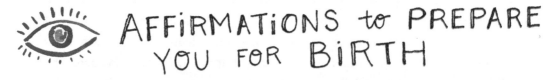

I BELIEVE IN MYSELF, and I HAVE NOTHING to FEAR.

THE UNIVERSE LOVES ME and SUPPORTS MY BABY and ME.

I AM WILLING and OPEN TO MY SENSUAL BIRTH EXPERIENCE.

MY BODY WAS MADE FOR THIS.   I LISTEN to MY BODY.

I AM CALM and RELAXED.

MY BABY and I ARE RESTED and READY for THE WORK WE WILL DO.

Remember, Birth Is Part of Nature

While fear is natural, and even to be expected to some extent, I found it comforting to remind myself that childbirth is completely natural, too. One thing that comforted me was remembering that birth has been happening since humans first existed. Think about it: Generations and generations of women before you have gotten through it, and you can (and will!) as well.

Giving birth is as much a part of nature as high tide, sunsets, and rainstorms. Accepting that birth is part of nature's regular programming helps you surrender to it. And when you stop resisting the sensations that accompany birth, the tension they cause recedes, and that helps lessen your discomfort and pain. I'm not saying it goes totally away, but if you're panicked and bracing yourself through every contraction, that is going to make the whole experience more taxing and your perception of the pain more acute. Resisting them only saps your energy, while accepting it invites you to be present for one of the most miraculous experiences of your life.

Making Decisions on Behalf of Your Baby

I've already walked you through many of the seemingly countless decisions there are to make regarding early trimester screenings and diagnostics, as well as about the specifics of your labor and delivery. While these are certainly not easy conclusions to come to, many moms-to-be find them slightly simpler than the choices that have to do with their baby after birth. After all, the consequences of your actions are more "real" then: You can see and hear if your little one is upset over a test you opted to do, for example. If they're screaming and crying, you may begin to second-guess your judgment, and the mommy guilt can set in real quick. That's why it's a good idea to fully think over these decisions now, and prepare yourself for what can happen whichever route you settle on.

The Circumcision Conundrum

To circumcise or not to circumcise: If you're having a boy, it's one of the biggest questions you'll face. First off, it's important to know that circumcision is an entirely elective procedure. It is not required by any laws or hospital policies. And while it has long been the norm in this country—as well as in Canada and the Middle East—the tide may be shifting here. In fact, in 2013, the US Centers for Disease Control and Prevention (CDC) reported a drop in male circumcision rates for the first time: from 64.5% in 1979 to 58.3% in 2010.[25] It's likely rates have further decreased, as some health organizations are clarifying their positions on the practice and news outlets are increasingly reporting that the arguments for its health benefits may not hold up too well after all this time. That said, religious beliefs around it remain, of course, as do various other cultural and social considerations. The practice is not nearly as common in other countries throughout Europe, Central America, South America, and Asia.

Currently, the American Academy of Pediatrics (AAP) states that while the health benefits of newborn male circumcision outweigh the risks of the procedure, those benefits are not great enough to warrant a position that all newborn boys undergo it—just to recommend that it should be made available to parents making decisions on behalf of their baby and older children that want it done. The American College of Obstetricians and Gynecologists supports the AAP's position. The CDC also agrees with the AAP policy, but clearly affirms circumcision as an "important health measure."[26]

The benefits of circumcision these organizations cite include:

- Prevention of urinary tract infections in the first year of life

- Almost complete elimination of the risk of penile cancer in adult men

- Reduction in the risk of contracting some sexually transmitted diseases, including genital herpes, HIV, and HPV

There are some caveats to these potential benefits. Rates of UTI infection in male infants are low, and typically, UTIs are easily treated. Rates of penile cancer are also very low; in fact, it's one of the rarest forms. Studies from Africa do indicate that circumcision may help prevent men from contracting HIV through heterosexual sex—at least there, where the rate of infection is high; although, there aren't studies indicating it can do the same in this country. Some experts state that the studies suggesting lowered risk of contracting other sexually transmitted diseases may not be entirely statistically significant.

Potential risks:

Although health experts state that the risks are minimal, circumcision is a surgical operation and can present complications, some more common than others, including:

- Infection
- Bleeding
- Pain
- Removal of too much of the foreskin, which could cause pain with erection as an adult
- Meatitis and meatal stenosis, infections that affect urination

Some opponents of the practice believe that circumcision leads to reduced penile sensitivity, and thus sexual satisfaction, later in life. The likelihood of complications can be reduced if the circumcision is performed in a medical setting, and pain-relief methods can be implemented. Opponents also note that the foreskin serves other functions outside of satisfaction, including protecting the head of the penis, and should be left to do its job as nature intended.

Those against circumcision feel it really is an ethical, more than medical, dilemma. Your baby can't choose the procedure; you must choose to have a piece of their body removed for them. Some organizations feel making this choice is a violation against your newborn's basic human rights.

Ultimately, the choice is up to you and your partner. I encourage you to do your own research and decide what feels right for you and your family.

I've been completely open and honest with you throughout the book, and I won't stop now. While my husband and I opted to circumcise both of our sons, that decision is one of my biggest regrets.

With our first son, Hendrix, I went back and forth on the decision but ultimately chose to do it because it was the norm and I didn't want him to feel "different than." It was something I felt great about, but the process wasn't straightforward so I didn't have any occasion to seriously second-guess the choice. When I gave birth to our second child, Legend, also a son, we decided to go ahead, since our first son was circumcised. But when the rubber band that doctors typically use to keep the wound closed popped off, he ended up having to get stitches around his penis. The healing process was awful. It oozed blood for days. I felt incredible guilt for causing him that much pain over something elective. Whether he remembers it or not, I do, and it's an awful feeling. If I had it to do over, I would 100 percent choose not to circumcise, and just teach my boys good hygiene.

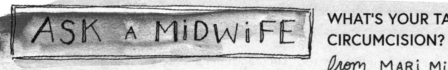

ASK A MIDWIFE

WHAT'S YOUR TAKE ON CIRCUMCISION?

from MARI MIKEL:

"I'll be very upfront about it: I am not a fan of circumcision. If it's part of your religion, or even if it's not but you feel very strongly that it is the right choice for your baby, I don't judge. But I think that we don't consider how painful it is to the baby and how much it impacts their sexual reality for the rest of their lives. The head of the penis is exquisitely sensitive, and without the foreskin to protect it, a lot of that sensitivity fades. Also, while some babies aren't all that bothered by the procedure, many babies scream bloody murder during it, and there's no way to tell what reaction your baby will have beforehand. It's a decision that is utterly permanent and that your baby has no say in. Really do some hard thinking about this one, and if you do choose to circumcise, have a stronger reason than, 'It's what everyone else does.' Your baby may grow up to be a man who will want to know why you made the choice that you did."

Other Newborn Procedures and Tests: Your Options

I mentioned lots of tests and screenings to consider back in Chapter 8. Well, there's more. Again, it pays to research your options and make choices now about those you want and don't want—or to simply familiarize yourself with what will happen if you opt for them all. Once your baby has arrived, you'll be exhausted and also elated holding your little one. You won't want to be surprised and worried by what's happening. And it won't be the time to make decisions, especially for those procedures or medication administrations that need to happen immediately after birth.

Screenings

There are several newborn screens that will be performed shortly after birth. There are national recommendations for these screenings, but states can decide individually which tests to include as part of the screening profile they offer. Though some of these screenings are considered required by law, you may be able to refuse them. But you likely won't want to. They test for genetic disorders, along with heart defects and hearing loss. And they're noninvasive or minimally invasive, without risk of negative side effects.

The Newborn Screen

This screening simply involves gathering a tiny bit of your baby's blood (through a prick on their heel) and sending it to the lab to check for genetic disorders, chiefly metabolic genetic disorders. There are no medications or shots involved. Conditions assessed by the test include phenylketonuria (PKU), cystic fibrosis, sickle cell disease, congenital hypothyroidism, and numerous others. It's important to repeat genetic screenings once your baby is born, because these disorders can be more easily detected at birth; most aren't detectable at all until this time.

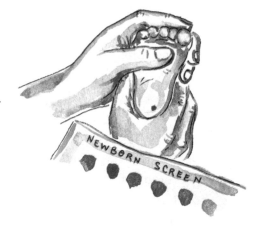

And although these disorders can be serious, many can be treated if and when they're discovered early—but you have to do the screenings in order to detect them. The heel prick usually happens within your baby's first 24 to 48 hours of life, typically in the hospital although it can occur at a doctor's office; there may be a follow-up blood test conducted by their pediatrician when they are just a week or so old. The test can be performed even if you don't give birth in a hospital: Your doula or midwife can easily collect a blood sample. Your baby may cry and experience some discomfort, but the procedure is very minimally invasive and safe.

Critical Congenital Heart Disease (CCHD) Screening

CCHD is a group of serious heart disorders present at birth that prevent the heart from pumping blood—and oxygen—to the lungs and throughout the rest of the body. About 200 out of every 10,000 babies have CCHD.[27] There are lots of different types of CCHD, but they can all cause major health problems and need treatment early on, whether surgery or medications, so screening is important. Like the heel prick, this screen is performed between 24 and 48 hours of age. Using a pulse oximeter, a health care practitioner will measure the amount of oxygen in your baby's blood. If it sounds like a scary machine, it's not: The provider simply places a small, soft sensor on your baby's skin (on their hand or foot), and the device measures oxygen levels. Low oxygen indicates a higher risk of CCHD, and a need for additional testing. This screen is entirely noninvasive and totally risk-free.

Hearing Testing

Before your baby heads home from the hospital or birthing center, they can—and I believe should—have their hearing tested. Hearing loss is relatively common: Roughly two or three out of every 1,000 children in this country are born with some amount of hearing loss, in either one or both of their ears.[28] The screening is painless; your newborn may even sleep during it. The screen can actually be one or two tests:

- The otoacoustic emissions test uses a soft earphone and microphone that are placed into your baby's ear canal to see if the ear responds to sound waves. The tiny earphone plays sounds and looks for an "echo" response in the microphone to those sounds. This response occurs when hearing is normal; no echo may mean there's an issue.

- The auditory brainstem response test may provide the most reliable information about your newborn's hearing. It also uses earphones, which play clicks and tones. This time, though, electrodes on their head measure the brain's response to those sounds. The electrodes have a sticker backing and go on and come off easily.

Newborn Shots and Medications

There are a small handful of medications and shots that babies are typically given in a hospital setting as a standard procedure, including:

Hepatitis B Vaccine

This is the first vaccine your baby will be offered. The first dose is typically administered within 24 hours after birth; it is a multidose vaccine, with additional doses between one and two months and again between six and 18 months. It serves to protect against infection with the hepatitis B virus, which affects the liver and can ultimately lead to liver damage and failure, liver cancer, and even death. But it is not without controversy.

First of all, hepatitis B is typically contracted later in life—it is transmitted orally, although it can be passed from mothers to their children during childbirth and by other contact between a newborn and an infected person's bodily fluids. Proponents argue that while expecting moms can be—and routinely are—tested during pregnancy for the virus, they could also in theory still contract it after a negative test (or the test could have been inaccurate) and pass it along to their child, so better safe than sorry. Opponents argue that rates of transmission to newborns are low, and that the vaccine may not actually offer lifetime protection. And, they feel there are risks associated with the vaccine that shouldn't be ignored, citing instances of minor adverse reactions like headaches as well as the development of very serious disorders such as multiple sclerosis. The CDC stands behind it as a safe and necessary preventive measure that can prevent mother-to-baby infection and offer full long-term immunity, as does the AAP.

I opted to wait until each of my babies were a month old before getting them vaccinated, as I believe that a newborn baby's immune system is still developing and introducing a vaccine at that vulnerable point adds an unnecessary challenge, particularly for an infection that newborns have such a low risk of exposure to. For these reasons, Mari Mikel encourages all of her clients who are fully breastfeeding their babies to wait until two months before introducing any vaccines, as breastfeeding provides babies a natural immunity up until six months, at which point it is gone.

> "MARI MIKEL ENCOURAGES ALL OF her CLIENTS WHO ARE FULLY BREASTFEEDING their BABIES to WAIT UNTIL TWO MONTHS BEFORE INTRODUCING ANY VACCINES."

Vitamin K Shot

Vitamin K helps blood clot and therefore stops bleeding. Babies are born with very low levels of this vitamin and thus are at risk for severe, potentially life-threatening bleeding called vitamin K deficiency bleeding, or VKDB. This risk remains up until six months. A shot of vitamin K given at birth can eliminate this risk. Proponents argue that the shot is safe and is the very best way to prevent VKDB. Opponents worry it's too large of a dose of the vitamin for a baby's body and feel that it, like the hepatitis B vaccine, carries risks of unwanted side effects. Although an early study did suggest an association with cancer, it was just an association, and it has since been refuted. Some opponents are concerned about the preservative benzyl alcohol in the shot; the medical community stresses the amount in the vitamin K shot is too small to pose a danger. Proponents also counter that a large dose is necessary, since vitamin K does not cross the placenta and is present only in very low levels in breast milk.

The AAP has recommended the vitamin K shot be administered to newborns shortly after birth since 1961, never wavering on their position throughout the decades.

Antibiotic Eye Ointment

Although you can decline this intervention, most states mandate it very soon after your baby is born. Antibiotic eye ointment or drops, typically containing the medication erythromycin, are used to protect babies from bacterial infections in the eye that can be acquired during birth, chiefly from sexually transmitted diseases like gonorrhea, although it may also protect against other infections by bacteria naturally present in everyone's genital area. (They can occur in babies delivered via Cesarean as well.) These infections can cause blindness and can be easily prevented with antibiotic treatment.

Many moms argue the treatment is unnecessary, as they know their sexual health status. But again, an infection can occur from other "healthy" bacteria as well. The ointment might make your baby's eyes look cloudy, and even a little red and swollen, although anything other than cloudiness is rare. These effects are short-term. The AAP, CDC, and other organizations stand by the recommendation. Some opponents believe it can make your newborn's vision blurry and contribute to difficulty breastfeeding. You can choose to delay the application for a few hours, until you and your baby have had a chance to bond and your baby has latched onto your breast and breastfed successfully for the first time. (This is what I did.)

I encourage you to do more of your own research and talk with your health care practitioners about these newborn shots and medications. This isn't an exhaustive list of all the interventions that may be performed shortly after your baby is born.

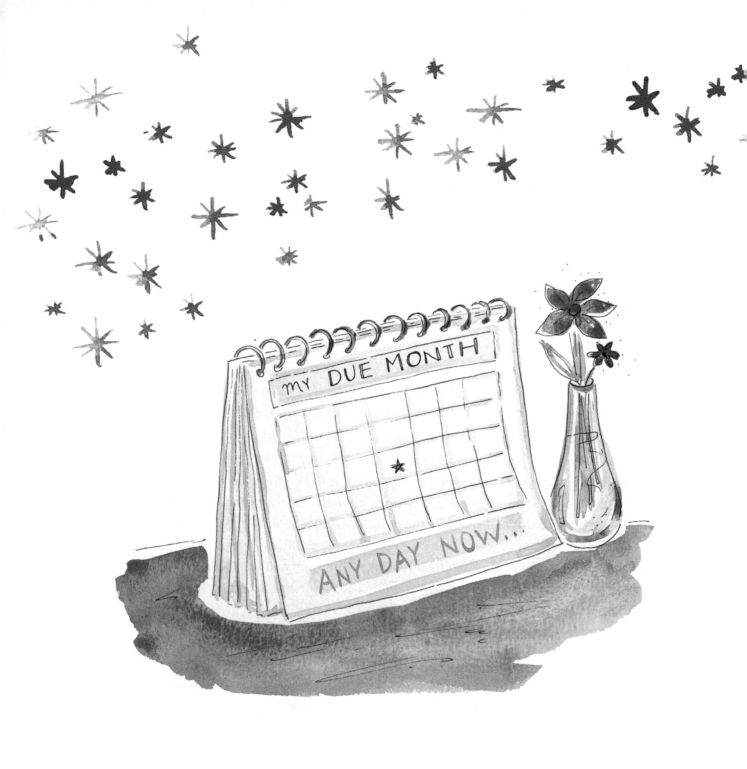

Chapter 16

YOUR DUE DATE IS NOT YOUR EXPIRATION DATE

Right about now, you are probably experiencing people—whether they're friends, family, co-workers, or strangers on the street—looking at your belly and then asking, "When is the baby due?" We place a lot of emphasis on this date, but the truth is, it is just a guess. As the title of this chapter says, it is not your expiration date. Your baby is not a container of milk that will go bad after the date stamped on the carton. In fact, it can be completely normal for you to remain pregnant up to two weeks beyond your due date (and for you to deliver several weeks before it as well). Did you hear me? Entirely normal and a-OK!

The trick, then, is to remind yourself of this—daily, if needed—and to stay rooted in your confidence that the baby will come at the exact right time. Even many Ob/Gyns will get focused on this date and start suggesting that you schedule either a Cesarean or an induction before it even arrives. But when you give birth shouldn't be dictated by the calendar. Your body and your baby should call the shots.

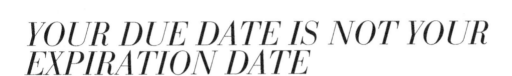

> IN FACT, iT CAN BE COMPLETELY NORMAL for YOU to REMAIN PREGNANT UP to TWO WEEKS BEYOND YOUR DUE DATE (AND for YOU TO DELIVER SEVERAL WEEKS BEFORE iT AS WELL).

There's still so much development happening with your baby—every day they're in the womb makes a difference in the development in their gut, organs, lungs, and brain.

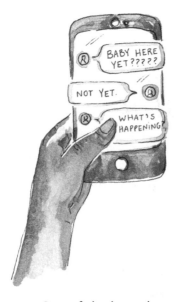

The more developed their gut is, the better they'll be able to absorb the nutrients they need to grow once they're out, and the less likely they'll be colicky. The more developed their liver is, the less likely they'll be to get a little jaundiced once they're born. And the more their brain is developed, the better they'll be able to bond with you and establish breastfeeding.

So long as you are eating healthy foods, staying hydrated, getting exercise, and aren't crazy stressed, your baby is probably best served by being inside a little while longer. Both my children were born in the 42nd week. I know firsthand how hard it can feel to wait, but you can count on your body to do a good job.

One of the best things you can do to manage other people's expectations is to hold back on sharing your due date. Instead, tell them the baby could come anytime between 39 and 42 weeks. You can figure out the dates that correspond with these ranges based on your due date, which is 40 weeks, but you really do want to refrain from telling them what that actual due date is. People can get really focused on that date and start texting you and asking you if the baby has come yet. And then you have to not only tell those folks that the baby's not here yet, but you also have to reassure yourself that everything's happening exactly as it should. Staying focused on a three-week window instead of on a specific date is easier on everyone—most of all, you.

If you have gone past your so-called due date without going into labor, your labor is not "late." Your body is not betraying you, even though I know it may feel that way. In fact, it's just working that magic I've been talking and talking about all this time. Your baby has a say in the whole thing, too. And if they aren't ready, well, they aren't ready! When they are ready, their body will let your body know.

In fact, researchers think that labor begins when your baby releases cortisol and your production of estrogen increases.[29] They also speculate that it's your baby who gives labor the green light by releasing a protein that acts like a hormone and cues the hormone symphony to sound its first note.[30]

To reiterate, the takeaway here is that your labor will start when you (and your body) and your baby are ready. It's a magical thing to let happen on its own and, according to health experts, the best way to know that everyone really is ready for birth and the best way to ensure everyone has a healthy labor and delivery.

> "STAYING FOCUSED on A THREE-WEEK WINDOW INSTEAD OF ON A SPECIFIC DATE IS EASIER on EVERYONE - MOST of ALL, YOU."

What to Do If You Go Past Your Due Date

You may have heard that it's inadvisable or even dangerous to go too far past your due date because your baby could get too large, but I'm here to tell you that's not really a concern. In fact, several studies have shown that inducing because a baby is suspected to be large increases chances of Cesarean and doesn't actually lead to any improved health outcomes for the baby either.[31] What's more, it's difficult to know if your baby is in fact larger than average, and mothers who are told their baby is—to use the fancy medical jargon—*macrosomic* may actually be carrying a totally normal-weight child. The truth is, ultrasounds and even hands-on examinations are often off base.

That said, there are medical reasons why health care professionals may need to intervene if your little one just doesn't seem to want to come out. One way doctors can tell if labor intervention is necessary is by performing what is called a nonstress test. It may be a little stressful for you, since you of course want to know if everything is okay and if anything is wrong. But it won't cause your baby any stress at all, thus the name.

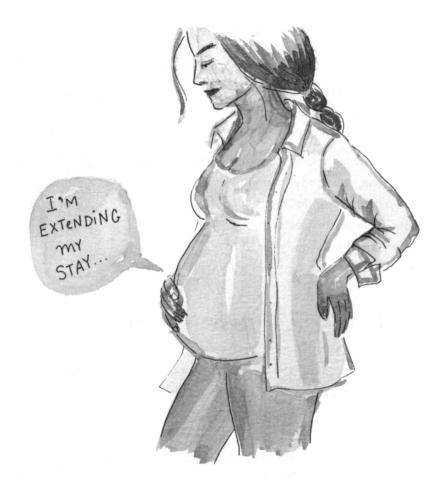

It measures their heart rate and how they respond to movement, and can tell your health care provider if your baby is getting adequate oxygen inside your womb. It's performed while you're lying down comfortably. You'll have two straps or belts around your belly that act as monitors and measure your baby's heartbeat and any contractions you may be having. When you feel your little one move, you'll likely be asked to press a button, although not all monitors are the same. The test typically lasts around 20 or 30 minutes.

If your baby's heart rate is normal and they're moving around a lot, they'll be classified as "reactive." That means they're healthy and fine where they are. If things are off with their heart rate or they're not moving around as much as they should, they'll be classified as "nonreactive." That doesn't necessarily mean they're in any

> "ONE INTERVENTION MAY MEAN YOU END UP NEEDING ANOTHER and ANOTHER, and THEY AREN'T WITHOUT SIDE EFFECTS and SOMETIMES UNDESIRABLE CONSEQUENCES."

serious danger (they could just be snoozing). But, it could mean they aren't getting ample oxygen, and it will usually mean the nonstress test may need to go a little bit longer while care providers try to get your baby to move (by giving you foods or sugary drinks or playing sounds by your belly, for example). You may also need more testing to determine if it really is time to induce or deliver through a Cesarean.

There are other reasons you may need a nonstress test, or repeat nonstress tests, such as if you have a high-risk pregnancy. Testing will still start later in your pregnancy though, after 28 weeks, as it isn't accurate before that time. Once you hit the 40- or 41-week mark, your health care provider may want to do a nonstress test more than once.

The Truth About Hospital Interventions

I shared a little bit of information on some of the following interventions in Chapter 8, when we talked about writing your birth plan. But now's a good opportunity to devote some time to thinking through whether you want a few, all, or none of the barrage of interventions you'll be offered by medical staff if you give birth in a hospital. (Note that some may be offered at birthing centers, although all centers may not provide them; typically, midwives do not provide them at home births.)

Even if you're planning a home birth, you still want to research these interventions and decide how you want to handle them in the event that you end up transferring to the hospital for a medical reason.

These interventions are often thought of as standard or routine in a hospital setting, but that doesn't mean you have to agree to them. After all, while they can be helpful or even necessary in some instances, they aren't benign: One intervention may mean you end up needing another and another, and they aren't without side effects and sometimes undesirable consequences. Read through the overviews shared here, do your own research, and talk with your care providers to decide what is right for you and your baby.

The most common hospital interventions include:

Routine IV

Many hospitals will hook you up to an IV the minute you walk in their doors. It's typically there as a precaution, usually to administer fluids to prevent dehydration—because some hospitals don't allow eating or drinking during labor—and to be there should you need medication, decide you want an epidural later, or in case of an emergency. (Note that the American College of Obstetricians and Gynecologists's guidelines are against the restriction of fluids by mouth during labor.) IV fluids are given before an epidural to help control blood pressure and are the way to administer Pitocin, for example, to speed labor along.

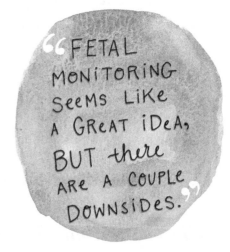

"FETAL MONITORING SEEMS LIKE A GREAT iDeA, BUT there ARE A COUPLE DOWNSIDeS."

What's the downside? An IV tethers you to either your bed or an IV pole, which limits your ability to move during the laboring process and might just make you more uncomfortable. It's also possible you could receive too many fluids if you're in labor for a long time, leading to complications. The intervention may have negative impacts on breastfeeding—too high a volume of fluids can cause the breasts to swell and become painful.

You may be able to ask for a heparin lock or saline lock instead. In both cases, you're not attached to your bed or pole; rather, a flexible catheter is placed in your vein with either saline or heparin (a blood thinner) to prevent any clotting, and then the catheter is "locked" off. Doctors and nurses then have easy access to an open vein if there's an emergency, but you can still move around.

Continuous Electronic Fetal Monitoring

During this intervention, special equipment measures the response of your baby's heart rate to your uterine contractions. While minor fluctuations in your baby's heart rate are normal, fetal monitoring's goal is to detect major changes in a normal heart rate pattern that could indicate fetal distress, so that steps can be taken to help treat any underlying problem or prevent unnecessary treatments.

Fetal monitoring seems like a great idea, but there are a couple downsides: It has a tendency to set off false alarms since, again, some fluctuations are normal. Continuous electronic fetal heart rate monitoring has been associated with both an increase in instrumented-assisted births (see below) and Cesarean births. What's more, it can require you to be tied to your bed and to lie flat on your back, which can present complications in addition to provoke general discomfort.

As an alternative, you can ask for intermittent electronic monitoring; you may still have limited mobility, but there could be less chance of false-positives. Or, you can request what's known as intermittent auscultation. The baby's heartbeat is checked periodically throughout labor using a handheld instrument called a Doppler, which allows you to maintain your mobility. If laboring in a hospital with a shower or tub, you'll want to make sure they have a waterproof monitor or they will limit your time in the water.

Labor Augmentation

If you're in labor but things have stalled—your contractions are irregular or have stopped altogether, you're not dilating, etc.—or if your due date has come and gone, or if your doctor feels your baby isn't growing enough inside you, doctors often suggest a medical intervention to either get things going or keep things moving. And their primary recommendation is the administration of Pitocin, a synthetic form of the hormone oxytocin, which your body produces naturally and causes uterine contractions.

Although it is generally considered safe, Pitocin can potentially overstimulate your uterus, making your contractions come too fast or too frequently. That can cause a whole host of problems, from changes in fetal heart rate to uterine rupture. Not to mention, it can just make your labor feel that much more intense and painful. Thus, it may make you more likely to opt for an epidural to relieve that pain.

There are natural ways to get labor going, which we'll cover in Section 5.

Assisted Labor

To help move your baby down your birth canal, some doctors may use a vacuum extractor; a small suction cup is attached to your baby's head to help guide them out. Forceps can also be used to help bring your baby down the birth canal. This metal instrument looks like two large metal spoons or a big pair of tongs. These tools are often used when there is a strong desire for a vaginal birth but assistance is needed, rather than going for a Cesarean.

Their use can result in some bruising or swelling. Rarely, scalp lacerations and brain hemorrhage could result from the use of a vacuum, while forceps could pose a risk for skull fracture.

Episiotomies can also be used to speed up the birthing process, and to prevent tearing. An episiotomy is a small incision in the perineum that opens up the vagina. Women who have an episiotomy may actually be more likely to spontaneously tear. The incision can also take a while to heal and thus up your risk of complications.

An epidural is an extremely common medical intervention—chosen by more than 70 percent of pregnant women, according to a 2018 study[32]—but it may or may not be right for you. It blocks nerve signals, and hence the feelings of pain (you may hear it called an epidural block) from the lower part of your spine: An anesthetic medication (or medications) is administered through a catheter that is run through a large needle inserted into the space around your spinal cord. It stays there, delivering you pain-blocking medication, during your labor and delivery. You can ask for an epidural at any time during labor. Meaning, you may decide you don't want one on your birth plan but change your mind once you're in the delivering room or labor is under way. Or, vice versa: Maybe your birth plan includes an epidural, but you feel differently when the day comes.

The pain relief it provides can allow you to rest and relax during your birth experience. But there are cons. Like the other interventions, it limits you to laboring from a bed on your back. You may experience side effects, from fever to headache, nausea, and localized soreness. Though rare, nerve damage is possible from insertion of the needle or catheter. An epidural may also stall contractions, requiring administration of Pitocin. (This happens because it interferes with your body's production of the hormones that bring on labor.) Or, it can make it more difficult for you to push, or even stall contractions and slow down labor, either of which can increase your chances of needing an assisted vaginal delivery or Cesarean. It can also increase your risk for perineal tears, and some studies (but not all) show an increased risk of respiratory distress for your baby.[33]

A lot of times women want an epidural because they are very close to giving birth and the sensations have intensified, and if they just held out a little longer they wouldn't need it.

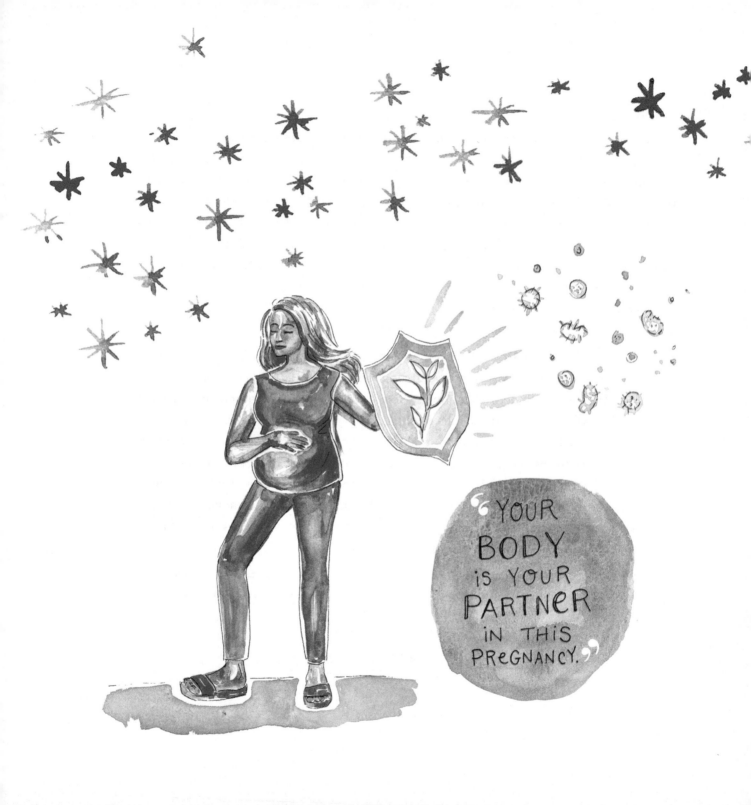

"YOUR BODY is YOUR PARTNER IN THiS PREGNANCY."

Chapter 17

NATURAL REMEDIES FOR THIRD TRIMESTER CHALLENGES

As your baby and your belly grow bigger by the day, it might feel like the symptoms are piling up. For most third trimester challenges, an ounce of prevention is worth a pound of cure, but in this chapter we'll talk about both how to keep common ailments at bay as well as how to treat them if they show up anyway (or are already have). Just remember that unpleasant symptoms aren't a sign of weakness, or that you're doing anything wrong. They're simply pointing out an area where your body needs a little more support. Even catching a virus can be your body's way of indicating that it needs more rest—and stopping you in your tracks to make sure that you get it. Your body is your partner in this pregnancy. Approaching it with love and care (instead of disappointment or even distrust) will help you heal and be even more prepared for birth.

Trouble Sleeping

As your belly grows and your symptoms intensify, it can be hard to find a comfortable position to sleep in. You've also probably got plenty on your mind as you're prepping for your baby's arrival and trying to finish up things, whether at work or at home or both, before you go into labor.

I highly recommend investing in a big body pillow to throw your top leg and arm over when sleeping on your side, and/or a foam wedge to place under your belly so it's not pulling on your back muscles as you sleep. It's worth some trial and error to find the pillow situation that will help you get your rest.

> *"IT'S ALSO IMPORTANT to MAKE SURE YOU'RE GETTING ENOUGH MAGNESIUM."*

It's also important to make sure you're getting enough magnesium, which, as I covered in Chapter 12, is a relaxant and has been shown to help promote deeper sleep in people with restless legs syndrome or who sleep fitfully. Foods that are high in magnesium are dark leafy greens, seeds, nuts, legumes, unprocessed whole grains, and chocolate.

Finally, make sure you're getting enough exercise. If you already have kids, you know that wearing them out physically helps them sleep better, and the same goes for you, too. You're in training for the athletic event of your life (i.e., birth), remember? Make sure you get plenty of movement.

Swollen Ankles

It's really amazing to see just how much fluid can build up in your ankles at the end of pregnancy. I remember taking my socks off and seeing a dent in my legs where the top of my socks were—not a great look!

Swollen ankles are a common side effect of pregnancy because you have extra fluid in your body—such as blood and lymphatic fluid—and the baby's growing weight exerts downward pressure, which can send some of that excess fluid down toward your feet.

The best way to treat swollen ankles is to prevent them from happening in the first place, and the way to do that is to avoid eating salty foods, because salt is the most common cause of swelling. That means taking it easy on things like chips, salsa, bacon, barbecue, and all processed and packaged foods. Make sure you're continuing to drink three to four quarts of water every day so that you can flush away any excess salt that you do eat.

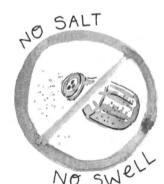

Elevating your feet by resting them on a stool or ottoman whenever you're sitting can also help, as can sleeping on your left side and avoiding standing for long periods of time.

Putting on compression socks or tights before you get out of bed in the morning can also help keep fluid from moving down to your lower extremities. I also enjoyed using a chi machine, which is small appliance about the size of a toaster that you use by lying on your back and resting your feet on top of it. Then the machine sways your feet back and forth, which helps increase oxygen in your blood and move your lymphatic fluid around. It's a great way to get the benefits of movement on those days when you don't have time or energy to exercise, and it's helpful for reducing edema (the medical term for swelling).

You can also drink nettle or dandelion tea, both of which aid detoxification. And if you get uncomfortably swollen, liquid chlorophyll is a great diuretic. Chlorophyll is the substance that makes plants green; it's basically the blood of the plant, and it's a great blood builder and detoxifier for humans. To use it as a diuretic, put 10 tablespoons (I like the mint flavor) in a quart of mint tea, sweeten it with honey to taste, and divide it into five portions so that you're getting approximately two tablespoons per dose; drink throughout the day until it's finished. The tea will be deeply green, and it might make your stools green, but it will help usher excess fluids out of the body.

Just one note: If your swelling is sudden, it could be a sign of preeclampsia, a potentially dangerous form of high blood pressure experienced by a very small amount of pregnant women. Reach out to your care provider to tell them about your symptoms so they can monitor you.

Bladder Infections

There are a few reasons why you're more likely to get bladder infections—which can show up as cloudy urine, painful urination, the feeling that you need pee frequently although you may not actually pass urine, pelvic or lower back pain, fever, and even nausea or vomiting—now. Yep, you can thank the baby and the pressure they're causing for this one, too, because

> "REALLY, THERE ARE SO MANY REASONS to DRINK A CUP OF WATER for EVERY HOUR YOU'RE AWAKE — MAKE SURE YOU ARE DOING iT."

they are pressing on your bladder and forcing more urine into your urethra, which is also larger now than it is when you aren't pregnant. Once the urine is in there, it's likely to hang around. On top of that, your urine has more sugar in it than normal. All these things encourage the growth of bacteria that can lead to infection. Having sex can also cause bacteria that's normally in the vagina to get into the urethra, where it can travel up into the bladder and cause infection.

Again, drinking three to four quarts of water per day helps prevent this particular pregnancy symptom from happening in the first place. Really, there are so many reasons to drink a cup of water for every hour you're awake—make sure you are doing it! You also want to be sure that you pee after sex, every time. (If you are drinking this much water every day, you will need to pee after sex because you need to pee after everything.)

If you're prone to bladder infections, keep CranActin on hand—it's a supplement that contains cranberry extract. Look for the version that also contains D-Mannose, which is a form of sugar. Together, these two natural remedies help strengthen the membrane that keeps urine in the bladder and out of the urethra and makes it less permeable to bacteria. Take it at the first sign of discomfort to keep the infection in check, but still tell your care provider about any symptoms you might be experiencing; left untreated, bladder infections can migrate and become a kidney infection, which is serious.

Illness

The baby can lower your immunity as they're taking up more of your inner resources. If you come down with any sort of bug, first, stop everything you can stop—work, exercise, housekeeping—so you can let every bit of your body's vital life force go to healing. A lot of the times when you catch an illness it's a sign that you've been pushing a little or a lot too hard. Second, be sure to tell your care provider so that they can keep an eye on you. Third, really clean up your diet and stick to only easy-to-digest, highly nutritious foods, such as quinoa, vegetables, brown rice, fish, chicken, soups, and smoothies. That also means minimizing or altogether avoiding wheat, meat, dairy, and sugar, which can be difficult to digest and can divert too many of your resources away from healing.

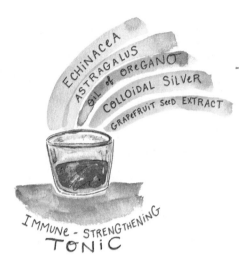

ECHINACEA
ASTRAGALUS
OIL of OREGANO
COLLOIDAL SILVER
GRAPEFRUIT SEED EXTRACT

IMMUNE - STRENGTHENING
TONIC

Try this Immune-strengthening tonic:

To a small glass of strongly flavored juice (like tart cherry or pomegranate), add six drops of echinacea, astragalus, oil of oregano, colloidal silver, and grapefruit seed extract.

It will taste horrible, so shoot it back as fast as you can. Take it every four hours if you're already feeling sick, or every six hours if you're trying to ward off something. These herbs have powerful antibacterial and antiviral properties. If you don't feel noticeably better in 24 hours, get in to see your care provider.

Hemorrhoids

You can thank your baby for putting pressure on your rectum and anus, too, which can lead to the swollen veins known as hemorrhoids. They can be painful or itchy or even bleed. Prevention is the best approach. Cut way back on the amount of wheat you eat because it can really slow down your digestion. (Think about what happens when you combine flour with water—it turns into paste, and it can do the same in your intestines.)

Keep drinking your water. And take plenty of vitamin E and vitamin C to keep your vascular system and capillary system strong—it will also strengthen the placenta and the baby's vascular system.

If you're prone to hemorrhoids, Mari Mikel recommends taking the herb white oak bark (one or two capsules in the morning and one or two capsules at night) to firm up

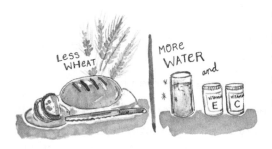

the capillary walls, and avoid taking evening primrose oil—which can soften all your tissues and comes in handy for getting your cervix ready for delivery—until the very end of pregnancy.

If you already have hemorrhoids, a great home remedy is to grate a russet potato (the kind typically served baked) and put it right on the hemorrhoid. It will help soak up the excess fluid. You can also wet a cotton pad with witch hazel and then put it in the freezer. Once it's nice and cold, put it right on the affected area for pain relief. If you're uncomfortable throughout the day, put a couple of sanitary pads in your underwear and nestle them right up against the painful area so that they apply pressure to it and keep it supported.

Stress

It's super important that you reduce your stress as much as possible, especially the closer you get to your due date. If you're stressed, so is your baby. And just like you want to be as healthy and strong as possible for labor and delivery, you also want your baby to be at their best, because it's just as hard to be born as it is to give birth.

As I introduced in Chapter 14, I know it's tempting to work right up until you go into labor so that you have more time off with your baby after they're here, but being stressed and tired going into delivery is an invitation for a more difficult birth.

Take more off your plate now. Don't volunteer for anything new. Don't take on more at work. Don't push yourself. Be in nature and in water as much as you can. Spend time talking to your baby and telling them that you're in this together and you can't wait to meet them. It's not too early to start bonding! Put your energy into nesting and daydreaming about what life will be like after your baby is here. If you can—and even if at first you think you can't—stop working at 38 weeks. Read what Mari Mikel has to say...

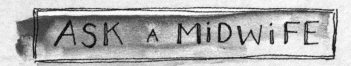

IS IT OK TO WORK UP UNTIL I GO INTO LABOR?

from MARI MIKEL:

"I tell all the women I see in my practice to stop working once they get to 38 weeks. I know how difficult that sounds, and the first thing these women say to me is, 'I couldn't possibly.' The second thing they say is, 'I'd rather have time with the baby after the birth—if I take time off now I'll have less time to spend later.' I know that what I'm proposing sounds radical in our productivity-obsessed culture, but the truth is, you are in training for the Olympics. If you knew you had the Olympics coming up, you would do everything you could to be in the best mental and physical state possible. You'd take your vitamins, drink your water, and eat perfectly. You wouldn't be logging eight hours a day in a desk chair, stressed out, trying to get work done. You wouldn't want your body aching and your mind fatigued. Any day now, your Olympic event will happen. You don't want the day before that event to be a bad day.

"Ninety-seven percent of my clients stop working at around 38 weeks, and they say it's the best thing that ever happened to them. I have to give 100 percent of my clients a big speech about how important it is to go into labor rested and refreshed. If you're still doubting whether this is a good idea, consider this: When you are working, your baby is working. When you are stressed, the baby is stressed. When you are tired, the more likely you are to have a difficult birth.

"It's not easy to be born. You want your baby to be as strong as possible. When you are peaceful and rested, you have the deepest reserves of strength, and so will your baby. Every day, act like your Olympic event could happen the next day and take exquisite care of yourself. By the time you really start to go out of your mind with boredom, birth will start to sound like a great idea, and the baby will come. And you will be ready for it."

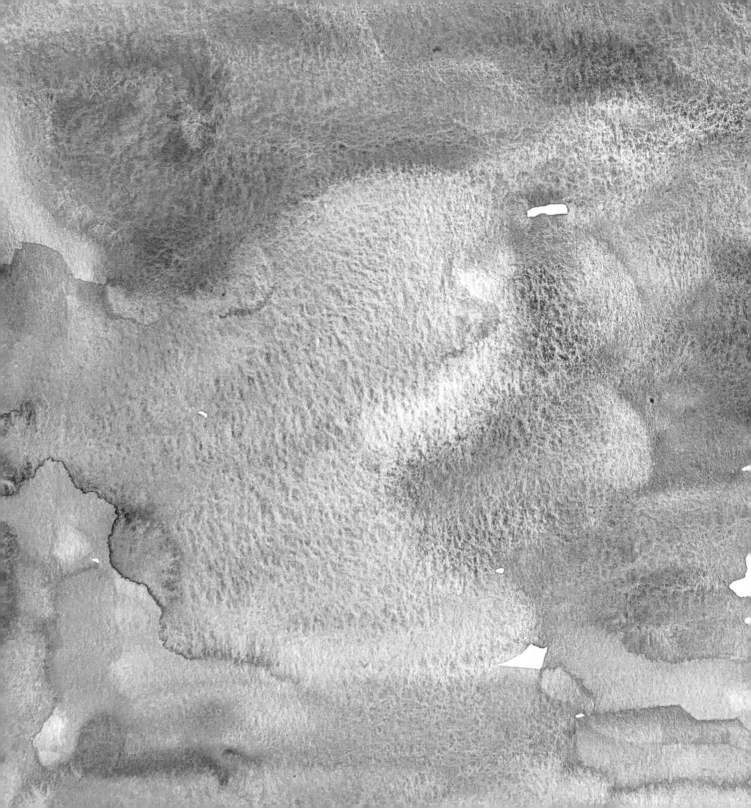

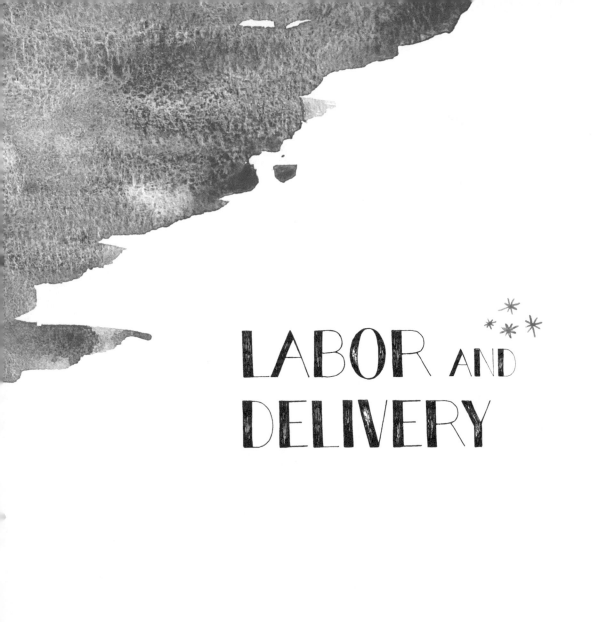

LABOR AND DELIVERY

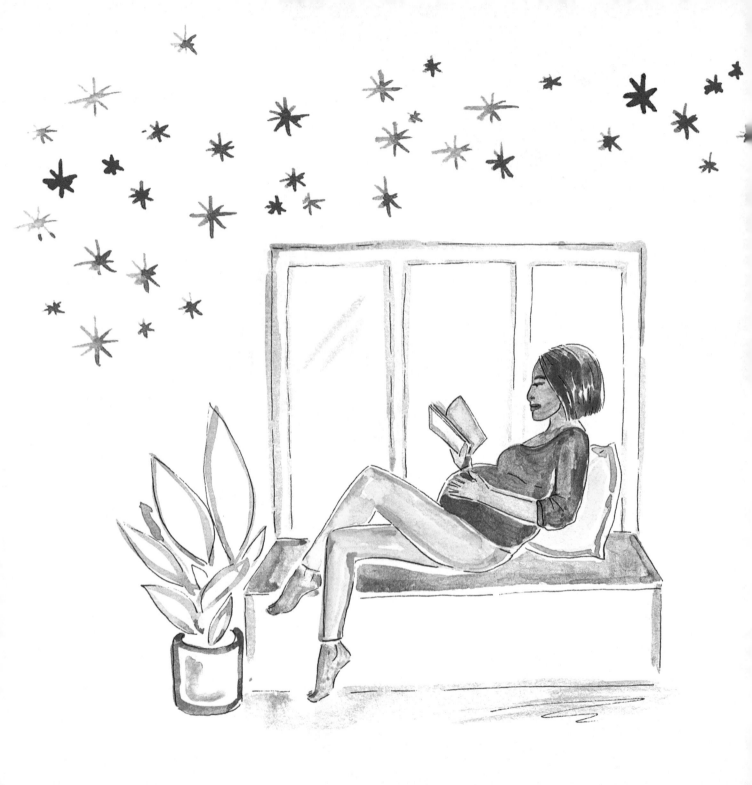

Chapter 18

WHILE YOU'RE WAITING

Once you're within what I like to think of as your "due range" (two weeks before and after your due date), it's hard to be patient. Extremely hard. Trust me, I know—I went well past my due date with my first birth.

In this chapter, I'll cover things you can do during this funny little pocket of time when you're basically just waiting for labor to start.

My First Birth Story

After each of my children was born, I wrote them a letter to tell them about how they came into this world and how much I love them. I'm sharing the letters here, in the pages of this book (the other stories will come later), to show you how different each birth can be and to give you a glimpse at the difference between a home birth (which I had with my two boys) and a hospital birth (which is how my girls were delivered). I'm going in chronological order, starting with my oldest son, Hendrix.

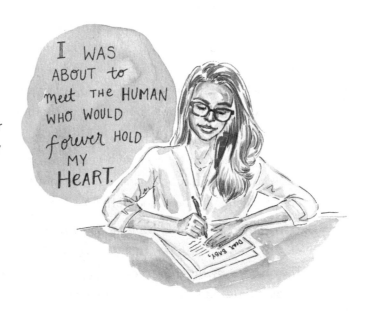

Dear Hendrix,

It was important to me that I write your birth story down so that not only can you read it one day but also because it's a day I never want to forget.

I impatiently waited all of December for you. My Ob/Gyn had told me that, according to the measurements from the ultrasound, you were due on December 7. My midwife maintained that you were going to come a week after my due date, which she had estimated to be December 12.

My water finally broke at 1:30 am on December 18. I woke up to use the restroom and felt a slight trickle and pop. I knew immediately that it was my water breaking, and I excitedly starting prepping for your birth. First I called my midwife to tell her you were coming. She wasn't too concerned since I wasn't having many contractions and she said she could tell by my voice that true labor hadn't started yet. She told me to try to go back to sleep so I would have both strength and energy when labor started. So, I did what every laboring woman does... I got in the shower, washed my hair, applied a hair masque, shaved, blow dried my hair, and curled it in big bouncy curls. I wanted to look good for you and I was too excited to sleep. In the middle of this your Dad sleepily woke up and asked what was going on and would I please come to bed? There was no way I was sleeping. After all, I was about to meet the human who would forever hold my heart.

I fell asleep around 6 am and slept until 11 am. After I awoke, Mari Mikel came over and did a bacteria test to make sure I could keep laboring and waiting for you at home. Since I still had no contractions, she also brought over a breast pump to try to stimulate the onset of labor. I used it and nothing.

The day passed and I went to bed wondering if I'd be the only woman on earth who stayed pregnant forever. Then it happened. I woke up at 1:24 am with REAL contractions. They were very different than my practice contractions that had gone on for weeks leading up to this day. I knew this was it so I woke your Dad and he called the midwife. I turned on every light in the house and went and sat in the living room, and I opened up my laptop and searched for psychedelic videos on YouTube (I wanted something to help me focus, and these are known to be mesmerizing). I watched videos of circles expanding for about 45 minutes. During this time contractions were steady.

Mari Mikel and her apprentices arrived one by one and started setting up. As they did, I walked the hallways, hung out on the floor on my hands and knees, and roamed the house trying to stay active. During contractions I would brace myself against a wall or, as they progressed, go to the ground on my hands and knees. It was clear to me that neither my midwife nor your Dad would be able to help me and I was on my own.

The first time Mari Mikel checked me I was six centimeters dilated. By this time contractions were intense, and she suggested that now would be the time to get in the birthing tub. I had written my birth mantras on poster board and displayed them near the bathtub and in our bedroom. As ridiculous as I thought the breathing exercises that Mari Mikel had made me practice were, they were the only thing that kept me focused and able to get through each contraction. Anytime someone talked to me or made me think it was 100 times more painful. Mari Mikel came and checked my progress often, but let me have privacy to go to the bathroom, be in the tub, and be with myself. Your Dad sat quietly in the corner.

Regularly and increasingly Mari Mikel wanted to check your heartbeat and occasionally do a vaginal exam to assess progress. To do that, I had to lie on my back and I will tell you that made the contractions SO much worse. Finally after getting sick three times and going through the most intense feelings of pressure, release, and tightening over and over again I told her it was time to push. The pressure and contractions were so intense I knew pushing you through the birth canal would be worth it (something I had always been scared of doing, ever since I was a little girl) because it meant that labor would be over and you would be here.

When it was time to push I got into a squatting position and did it with all my might. When you were about to crown the team picked me up and put me on the bed. From here

Mari Mikel starting using hot packs with sterile water and sterile gauze to prevent tearing. With each contraction I would push and between each contraction she would used olive oil to guide your head out and prevent tearing.

After 50 minutes of pushing, you were here! There was meconium in the bag so Mari Mikel put you on my belly and suctioned your airways. I held you, in shock of what had just happened and in awe that you somehow had fit inside of my body. You were a beautiful gray color and slowly getting pink. About five minutes into cuddling, your Dad asked, "Well, what is it??" To me you were so perfect I forgot to check! "A boy!!!!" I cried. I was so happy and so thrilled it was over and life with you was now beginning.

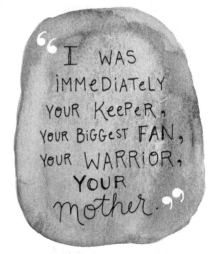

You are the child I always dreamed of. You chose me and I will do anything I have to do to make you not regret that decision and not mess this opportunity up. I was immediately your keeper, your biggest fan, your warrior, your mother. Not only were you born that day, but I was born as a mother. I existed before you, but my new and most important role in life had just begun.

My role as your mother is to raise you to be strong, independent, and capable so that you may one day successfully leave the house. When you were just two days old you looked at me and I swear I heard you communicate, "I am a much older soul than you; just get me up and moving and I will be fine." It was clear as day. I still feel it in my bones. You are a deep thinker already and love to study things. You are determined, focused, observant, energetic, and absolutely delightful.

You are life's gift to me. I thank you for choosing me to be your mother. Let's live a life of adventures together. I love you. *Mommy*

Figure Out Your Food Strategy

Once the baby is here, you're really going to want to rest as much as possible—Mari Mikel suggests staying in bed as much as you can for at least those first two weeks (more on this in Chapter 23). While I know that's not always easy to do, especially if you've got older kids, if you have your meals and snacks planned out—and ideally, even waiting for you in the freezer—it makes those precious early days that much less stressful and more restorative.

Also, planning out those two weeks of meals and snacks is a great thing to do now, while you're waiting for the baby to come. And cooking them in advance is a perfect activity to keep your mind off wondering when your labor will start. I did a lot of cooking with my mom and sister in weeks 40 and 41 of my pregnancy; it was a lot of fun.

If your baby ends up coming before you have a chance to think out your food strategy for those first several days, it's a great thing for your partner to do. Although, most often, women can figure out what to make, what to shop for, and how to make it with their eyes closed, while in my experience the task can really throw men for a loop. Maybe it's something you could work on together.

Because you'll be recuperating from the athletic event of your life and providing your baby's sustenance (assuming you choose to breastfeed and all goes well), you want to choose foods to have on hand for their nutritional value as well as their taste—and not just on their taste alone. Think of 10 great breakfasts, lunches, and dinners and 20 great snacks. Then you can make a shopping list and go get everything you need in one trip to make and freeze ahead as much as you can. (I share recipes for some of my favorite freezable meals to help jump-start the process for you in this chapter.) But before we get there, it's important to know about the foods that you might want to consider steering clear of, at least in those first few weeks—either because they're hard for you to digest, especially after your abdomen and all the organs in it have just been through a major trial, or because they're hard for your baby to digest (components of the food you eat make their way into your breast milk, so essentially the baby is eating the same things you are).

Some babies are very sensitive to some of the harder-to-digest foods, such as beans and legumes, and you just don't know if your baby will be until they are here. So if you'll be breastfeeding, you'll want to make a meal plan that doesn't include these foods. That way, you don't have a newborn with an upset tummy because you ate hummus. You'll also want to make sure that you get plenty of the foods that will help you heal, deliver nutrients to your body and to the baby, and that will help you begin your new reality as a mom on the right foot.

Foods to Avoid in Your Post-Baby Meals

- Beef (it's common to be constipated in the few days after birth, and red meat is tough to digest)

- Wheat (for the same reasons as beef)

- Broccoli, cabbage, Brussels sprouts (because these cruciferous vegetables contain a sulfur compound that can cause stomach upset in the baby)

- All beans and legumes (they don't call them the magical fruit for nothing; this includes chickpeas)

- All soy products (soy milk, tofu, tempeh—soy is a bean, and can therefore be gas-producing)

- Any food that's ever made you bloated or gassy

Great Foods to Eat Those First Few Days

- Roast chicken
- Grilled or baked fish
- Brothy, non-creamy soups
- Salads
- Fruit

- Quinoa
- Brown rice
- Smoothies
- Oatmeal

Recipes for Make-Ahead, Freezable Meals and Snacks

Gluten-Free Coconut Chicken with Sweet Orange Dipping Sauce

These chicken strips are so tasty they'll make you feel like you're eating takeout. Using gluten-free flour and breadcrumbs helps you avoid wheat, which can constipate you and might upset the baby's stomach.

Ingredients | Chicken

- 1½ pounds chicken breasts or tenders
- 1 cup shredded coconut
- ¾ cup gluten-free Panko-style breadcrumbs
- ½ cup Bob's Red Mill Gluten Free 1-to-1 Baking Flour
- 1 teaspoon salt
- ½ teaspoon ground black pepper
- 2 large eggs
- ¼ cup coconut oil

Sweet Orange Sauce

- ½ cup orange marmalade
- 3 tablespoons Dijon mustard
- 1 tablespoon honey
- salt and pepper, to taste

Instructions

1. Preheat oven to 400°F.
2. If using whole chicken breasts, use a mallet or heavy saucepan to flatten, then cut into strips. If using tenders (the little strips of meat that are attached to the underneath of the breast), cut in half lengthwise.
3. If your coconut isn't already shredded fine, chop it with a chef's knife to make the pieces smaller, then combine it with the breadcrumbs in a shallow bowl.
4. Whisk the gluten-free flour, salt, and pepper together in another shallow bowl.
5. Whisk the eggs together in a third shallow bowl.

6. Dip each piece of chicken in flour first, then the egg, and finally in the coconut mixture, shaking off any excess after each step. Plop each chicken strip onto a sheet pan that's been covered in parchment, foil, or a silicone baking mat.

7. Pop the baking sheet in the freezer for 2-3 hours until chicken is frozen solid.

8. Put the chicken strips in a freezer bag and seal, squeezing out as much air as possible.

Store in: A plastic freezer bag.

Lasts in the freezer: Up to four months.

How to defrost and cook: Chicken can go straight from the freezer to a 350°F oven, placed on a baking sheet that's been covered with parchment paper, foil, or a silicone baking mat. Bake for 30 minutes or until they read 165° on a meat thermometer. While the chicken bakes, mix together the sauce ingredients in a small bowl.

Before You Get Busy Cooking

Make space in your freezer. There's no sense in precooking a bunch of meals if there's nowhere for them to go. Get rid of the food that's been in there so long you no longer remember—or can tell—what it is.

1. Get the right containers. Zip-top freezer-safe plastic bags are good for bars, muffins, and soups. Some reusable aluminum pans for casseroles and lasagnas also come in handy. Plastic, freezer-safe containers that easily stack or stand on their sides are also great to have on hand.

2. Think about freezing some smaller portions. If you make a pot of soup, freeze it in two portions so that you don't get sick of it.

3. Accept what you can do. If you planned to make 10 meals and five snacks but only got a couple things put away, it's still way better than nothing. Don't be hard on yourself.

Gluten-Free Zucchini Noodle Lasagna

I know you want comfort food. Here's a way to enjoy a bowl of cheesy goodness without the pasta (and the wheat it contains). If you want to make it vegetarian, either omit the turkey or try Quorn meatless grounds—my family can't tell it's not meat!

Ingredients

- 4 large zucchini
- 2 pounds ground turkey optional, or 2 packages Quorn meatless grounds
- 24 ounces pasta sauce
- 15 ounces ricotta cheese
- 1 cup shredded Parmigiano-Reggiano
- 1½ cups shredded mozzarella
- 1 egg
- salt and pepper, to taste
- fresh parsley and basil, chopped, to taste

Instructions

1. Preheat the oven to 400°F.
2. Slice the zucchini lengthwise into thin slices—using a mandoline or vegetable peeler can help make them more uniform.
3. Brown the turkey in a large pan over medium-high heat, breaking up with a spoon, until cooked through.
4. Take the pan off the heat and pour all but about a ½ cup of pasta sauce into the pan and mix with ground turkey.
5. In a medium bowl, stir together ricotta, Parmigiano-Reggiano, egg, salt, and pepper.
6. Spread reserved ½ cup of pasta sauce in the bottom of a disposable foil 9x13 pan.
7. Make a layer of zucchini slices on top of the pasta sauce.
8. Add ½ the turkey-sauce mixture on top of the zucchini.
9. Spread half the ricotta mixture on top of that.

10. Sprinkle ½ cup mozzarella on top of the ricotta.

11. Add some chopped parsley and basil to the ricotta.

12. Repeat layers of zucchini, turkey-sauce, ricotta, mozzarella, and herbs.

13. Add a final layer of zucchini. Then top with remaining herbs and ½ cup mozzarella.

Store: Right in the pan you assembled it in, wrapped tightly in foil.

Lasts in the freezer: Up to four months.

How to defrost and cook: Defrost in refrigerator overnight, then bake (with the foil still on) in a 375°F oven for 45-50 minutes. Remove foil and bake for another 10-15 minutes until fully heated through. For an extra bubbly top, broil for 2-3 minutes at the very end.

Zingy Chicken Quinoa Soup

Long heralded as a go-to meal any time you're sick, chicken soup really does have restorative properties. And the lemon in this one makes it extra enlivening. Bonus points for using homemade stock—I make mine by saving the carcass from a roast chicken and simmering it with some celery stalks and a chopped onion for a couple of hours—otherwise, canned or boxed stock is fine.

Ingredients

- 2 tablespoons olive oil
- 1 yellow onion, diced
- 2 cups carrots, peeled and chopped
- 4 stalks celery, diced
- 6 cups chicken stock
- salt and pepper, to taste

- 2 bay leaves
- ½ cup quinoa
- 1 lemon, zested first and then juiced, to taste
- 2 cups chopped chicken—leftover cooked chicken or raw both work

Instructions

1. In a large pot, sauté onion, carrot, and celery in olive oil over medium heat for 5 minutes, until soft.

2. Add chicken stock and bay leaves. Add salt and pepper to taste. Bring stock to a boil, then pour in the quinoa and add the chicken (if using raw). Cook 20 minutes or until tender.

3. Stir in lemon zest, lemon juice to taste, and cooked chicken if not using raw.

Store in: A plastic freezer bag.

Lasts in the freezer: Chicken soup can be kept in the freezer up to six months for best quality—you can keep it and eat it safely for longer, but it may start to taste more like your freezer than your delicious soup.

How to defrost and reheat: If you let it defrost in the refrigerator (it will take a day or two), it can last up to four days before you eat it. If you defrost it in the microwave or in a pot on the stove, you should eat it all and not store leftovers in the fridge.

Savory Breakfast Casserole

You can really use whatever you have on hand to round out this baked egg-y dish. It's hearty enough to refuel your stamina after a sleepless newborn night.

Ingredients

- ¾ pound uncooked sweet Italian sausages, casings removed

- salt and fresh ground black pepper, to taste

- ½ cup milk (or non-dairy milk of your choice, so long as it's unsweetened and unflavored)

- ½ cup shredded cheese (of your choice, or whatever you have on hand)

- 4 slices day-old bread (whatever you have on hand—gluten-free is best for those early days, as wheat can be hard to digest for you and the baby)

- 2 bell peppers, diced
- 1 cup mushrooms, sliced
- 10 large eggs
- 1 cup fresh spinach, chopped
- ½ medium yellow onion, diced
- 1 garlic clove, minced

Instructions

1. Sauté sausage in a drizzle of olive oil over medium heat, breaking up with a spoon until cooked all the way through. Pour sausage into a bowl.

2. Add another small drizzle of oil to the pan and sauté the peppers, mushrooms, and onions. After 5 or so minutes, when the vegetables have softened, add the spinach and garlic. Season with salt and pepper. Continue cooking until all veggies are soft and starting to brown.

3. Butter an aluminum foil 9x13 baking pan.

4. Tear the bread into pieces and place in the bottom of the pan to form an even layer.

5. In a mixing bowl, stir together the eggs, milk, and ¼ cup shredded cheese.

6. Pour half egg mixture over the bread, then add the sausage and vegetables, then pour the rest of the egg mixture over the top.

7. Sprinkle with remaining cheese and salt and pepper to taste.

8. This casserole can go straight into the freezer for cooking later; just cover it tightly with plastic wrap and foil.

Store in: Aluminum pan covered in plastic wrap and foil.

Lasts in the freezer: Up to three months.

How to defrost and reheat: Thaw overnight in the refrigerator. Bring to room temperature just before baking (don't let it sit on the counter for more than 30 minutes) in a 375°F oven for 40-45 minutes, until golden. Let cool for a bit before cutting into slices and serving. Garnish with some fresh-cut herbs if you like for an extra taste boost.

Gluten-Free Pumpkin Muffins

Ingredients

- 1 cup pumpkin puree
- 2 cups Bob's Red Mill Gluten Free 1-to-1 Baking Flour
- ½ cup almond flour
- 2 teaspoons pumpkin pie spice (or substitute 1 teaspoon cinnamon and 1 teaspoon allspice)

- ⅛ teaspoon salt
- 1 teaspoon baking powder
- 1 teaspoon baking soda
- 1 teaspoon vanilla
- ¼ cup water
- ½ cup chocolate chips (optional)
- ½ cup brown sugar
- ½ cup plain or vanilla yogurt
- 2 large eggs, room temperature
- ½ cup coconut oil, melted

Instructions

1. Preheat oven to 350°F.
2. Place liners inside a 12-cup muffin tin.
3. In a large mixing bowl, add all dry ingredients and whisk to blend.
4. In a medium bowl, add all wet ingredients and whisk to blend.
5. Pour the wet ingredients into the dry and mix gently, taking care not to overmix.
6. Pour batter into muffin liners, filling only about ¾ of the way, as the muffins will expand when they bake.
7. Bake 20-25 minutes until a toothpick comes out clean. Cool on a wire rack.

   Store in: Freezer bag or freezer-safe food storage container.

   Lasts in the freezer: Up to four months.

   How to defrost and reheat: Put them in the fridge overnight, then either allow to come to room temperature by putting them on the counter for an hour, toasting in a toaster over, or, for a real treat, slicing in half, slathering each half in butter, and putting the buttered-side down in a pan over medium-low heat for a few minutes until browned.

Delish Granola Bars

Granola bars are great snacks, but most of the ones you buy at the store are loaded with added sugars. These get their sweetness from dates and honey, which have a lower impact on blood sugar than table sugar, and come with nutritional benefits of their own. The nuts, seeds, and nut butter also deliver plenty of healthy fats and protein.

Ingredients

- 1 cup rolled oats
- 1 cup puffed rice
- ½ cup chopped almonds (or pecans, or cashews)
- ½ cup pumpkin seeds
- ½ teaspoon salt

- 9-10 Medjool dates, pitted
- ⅓ cup honey
- ⅓ cup nut butter (such as peanut, almond, or sunflower)
- 2 teaspoons vanilla

Instructions

1. Combine the dry ingredients, including the salt, in a large bowl.

2. Either pulse the dates in a food processor or chop them up fine with a knife.

3. Incorporate the dates into the dry ingredients—it works best if you use your hands instead of a spoon, and wetting your hands can help keep ingredients from sticking to your fingers.

4. Combine the nut butter and honey either in a small saucepan or a microwave safe bowl, and heat gently until you can easily stir them together.

5. Add the vanilla to the combined nut butter and honey, then pour the mixture over the dry ingredients and stir to combine.

6. Transfer the combined ingredients to an 8x8 pan that you've lined with parchment paper. Use your (slightly wet) hands to press the mixture down so that it's evenly compressed.

7. Pop the pan in the freezer for 30 minutes, just to harden the mixture up enough to make them easy to cut, then cut them into bars.

Store in: Freezer bag.

Lasts in the freezer: Up to four months.

How to defrost: Take as many bars as you'd like to eat right then out of the freezer and allow to come to room temperature for about 15 minutes (or pop in the microwave for 30 seconds) before eating.

Gather Food and Drink for Labor

Now is also a great time to assemble the things you'll want to eat and drink before, during, and after your labor, because it's super important that you stay fed and hydrated. As for food, you're going to want to eat as much as you can during early labor, because you'll need those calories when you're in active labor, and by then you probably won't feel like eating, or, if you're in the hospital, they likely won't let you. (I'll cover more about the stages of labor in Chapter 19, so if you're wondering what I'm talking about, stay tuned.)

You also want to think about what you want your first meal to be after the baby is here. I remember being so hungry after birth that I ate three plates full of food—don't leave this important refueling to whatever you happen to have in the fridge!

"I REMEMBER BEING SO HUNGRY AFTER BIRTH that I ATE THREE PLATES FULL of FOOD — DON'T LEAVE THIS IMPORTANT REFUELING to WHATEVER YOU HAPPEN TO HAVE IN the FRIDGE."

Here are some suggestions of things to have on hand for labor and post-delivery:

- **Coconut water** is a great source of electrolytes. You can mix it with liquid chlorophyll—30 drops in one cup of coconut water—for extra energy, and add some pineapple juice to it—which contains enzymes that are thought to help soften the cervix—or just sip it plain.

- **Red raspberry leaf tea** is great for strengthening your uterus. And, thanks to the ellagic acid it contains, it appears to increase oxytocin (the hormone that plays a big role in the start of labor) as well. Make a big pitcher of it and keep it in the fridge so that it's ready to enjoy whenever your labor starts: Bring loose red raspberry leaf to a boil in water, at about a 1:4 ratio. Then, let it simmer for approximately 20 or 30 minutes. You can add honey to sweeten it if you like.

- You can also make **ice cubes out of coconut water or red raspberry leaf tea**—they can be handy to have later in labor when you may not feel like drinking but still need hydration. Just only fill the ice cube trays up about halfway so that you don't have to negotiate a full-sized cube.

- As for food, you want to have things on hand that are an even mix of protein, carbs, and fats—like a chicken and avocado wrap, or chickpeas and quinoa. I remember eating some chicken wings we made in our air fryer that were delicious. You want to eat anything that sounds good and that offers up nutrition, as you want a lot of stamina. It's not the time to eat Doritos.

Strategies to Encourage Labor to Start

Now that we've covered food, let's talk about what to do when you're really feeling like you're ready for the baby to go ahead and get here.

While your doctor can use conventional pharmaceutical, and even manual, approaches to induce labor, there are a variety of ways you may be able to kick-start labor naturally. Midwives have been using and standing by these strategies for quite some time, and anecdotal evidence is compelling. Of course, talk with your doctor *(continues on page 292)*

Things That Keep You Busy and Can Nudge Your Body Toward Labor

While you don't want to do anything physically exhausting now (because you want all your energy available for labor, once it starts) it is helpful to keep your body in motion—it occupies your mind and helps your body find a rhythm.

I'm not trying to say you need to be productive. This isn't about checking things off your to-do list; it's just about filling the time in a way that also helps you stay in a mentally and physically primed state.

- Bounce on an exercise ball

- Slow dance, swaying hips side to side

- Practice diaphragmatic breathing

- Take a nap

- Organize drawers and cabinets

- Declutter your closet

- Clean out the fridge and freezer

- Wash and fold all those newborn clothes and bedding

- Go get fitted for nursing bras (in a size or two bigger than your current size, as your boobs will be larger once your milk comes in—yes, even bigger than they are now)

- If you already have kids, go and buy a gift for each of them from the baby, and pick up some activities you can do with them in bed, like books or games

- Find all your device chargers and put them near your bed

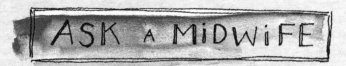

WHAT ABOUT TAKING CASTOR OIL TO STIMULATE LABOR?

from MARi MiKeL:

"I say do not take castor oil unless your health care provider has a very good reason for telling you to do it. First off, taking castor oil can cause terrible diarrhea. The diarrhea can contribute to dehydration, which can cause fatigue. And you really don't want to be fatigued during labor! Also, the castor oil can reach the baby through the placenta and cause the baby to poop, too. This first poop, called meconium, then goes into the amniotic fluid.

"Having meconium in the water is very common and normal—one in 10 of my patients has it. But if there's a lot of it, it could block the baby's airways, or expose them to unfriendly bacteria. Having meconium in the water is a complication of labor—and why would you want to invite a potential complication into your labor?

"The urge to use castor oil to try to bring baby usually stems from impatience and fear. You need someone to talk you through and talk you down. It's completely normal to feel impatient and to experience some fear. But you want to keep your wits about you enough to make the decisions that are best for you and the baby.

"Waiting for labor to initiate is a great preparation for dealing with kids. They take so much patience. Luckily, the same hormones that bring on labor also encourage bonding, which makes you happy to do things for your precious baby. Those hormones will get you into labor too. They are worth waiting for. Let the process unfold. Trust that the baby knows when to come.

"Just do all the things you are in control of—eat well, drink your water, get regular exercise, get good sleep, and do things to manage your stress and your fear. When you've done all that, that's all you can do. You can relax. Don't sit there and ponder when's the baby coming. Every day it becomes more likely that you'll have the baby the next day. You just don't know when that day is. You have to act every day like you're going to have the baby the next day. Have faith. Gather intellectual information to answer the questions of your head (like the information you'll find in books) but also tend to your emotional self. Talk to friends or family who will comfort you and let you cry. If you have a faith, or even if you think you don't, pray. Giving birth is a spiritual journey as much as it is a physical event. It's not a problem that can be 'fixed' by drinking castor oil. Make sure you are being followed by a care provider, who is monitoring things like your blood pressure, the sugar in your urine, your cervix, and the position of the baby. And then have faith."

Things That Keep You Busy and Can Nudge Your Body Toward Labor

- Walk
- Swim
- Do gentle yoga
- Climb stairs
- Run errands
- Have sex
- Iron
- Sweep
- Rake

or midwife, as there may be reasons the following recommendations are not right for you. And they're not without risks. Remember, only employ most of these strategies in the latest stage of your pregnancy and not earlier (although some things, like exercising and having sex, are things you've hopefully been doing all along!).

Get Moving

Moderate, low-impact exercise—like walking—is great for reducing stress hormones. And it's so important that you don't feel stressed now, because your body won't want you to go into labor if it senses you're in any danger (and it can't tell the difference between being chased by a bear and worrying that you don't have the nursery put together yet).

Exercise also releases endorphins, the happy-making, pain-relieving hormones that produce a runner's high. Endorphins are at their highest right before women go into labor. Moving more will help you stay relaxed, which helps invite labor to start, and then once you're in labor, movement helps you feel the pain a little less intensely.

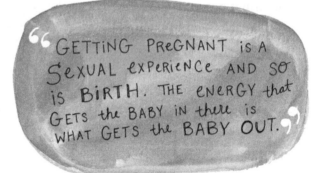

"GETTING PREGNANT is a SEXUAL experience AND SO is BIRTH. THE ENERGY that GETS the BABY IN there is WHAT GETS the BABY OUT."

Get Busy

Intercourse, nipple stimulation, and orgasm are also great at producing oxytocin. Semen also contains prostaglandins, hormone-like compounds that ripen the cervix. In fact, it contains the same prostaglandins found in cervical-ripening medications, which are of course synthetic versus natural. Why take them when you can just have fun having sex?

If your partner doesn't feel comfortable having actual intercourse at this stage of your pregnancy, there are lots of other aspects of sexual intimacy you can explore, either with your partner or on your own. Cuddling also gets oxytocin going, if you're just not feeling in the mood. But if it's at all possible, do what it takes to get in the mood—getting pregnant is a sexual experience and so is birth. The energy that gets the baby in there is what gets the baby out.

Get Pumping

When you're really serious about wanting labor to come, using a breast pump can help jump-start things, because it is all about nipple stimulation. The only catch is, your standard home breast pump won't do—you want a hospital-grade pump, because it is much more effective at stimulating oxytocin. You don't need to buy one; you can rent them from maternity stores, some pharmacies, and medical supply companies. The Medela website (www.medela.us) has a search function to help you find a place that rents pumps.

Mari Mikel suggests using the pump on the following schedule for trying to get labor started:

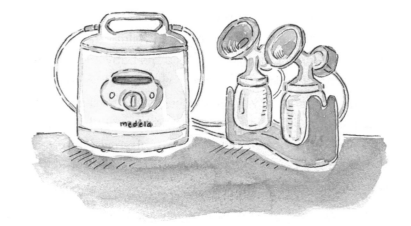

5 minutes right breast

5 minutes left breast

5 minutes rest

5 minutes right breast

5 minutes left breast

10 minutes rest

5 minutes right breast

5 minutes left breast

20 minutes rest

Take a long walk

Take a nap

You can repeat this process up to three days in a row (and under the advisement of your care provider, of course).

Get Real About Who's Invited into the Labor Room

Speaking of the sexual energy of birth, think long and hard about who you want to invite into the room when you do go into labor. Because it's so intimate, you really don't want anyone in there with you that you wouldn't be comfortable having in the room when you're having sex. If you're on the fence about inviting your mom or your mother-in-law in, trust your gut and ask them to respect your wishes for privacy. You need to feel safe in order to give birth, and if someone is making you feel judged or even just observed, it may make your labor slower, and therefore harder. It's not worth any worries you may have about ruffling feathers.

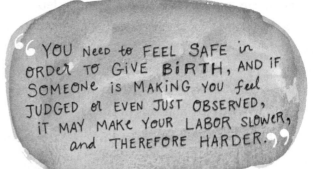

" YOU Need to FEEL SAFE in ORDER TO GiVE BiRTH, AND iF SOMEONe is MAKiNG YOU feel JUDGED or EVEN JUST OBSERVED, iT MAY MAKe YOUR LABOR SLOWeR, and THEREFORE HARDER. "

Get Your Cervix Ready

Throughout most of your pregnancy, your cervix—the lower, narrow end of your uterus, which the baby passes through during childbirth—can be described as "hard." And that's a good thing. That means it can hold the baby and placenta snuggly and securely in place for nine months. However, there is one time when you want a "soft" cervix: toward the end of your pregnancy, when it is necessary to allow the birth to occur. As your cervix gets softer, it thins out (effaces) and dilates until you're ultimately ready to deliver. The softening of your cervix before labor is often also referred to as cervix ripening. (See box on page 316 for more info.) That said, you don't want your cervix to get too soft too early, which could cause premature labor.

After 38 weeks in both my pregnancies, I inserted evening primrose capsules vaginally, because the herb helps soften the cervix—a key thing that helps send the signal to your body that it's OK for labor to start. Also, a thinner cervix equals a shorter labor. This is one of the most commonly recommended options to naturally soften the cervix by midwives and holistic practitioners. It comes from the plant *Oenothera biennis*, which has yellow flowers that bloom, not surprisingly, in the evening time. It has many traditional uses as a healing plant among Native Americans. According to some sources, it should be thought of as a last resort, because it can cause your water to break before your contractions have started (which is what happened to me).

Some evidence points to eating dates late in your pregnancy for helping with cervical ripening and dilation, and to reduce the need for medical intervention in labor. Studies suggest eating around 60-80 grams of the fruit a day.

Get Rubbed

Massage can help increase your oxytocin levels, not to mention relax you, and relaxation is said to boost oxytocin as well. Massaging certain areas, or applying pressure to these places using acupressure techniques, may be the most helpful. These areas include your shoulders, at the top of your trapezius; the inside of your lower leg just a little above your ankle bone; the ball of your foot; your lower back, between your tailbone and hip bone; and the webbed space between your thumb and index finger.

How to Get Ready for a Home Birth

If you're planning a home birth, there are a few things you need to do that someone who's planning a hospital birth doesn't.

An important thing to do if you're planning a home birth—and nice to do even if you aren't—is to have your home thoroughly cleaned. This isn't about making things picture-perfect; it's about creating a sanitary environment for you and your newborn so that you aren't exposed to germs during labor, delivery, and those first few days. Notice I said have your home cleaned: This is a job for your partner or a cleaning professional, not you. You do not need to be scrubbing the toilet at nine months pregnant!

- **Dust and vacuum.** Dust often hides bacteria and viruses as well as pet dander and dust mites, which many babies are allergic to.

- **Sanitize the bathroom.** Germs from the toilet get sprayed around the bathroom with every flush, so scrub the toilet, sink, counter, tub, and floor.

- **Groom and bathe your dog.** Keep that dander to a minimum by having your dog groomed.

- **Stock up on disinfectant (or make your own).** Keep a bottle of cleaner in each bathroom and in the kitchen and spray the sink, handles, and doorknobs throughout your home every few days to keep germs off of high-touch spaces.

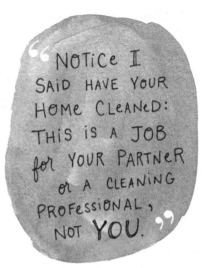

Other things to do to prepare your home for your birthing process include:

- **Make sure you've ordered your birth kit**—a package of medical supplies, such as sterile gloves, a thermometer, and a syringe for suctioning out the baby's airways. Your midwife will tell you how and when to order one; it costs about $100.

- **Sterilize several towels and two sets of sheets.** Your midwife will likely give you these instructions, but the basic idea is to wash, dry, and fold your towels and sheets, then put them in brown paper bags. Then place the bags in the oven at 250 degrees for one hour each. (You may need several bags, and to rotate one or two bags at a time in and out of the oven.) Once they're out, don't open the bags—store them in a plastic trash bag or bin in the room where you're planning to give birth.

- **When you go into labor, have your partner clean the toilet** with a Clorox bleach solution so that the toilet stays germ-free, as you'll likely be using it to relieve yourself—and maybe even as a place to labor, since you're already accustomed to relaxing your abdominal organs and pelvic floor on the pot.

DIY Disinfecting Spray

By now you know I love to DIY all kinds of cleaning and personal care products, and disinfecting sprays are no exception. I first made this during the early 2020 quarantine and sprayed it on everything that stood still.

Ingredients

- 16-ounce spray bottle

- 70% or higher rubbing alcohol

- ½ teaspoon hydrogen peroxide

- 30 drops tea tree oil

- 15 drops other essential oils of your choice, such as rosemary, lavender, lemon, orange, or eucalyptus

Directions

1. Fill the bottle almost up to the top with rubbing alcohol.

2. Add the hydrogen peroxide and essential oils.

3. Gently shake to combine before using.

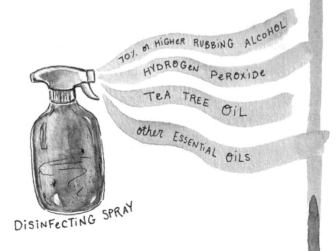

You can either spray this directly on surfaces, or I like to spray it on a clean rag and then wipe the object (like your cellphone, or a doorknob) with the moistened rag. Let air dry.

- **Secure and set up a birth tub**—basically an inflatable pool you can set up inside your house that is big enough for you to submerge yourself in and easily change positions. You fill it up by connecting a hose to a faucet or water heater. I loved being in the tub during my first birth, but spent a lot of my second birth in the shower—the tub didn't appeal. You may not use it at all, depending on how you feel in the moment, but floating in warm water can be very relaxing, which helps labor move along, and can also lessen the experience of pain. For only about $100, it's worth having that option available to you. Your midwife or doula can connect you to a place to rent one from.

What to Pack in a Bag for the Hospital

If you're planning a hospital birth, now is a great time to get a bag ready so that you can just grab it and go when the time comes.

   If you're planning a home birth, you don't need to pack a bag unless it comforts you to do so—if it only makes you worry about what could possibly go wrong, just make a list of what you'd want to have with you. That way, it will be out of your head, and it will be easier for your partner, doula, or midwife to pull it all together for you.

- Copy of your birth plan
- Paperwork—copies of your insurance card, photo IDs for you and your partner, hospital pre-registration forms
- Snacks and beverages
- Electric candles (to set the mood)
- Change of clothes (for you to wear home)
- Change of clothes for your partner
- Something to labor in (you don't have to wear the hospital-issued gown)

- Nursing gowns (something that opens in the front so you can have the baby skin-to-skin on your chest and breastfeed without having to be fully exposed)

- Nursing bras

- Slippers and/or warm socks

- Chargers for various devices (cellphone, Bluetooth speaker, etc.)

- Ear buds

- Depends or adult diapers (can be easier than dealing with pads)

- Nipple cream

- Cotton breast pads

- Hair care products if you're there longer than **24 hours**

- Face care products

- Toothbrush, floss, and toothpaste

- Moisturizer for you and the baby

- Comfortable pillow and blanket

- Sleep mask

- Reading material

- Notebook and a pen

- Snacks

- Large jug of spring water

- Clothes and hat for the baby

- Car seat for the baby (unless you live within walking distance, you can't bring them home from the hospital, or to their first pediatrician's appointment, without it)

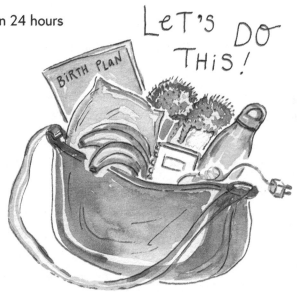

Other Things to Take Care of Now

I know I've included plenty of things to keep you occupied in this chapter. When you're not prepping, here are the very basic things you can do to make the most of this time.

- **Go on dates with your partner.** You may not feel like it, but you will appreciate these times together, without kids, so much later. The early days of parenthood can be challenging on a relationship, especially because the baby will need you so much, that anything you can do to feel connected to your partner now will go a long way.

- **Keep taking your prenatal vitamins.** Once the baby is here and you're nursing, your nutritional needs will only increase, not decrease. The only difference is that you don't call them 'prenatal' anymore.

- **Rest.** Take naps. Go to bed early. Trust me, you will be so glad you did whatever you could to fill up your sleep tank!

- **Take a CPR class.** It's a skill that will last you a lifetime.

- **Take a breastfeeding class or find a breastfeeding support group nearby.** In earlier times, everyone breastfed and we all grew up seeing women breastfeed, and it made the whole process more intuitive. Today, it can be hard in the beginning. Having information and support makes it much more doable and much less daunting. Do what you can to get that support in place before the baby's here and you're panicking that they're not getting enough milk.

- **Make an emergency plan.** I don't believe in rehearsing unhappiness, but you should also think through what would happen if, say, you're planning to drive to the hospital but your car is in the shop, or you're planning a home birth but you need to get to the hospital—how would you get there? What hospital entrance would you drive up to? Who will stay with your older child or children if you have them?

- **Decide on a pediatrician.** The American Academy of Pediatrics says every baby should see their pediatrician within three to five days of birth—I would add that this is if you've had your baby in the hospital. If you've had a home birth, your midwife should come check on you and the baby in the first few days after birth so that you can stay down and recover. Either way, you want to have your pediatrician already picked out so that you don't have to scramble to find one while you're recovering from labor. Ask your friends with kids for referrals, make sure the office is convenient to you and accepts your insurance, and then call and ask for a consult, or prenatal, appointment (although these may or may not be covered by your insurance). You want to ask them about their views on breastfeeding, vaccinations, circumcision, as well as how things work after-hours—if your baby starts projectile vomiting at 2am, who might pick up the phone if you call? You really want to feel a connection to your pediatrician, so if you don't feel it, keep looking.

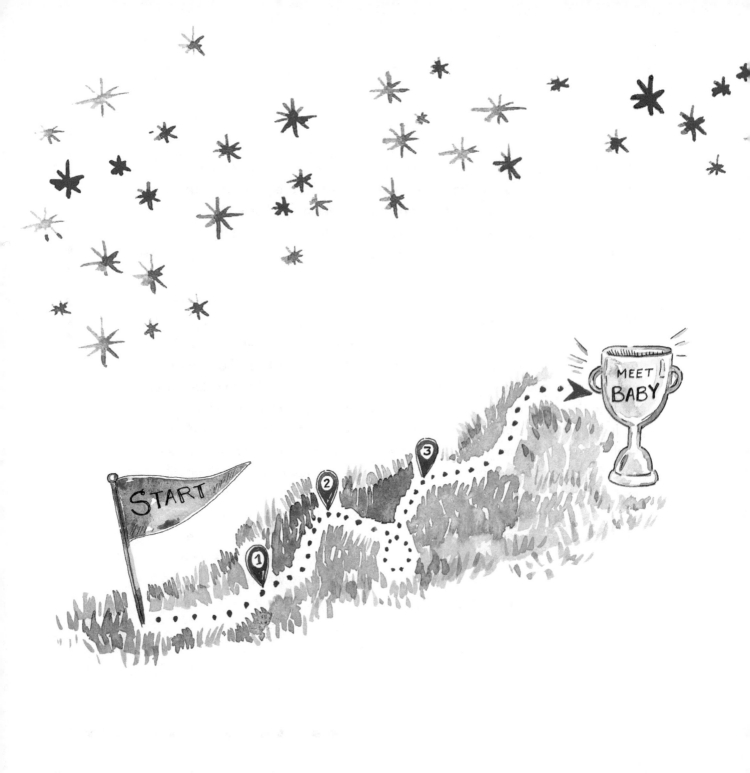

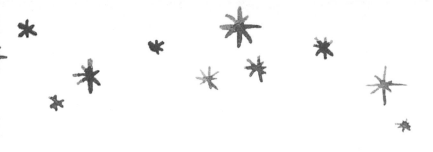

Chapter 19

THE PHYSICAL WORK OF LABOR AND DELIVERY

No matter when it happens, or how it happens, giving birth to your baby is an epic achievement, a massive transformation, and nothing less than a miracle. At the same time, it's also a bodily function—one with a fairly predictable path that has been traveled by billions of women throughout the thousands of years of human history.

Even still, especially when you are a first-time mom, it's really hard to wrap your brain around the fact that labor will result in the creation of a new human—a new human that emerges from inside your own body.

Knowing the landmarks along the path helps make this huge event in your life more manageable. Here is a tour through the physical aspects of labor. (We'll cover the mental aspects in the next chapter.)

When Do You Know You're in Labor, Exactly?

You know how it goes on TV shows and in the movies: A woman's water breaks in dramatic fashion all over the floor. Everyone panics and rushes her to the hospital, because it means the baby is coming—and fast!

In reality, only about 10 to 15 percent of women have their water break, aka membranes rupture, before labor. What's more, only a fraction of those women actually experience a big ole gush of fluid running down their legs and all over the place. Plus, membrane rupture doesn't mean labor is exactly imminent: Most women, between 77 and 95 percent, will go into labor within roughly 24 hours of the rupture happening. Rarely, a woman's water can break several days before the start of labor.[34]

> "IN REALITY, *only* ABOUT 10 *to* 15 PeRCeNT *of* WOMEN HAVE ~~*their*~~ WATER BREAK, AKA MEMBRANES RUPTURE, BEFORE LABOR."

What's more likely to happen is that you'll start to feel contractions that aren't actually official labor—they are part of what's known as warm-up labor. (I don't call it false labor, because there's nothing false about it, and I never call them Braxton Hicks contractions, because that's the name of a man—John Braxton Hicks, a 19th century English obstetrician—and I don't want any man to claim ownership over any part of giving birth.) Warm-up labor is just that—it's strengthening your uterine muscles and basically rehearsing for when the baby comes.

You may hear women say that they were in labor for three days, but most likely, they were having warm-up labor. You can tell the difference between warm-up labor and early labor (the first phase of actual labor) because warm-up labor contractions, which may feel similar to the cramps you get when you are about to get or are on your period, will slow down, go away altogether for a while, or decrease in intensity. (When you are in true early labor, the contractions grow longer, stronger, and closer together—more on this in a moment.) Warm-up labor contractions also often lessen or slow to a standstill when you change positions—early labor contractions won't.

You can have warm-up contractions throughout your third trimester, increasing as your due date inches closer, but they can sometimes occur as early as your second trimester; they often occur later in the afternoon or evening on days during which you've been quite mobile.

As your delivery date draws nearer, your warm-up labor may feel very real, as the contractions may be fairly strong. I'm not trying to discount that—at all. I'm just saying let's not make labor any longer than it actually is. Don't tell yourself as soon as you feel contractions that "this is it," and stay up all night timing them or get frustrated if they stall out. It's probably just warm-up labor. Best to ignore it until you no longer can.

The Most Certain Sign: Consistent Contractions

The easiest and best way to know if you're in active labor is to pay attention to your contractions. Remember these indicators: stronger, longer, more frequent, and consistent. Active labor begins when your contractions start to get stronger, last longer, and occur closer together—they also typically won't stop or stall once they start; they will only intensify.

Early in labor, they may only occur every 30 minutes. But as you move toward active labor, the intervals decrease to, say, 10-15 minutes, and then down to five or less. Other hallmarks of early labor contractions include:

- They will occur in a regular, predictable pattern or fashion; in other words, they will be evenly spaced apart

- They won't stop when you change positions or engage in activity

- They usually start in your lower back and then move to the front of your abdomen, or vice versa

Other Clues Baby Is On Their Way

Contractions and membrane rupture aren't the only indicators you may be in labor. Others are:

- **Loss of mucus plug.** This is one of the earliest things that typically happens before labor—either a couple days or a couple weeks before. It doesn't mean labor is starting, but it's part of the warm-up process. It means things are moving along, but not necessarily imminent. You can think of your mucus plug as a cork. It seals off your cervix in order to protect your uterus and your baby while you're pregnant. You may not notice it unplugging or dislodging at all, or you may notice a passing of clear, sticky mucus, either as one big glob at once or as several little blobs over time.

- **Bloody show.** It sounds like something out of a horror movie, but it's not so scary. Bloody show is simply an increase in vaginal discharge before labor that is often pinkish or even brown-tinged because of blood. This happens because the blood vessels in your cervix are rupturing as you get ready to deliver your baby—it means the cervix is changing more rapidly than those blood vessels can stretch. If it happens close to your due date, all is normal and it's a sign things are about to happen. If you notice big changes in your vaginal discharge before 37 weeks, though, or if the discharge is bright red or you're noticing actual bleeding, do call your doctor. While bloody show means it's almost, ahem, showtime, labor could still possibly be a day or so away. Pay attention to those contractions to know when the time is truly here.

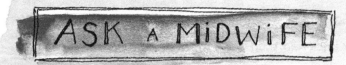

WHAT'S THE DEAL WITH WARM-UP LABOR?

from MARi MikeL:

"We've all heard the woman who says she labored for three and a half days—the mere thought of it is enough to send shivers down your spine. But typically, two of those days were all warm-up labor. They weren't the real deal. The problem with not recognizing those days as warm-up labor is that you can get so excited and amped up that things are finally happening that you don't get the rest you need to sustain you through those three and half days.

"Then you're exhausted, and that's an invitation for interventions—which are fine if they're medically necessary, but these aren't interventions that would have been needed if you were rested and ready to go. Also, if you're planning a hospital birth and show up at the hospital with warm-up labor that doesn't progress, you probably won't want to leave, and when they suggest starting a little Pitocin, you say yes, which is fine but then that can make contractions more intense so you'll probably want to get an epidural too, and every intervention increases your odds for the next intervention. Interventions, when medically necessary, are a godsend. But when they're not, they can get in the way of the biochemical wizardry of your own hormones—oxytocin kills pain, induces bonding, and causes orgasm in addition to stimulating uterine contractions. Pitocin only does the latter.

"Warm-up labor is a great thing: It gives you an opportunity to get used to the sensations of actual labor. It's the perfect time to practice your breathing, relaxation techniques, affirmations, and laboring positions with your partner. It's also a great time to rest and fuel up.

"You may be having contractions that are four or five minutes apart and one minute long and fairly intense, and it could still be warm-up labor; your contractions have to be getting longer, stronger, and closer before you are truly in labor.

"One reason to contact your doctor or midwife, even when you're only in warm-up labor, is if you think your waters may have broken. You may have heard a pop, or you may only be noticing that your panties are damp (and keep getting damp). Once the amniotic sac is broken, your baby is no longer in a sterile environment and they'll want to monitor you for possible infection."

When in active labor, you may also experience:

- Loose stools or diarrhea

- Nausea and occasional vomiting

- Loose, relaxed joints

- Fatigue

- The urge to be alone

- An increase in vaginal discharge

- A tiny bit of lost weight

- The baby may get very still (as the contractions get stronger and stronger, the baby can kind of freeze)

- Wanting to sleep more (honor that urge!)

- Your waters may break—you could hear a pop or just notice that your undies are damp and it keeps happening (meaning, it's not because you accidentally peed a little)

If you are experiencing any of these signs and think you're in labor, contact your health care provider. Don't be afraid to reach out, even if it ends up just being warm-up labor. They will appreciate a chance to hear how you're doing and get a heads up that the baby is getting closer to being born.

The Phases of Labor

Labor occurs in three phases or stages. For most first births, it lasts between 12 and 24 hours, although it can last longer—we've all heard the stories! Usually, labor is quicker if you've previously delivered a child.

The three phases of labor are:

1. Phase one, which is divided into early labor and active labor; it begins when you feel contractions that increase in intensity and don't stall out, and ends when your cervix is fully dilated

2. Phase two, the time to start pushing; it starts when your cervix is dilated fully, and ends once your baby is born

3. Phase three, which involves the delivery of the placenta

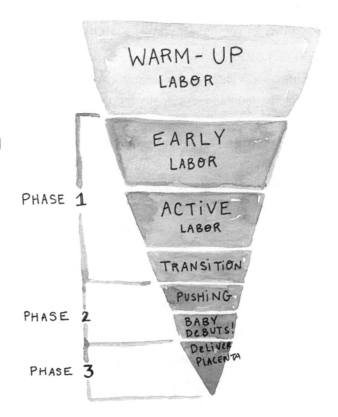

Feeling real contractions that keep growing in intensity and don't stop and start? You're in phase one, the longest of the three phases. During this phase, your contractions cause the cervix to dilate (or open) and efface (thin). (I talk more about these terms on page 313.) There are two distinct parts of Phase One:

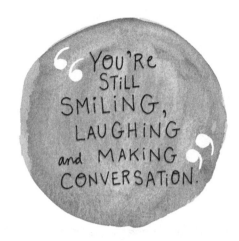

"YOU'RE STILL SMILING, LAUGHING and MAKING CONVERSATION."

Early labor (sometimes called the latent phase)

   In early labor, your cervix effaces and dilates between one and four centimeters. During this time, you'll likely feel tolerable contractions that you can easily talk through. You're still smiling, laughing, and making conversation. This is often when you experience a loss of your mucus plug, bloody show, and when your water breaks. How long early labor takes varies from woman to woman and can be highly unpredictable, lasting from hours to days. This is the time to relax, breathe, and rest in between your contractions. Try taking a leisurely walk, listening to soothing music, and using breathing and relaxation techniques to calm down and wait for the action to truly start. In this phase, the cervix dilates to four centimeters, and it can last as long as two days.

"DURING ACTIVE LABOR, YOU WANT to BE, WELL, ACTIVE."

Active labor (which ends with what is often referred to as transition or the transition phase)

   This is when you can start the clock on how long your labor is. During this part of phase one, your cervix dilates four to seven centimeters, and as its name indicates, things really get going. You're in true labor now, and it will likely start to feel like work: Your contractions will get stronger and much more intense, and occur more frequently and with more regularity. You may have heard of the 5-1-1 rule or the 4-1-1 or even 3-1-1 rule, which say that active labor starts when your contractions are either five, four, or three minutes apart, each lasting for a full minute and having occurred for an hour. The active part of phase one usually lasts between three and eight hours.

During active labor, you want to be, well, active. Mari Mikel advises being up for 40-45 minutes of every hour, and off your feet, resting, for 15-20 minutes of every hour. Getting on your hands and knees, or standing in a bent over position with your hands resting on your knees (like an athlete catching her breath after a sprint) makes the contractions not feel as strong—but it will likely make this phase of labor last longer. Standing up, or hanging off your partner's neck, or sitting on the toilet will all encourage the baby's head to press on your cervix and help the opening and softening process. Wherever you are, imagine relaxing all your muscles—especially your pelvic floor—with your exhales. Yes, you'll be efforting, but finding relaxation amidst that effort will help you progress. Getting in the bath, birthing tub, or shower now can help a lot with that relaxation.

Active labor generally takes one to three hours for every centimeter (three hours is more typical for first-time moms).

The transition part of active labor is when the cervix dilates from seven to 10 centimeters and your contractions become much more intense and closer together. If your water hasn't broken yet, it might happen now. You may also feel nauseated; that's because some women are sensitive to oxytocin, which is running high right about now. You might also have diarrhea, because the same nerves that enervate the intestines also enervate the uterus, and when the uterus gets stimulated, so can your bowels. Transition can be a scary time: You may feel like things are very

"TRANSITION is MAGICAL, BECAUSE iT MEANS YOU'RE GETTING VERY CLOSE to MEETING your BABY. THIS is the SHORTEST PART of LABOR."

out of your control and that delivery is going to be too difficult to manage. That is just part of it—most women have a moment when they think they can't go on, and generally midwives and doctors will get excited when you've reached this point because it often means you're in transition and you're almost ready to push. Transition is magical, because it means you're getting very close to meeting your baby. This is the shortest part of labor.

If you're delivering in a hospital or birth center, your doctor or midwife may advise you to head to the location where you've decided to give birth in early labor or to wait until active labor. If you're having a home birth, you get to rest in the knowledge that there's nowhere to rush off to.

Phase Two

Now, your baby has rotated and descended into the birth canal and into the proper position for delivery. Your cervix is fully dilated to 10 centimeters, and it's time to push! Luckily, you'll most likely feel a really strong urge to do so with your contractions at this phase. It can take a few hours or mere minutes to push your baby out and into the world. Your baby's head comes out first, in what is known as crowning. (The location of your baby's head as it descends is called its station, which can tell you how far along in phase two you are. Read more on page 315.) This stage continues until your baby has fully passed through the birth canal and your vagina and has been delivered.

Technically, you are done with labor now—because labor is the work needed to get you to this point. The only thing left to do is push the baby out. And you'll have a surge of oxytocin to reduce pain for both you and your baby, and to give you a euphoric thunderbolt of bonding when you get to lay eyes on one another.

Phase Three

Things aren't over yet! During the third phase—the shortest of the three—you'll deliver the placenta, often called afterbirth. This can take anywhere from a few minutes to a half hour or even an hour. You may still have some contractions in an effort to detach and push the placenta out so that the uterus can clamp down and cut off the big blood vessels that were feeding the placenta. You may need to focus and bear down to help get the placenta out. Soon enough, you'll have nothing to do but enjoy some skin-to-skin contact with your precious little one and try to encourage breastfeeding, all while bathing in a sea of oxytocin. You will be in a different realm with your baby. Revel in this time.

Terms You Need to Know: Dilation, Station, Effacement

There are three terms in particular that you're going to hear repeated over and over and over during labor and delivery: dilation, station, and effacement. I talked a little about them back in Chapter 17, because they pertain to specific changes within your body that indicate if you are in fact in labor, and that give clues as to how far along you are in the birthing process. Now's the time to dive in and define and understand these terms and body transformations a bit more.

Dilation

The word dilate means to become wide; to enlarge or expand. In pregnancy, it's your cervix—the opening to your uterus—that dilates. Normally, your cervix is closed up very tight to keep your baby inside your womb for nine months, and to keep anything harmful from the outside world from entering your uterus. But when it's time for your little one to arrive, your cervix has got to open up, and that's when dilation comes into play.

Dilation starts thanks to uterine contractions. They move your baby down and out of your pelvis and into your vagina, and then out into the world. Contractions put pressure on your cervix, which causes it to widen and expand over time so that your baby can journey through the birth canal.

As shared on page 310, dilation can begin in early labor. At this stage, your cervix will usually progress from zero centimeters dilated to about three or four centimeters dilated, becoming roughly the size of a quarter. But the bulk of dilation typically happens when

CERVICAL DILATION

the GRADUAL OPENING of the CERVIX
measured in CENTIMETERS from 0 to 10 CM

1 CM
BLUEBERRY

2 CM
GRAPE

3 CM
BANANA

5 CM
KIWI FRUIT

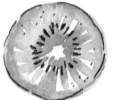

6 CM
TOMATO

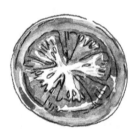

8 CM
APPLE

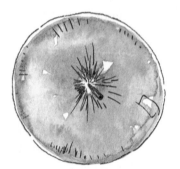

10 CM!
GRAPEFRUIT

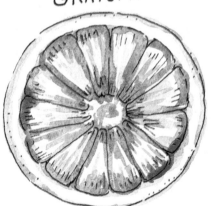

you're in the active labor stage of phase one. From early labor through active labor, your cervix dilates from zero to 10 centimeters; 10 centimeters is considered fully dilated, and 10 is the number needed for a vaginal delivery. Being fully dilated means your baby has the space it needs to be born and you're ready to start pushing. Ten centimeters is about the width of a softball or bagel, or, perhaps an easier to imagine and much more apt comparison, the diameter of your baby's head. Every woman dilates at a different pace. Again, you may be a few centimeters dilated in early labor, and this dilation can occur even a few days before you give birth. Or you may not dilate at all until your contractions really heat up and active labor gets underway. Your doctor or midwife will use their fingers to feel your cervix and gauge dilation.

Although dilation is important, it's not the only measure of how your labor is progressing—there's also station and effacement to consider (which I cover next). I'm pointing this out because it can be discouraging to go through multiple hours of contractions to find that you've only dilated an additional centimeter; you may feel defeated. But there is plenty of other important progress to be made, so try not to get too focused on this one number.

Station

Station tells you, in number form, how your baby is progressing through the birth canal. Typically, station refers to how far your baby's head has descended into your pelvis, as their head usually presents first. If your baby is not in a headfirst position, though, station could describe how far their buttocks or feet, for example, have descended. The distance is measured by the relationship of their head (or butt or feet, etc.) to the bony protrusions in your pelvis that you've probably heard a yoga teacher call sit bones. During a cervical exam, your doctor or midwife will feel for your baby and your sit bones and assign a station number from -5 to +5 to describe their positioning.

There are other words to know here, too. Before your baby has begun to descend into your pelvis, they're in a negative station. Usually a couple of weeks before labor, they drop down into the birth canal and become engaged, aka active participants in the labor and delivery process. (Dropping is also often called lightening.) When they drop, they are at a zero station; their head (or butt or feet) are now level with your pelvis. Station numbers then progress as positive digits per each centimeter they descend down into your pelvis. At +3 station, your baby's head is beginning to crown and emerge from the birth canal; at +5, their head is crowning or filling your vaginal opening and they are seconds away from being born. While a baby often drops and engages around 36 weeks, for some women this may happen later in their pregnancy or once labor has actually begun. You may realize you've "pulled into" station zero and your baby has dropped because you'll likely feel more room in your belly and like you're able to take bigger, deeper breaths. You may also need to urinate more often, as there will be increased pressure on your bladder at this point.

Effacement

In addition to widening in preparation for birth, the cervix also shortens and thins out, or effaces. You may also hear this process called cervical thinning or ripening. Effacement is measured in percentages. Just as you need to be fully dilated, or 10 centimeters dilated, for a vaginal delivery, you need to be 100 percent effaced for a vaginal birth. Your doctor or midwife will conduct a cervical exam to gauge effacement as they gauge dilation. Interestingly, first-time moms typically efface before they dilate, whereas women who have already given birth dilate before they efface.

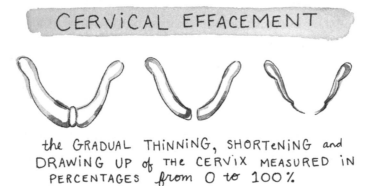

CERVICAL EFFACEMENT

the GRADUAL THINNING, SHORTeNING and DRAWING UP of THE CERVIX MEASURED iN PERCENTAGES from 0 to 100%

Ways for Your Partner to Support You in Labor

I'm writing this directly to you, partners and/or birth coaches. Of course, labor is most intense and challenging for the one who's giving birth. But it's not exactly a walk in the park for you, either… especially if you aren't sure how to be helpful. Here's a list to help you know what to do to be the best support for your partner.

- Time her contractions. You want to time both how long the contractions last as well as the length of time between when one contraction ends and the next one begins— this will be one of the first questions your care provider will ask when you call them to tell them that labor is starting.

- Call her care provider. Let them know what's happening (know the contraction times and any other signs of early labor).

- Manage any phone calls or texts from family and friends. Some people won't be able to stop themselves; they'll want to call and find out what's going on. You should be the one to field those calls—if your partner gets them, they may cause her anxiety (nothing like hearing "Where's the baby?" to think you're not doing it right), and anxiety slows down labor. You can also call the folks you know will want to know that things have gotten started.

- Set the mood. Darken the room, shoo people out so that she can have privacy, and make things quiet, except for any background noise that appeals to her (a favorite playlist or a white noise machine, as examples).

- Clean the bathroom and birth room. This is a must-do if she's birthing at home; even if you're planning a trip to the birth center or hospital, do this so that she can stay home as long as possible without unnecessary risk of infection.

- **Get out the birth kit and sterilized towels and bedding.** Time to get out all those supplies you've been stockpiling. Your home birth midwife may have additional instructions for you.

- **Eat something.** You'll need your stamina, too. Eat something and fix something for the birther while you're at it.

- **Rest.** If contractions are starting at night, try to get your rest (and encourage her to do the same).

- **Gather the devices you want to have on hand.** You'll want your phone and perhaps a portable speaker, camera, and possibly other devices nearby; don't forget to grab her chargers as well.

- **Provide emotional support.** Your most important job is to reassure your partner. Let her know you love and appreciate her. Tell her things like: "You're doing great." "You're amazing." "You can do this." "You're so strong." "I love you so much." "Everything is going great." "It's going to be OK." Feeling loved really does help. A lot.

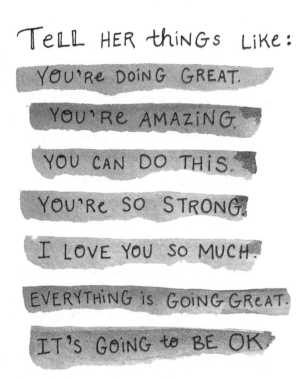

TELL HER things LiKe:
YOU'RE DOING GREAT.
YOU'RE AMAZING.
YOU CAN DO THIS.
YOU'RE SO STRONG.
I LOVE YOU SO MUCH.
EVERYTHING is GOING GREAT.
IT'S GOING to BE OK.

- **Lend physical support.** Help support her weight while she squats by standing behind her and lifting up an appropriate amount (that feels good to her) under her armpits. Or be more of a slow-dance partner, where you are facing each other, her arms around your shoulders so she can lean her weight either into you or downward during contractions. Suggest she change positions when the dynamic needs to be shifted, whether for emotional (fear or upset) or physical reasons (intense discomfort, trying to slow down and speed up labor).

- **Check in with her.** It's always best to ask her want she wants and be a good communicator. You may think she'll want a massage—maybe you've even discussed doing that beforehand—but then she may hate the feeling of being touched. It helps to ask.

- **Apply counterpressure or acupressure.** Your can press the palms of both your hands strongly on the area of her back that's experiencing pain—push in with the contractions and release in between. It can also be helpful during early labor to press strongly with your thumbs or even elbows into the places on either side of her neck where her neck and shoulders meet—this is an acupressure point for alleviating pain. Later, during active labor when the baby has moved down more, your can press your thumbs into the indentations along either side of her sacrum, the triangular bone at the base of her spine. Start by pressing your thumbs into the indentations at the top of her sacrum and wrapping your fingers around her outer hips; then as the baby moves farther down, you can move your thumbs farther down the sacrum. During each contraction press in with your thumbs and pull back with your fingers to help encourage the pelvis to open; release the pressure once the contraction ends.

- **Remind her to drink, eat, suck on ice chips, and try to pee.** She will most likely be on another plane for at least part of labor and won't remember to do these basic things.

Smart Strategies Once Early Labor Has Started

Once your contractions are growing longer, stronger, and closer together, you're out of warm-up and into official early labor. Here are some tips to keep your progress humming along.

- **Stay active.** Once you truly are in early labor, stay up and moving around; it will help your labor progress.

- **Eat.** Even if it's not normally a time when you would have a meal. You will need the energy! (And if you end up at a hospital, they won't let you eat once you get there until after the baby is born.) Keep in mind that it might come back up, so make everything you eat now very digestible, such as mashed potatoes, applesauce, fresh fruit, avocados, yogurt, miso soup, chicken broth, vegetable soup. If you become nauseated, stop eating.

- **Don't resist.** Remember that the strong sensations of your contractions are doing the work of bringing your baby into the world. Do everything you can to not resist them—you'll just be working against your own progress. Don't fight it. You are safe.

- **Keep drinking.** Make your birth partner help ensure that you drink at least 16 ounces of fluid per hour—only water or hydration tonic listed on page 288 (no soda, no coffee; nothing dehydrating).

- **Try to urinate at least once an hour.** We are trained to relax our pelvis and pelvic floor on the toilet. It will help the whole process. If you're drinking as much as you should, you will need to pee frequently.

Do what you can to make it easy for her. Put the cup of water or coconut water with a straw in front of her face. She should have a few sips of water every 10 minutes or so, and attempt to urinate once an hour.

- **Take care of your own needs.** You can take breaks to eat, pee, and rest, too. She needs you strong, aware, and awake for the duration.

- **Breathe with her.** You can either match your breathing to hers or start a breathing exercise you learned in childbirth education class to help her remember to do it too.

Possible Laboring Positions

Of course, if you find something not on this list that works for you, by all means, use it! But it's good to know your options in advance. Of course, you can also sit and/or recline in a tub or birthing tub. Water can be a wonderful way to make contractions more bearable. It can also slow labor down—this can sometimes be a good thing if labor is progressing quickly and you'd like to lower the intensity.

Walking, Standing, Leaning (either on a piece of furniture or your partner)

- Works with gravity
- Helps stimulate contractions
- Good for early labor

Kneeling (on hands and knees, or resting your torso on a chair, bed, or your partner's lap)

- May relieve back pain
- Helps baby rotate to most favorable, facedown position
- Relieves hemorrhoids
- Good for early/active labor

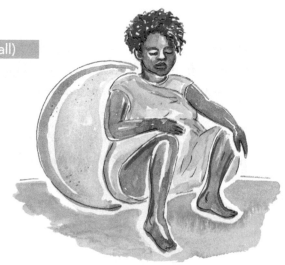

Sitting (in a chair, on the floor, on a birthing ball)

- Works with gravity

- Allows you to rest between contractions

- Good for active labor

Squatting

- Opens pelvis to provide more room

- Works with gravity

- Good for pushing (you can squat during the contractions and stand in between; have your partner stand behind you and use their legs to support you and help you stand back up—put rolled up towels or yoga blocks under your heels to make squatting easier)

One note: First-time moms may be more likely to tear when the baby crowns in a squatting position, so squat until just before that point, then lie down or get in a C-shape in bed

Reclining (either on your back propped up with pillows, or on your side)

- Allows you to rest

- Can be good for the final stage of pushing, especially for first-time moms (to prevent tearing, which can happen more in the squatting position)

Pushing Techniques

Once you're fully dilated and the baby is stationed, it's time to get the little darling out so you can finally meet them! If this sounds scary, know that by this point, the urge to push will likely be very strong. Also, the hormones that are cresting now are creating a bond between the two of you that will see you through the pain and make your meeting a truly transformational event.

- **Squat with contractions, stand up in between.** Your partner can sit on the bed and help you up and down.

- **Sit in a C position.** While sitting, curl your body into a C-shape; rest your chin on your chest, round your shoulders forward, curl your tailbone inward and upward.

- **Engage your abdominals.** All those core exercises you've done really pay off now—tighten and pull in your stomach muscles with each push so that the energy moves downward and not outward. Downward is what gets the baby out.

- **Use your breath.** If you've ever lifted heavy weights, you know that taking in a breath and holding it in while you lift gives you more power. The same goes for pushing: With each push, take a deep breath and hold it in as you bear down. Screaming or moaning will take away your air.

- **Push harder than it hurts.** This is how you get through the painful part faster.

Of course, labor isn't just a physical pursuit. It's an emotional, mental, and even spiritual journey, too—all things I'll cover in the next chapter so that you can get into the zone and stay there.

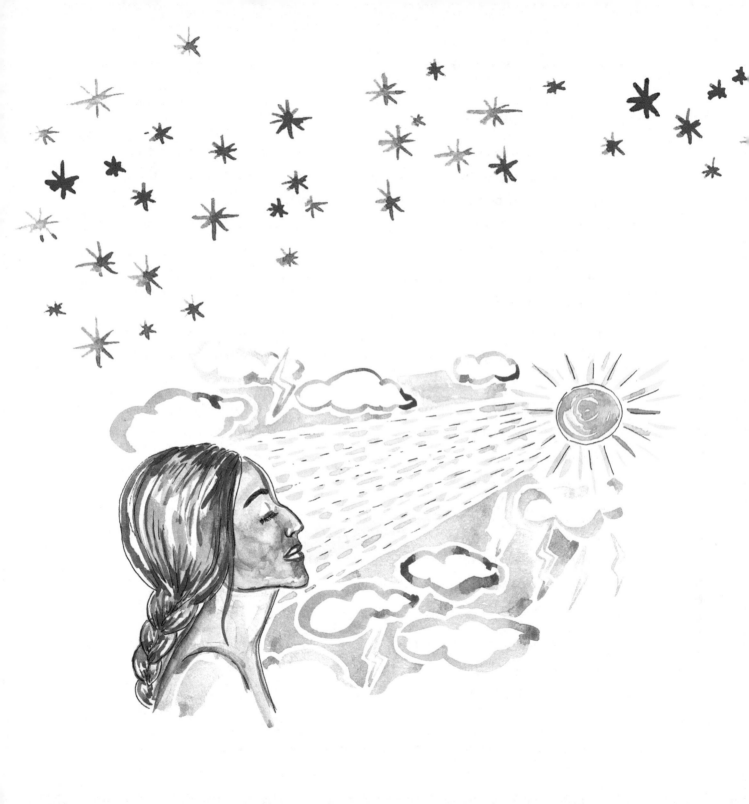

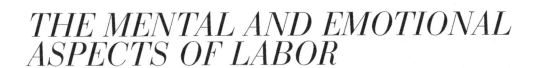

THE MENTAL AND EMOTIONAL ASPECTS OF LABOR

Yes, birth is an athletic feat. But there's so much more involved than just your body. It's an enormous workout for your mind, emotions, and spirit too. Not only are you performing a miracle by giving birth to another human—something that can't help but get you thinking about a higher power—but you are also going to be confronting fear and pain. Birth will bring up all kinds of emotions and thoughts for you, and you really want to have a plan for how you'll help yourself stay in a good mental place.

There's a cycle you don't want to get stuck in: fear leads to tension leads to pain. It's known as FTP for short. Interestingly, FTP is also a medical abbreviation for failure to progress in labor. In this chapter, we're going to cover the many tools you have to keep yourself out of FTP and stay in a zone where you are relaxed, in the moment, and present for the magic.

The Ability to Relax Is Your Super Power

When it comes to labor, relaxation is key. I know, it may sound like relaxation and labor are two words that don't belong in the same sentence—how can you relax when you're giving birth? But I don't necessarily mean that you are totally chill and kicked back. In labor, relaxation is more about what part of your nervous system is activated.

Your autonomic nervous system enervates your internal organs—including your blood vessels, your digestive organs, and your reproductive organs. It's divided into two main branches: the sympathetic nervous system, which is activated when you are stressed and rules your fight, flight, or freeze functions; and the parasympathetic nervous system, which comes online when you're relaxed and orchestrates your rest and digest functions. The more you are in the parasympathetic realm, the more relaxed your muscles will be and the easier it will be to move the baby out of your body. If you are stressed, it's almost like your body is working against you—it's going to go into protective mode and divert blood and energy away from your internal organs so that you can run away or fight.

On the other hand, the parasympathetic sphere is a healing realm. When you're in it, you're relaxed and calm. Your blood, and the oxygen it carries with it, is flowing easily to your baby. Your cervix will easily soften, and your uterus will be able to relax (which actually makes it stronger, because a tight muscle is a weak muscle). If you're in FTP, it's going to send your blood and oxygen to your limbs, your cervix will tighten, and your labor can stall.

Let's take a look at some of the tools you have at your disposal to help you get in—and stay in—the parasympathetic realm.

> " THE MORE YOU are in the PARASYMPATHETIC REALM, the MORE RELAXED your MUSCLES WILL BE and THE EASIER iT WILL BE to MOVE the BABY OUT of your BODY. "

Minimize Distractions (That Means People, Too)

Privacy is a big piece of feeling relaxed and safe—particularly when you're in a physically vulnerable position as you are when you're giving birth. This is a huge reason why I chose to give birth at home—you have so much more control over who's in your space at home than you do at the hospital. And that's not just about your comfort; it's about setting the stage for a positive birth experience.

One of the most important ways to create the safety of privacy is to be very, very thoughtful about who you invite into the room where you are laboring. Remember that birth is a sensual experience. Oxytocin, which is cresting in labor, is the orgasm hormone. I'm not saying your birth will be orgasmic (although it could be), but you want to have enough privacy to get into the same headspace that you are in when you're having great sex.

That means whoever's in the room with you needs to be able to let you feel unobserved, and certainly not judged. A lot of the ways we communicate are nonverbal, so even if someone promises to keep their mouth shut, they may broadcast things like fear, anxiety, or judgment that will impede your ability to relax. Even animals often choose a place to give birth where they're not being watched. Just keep this principle in mind: Birth is not a spectator sport. Privacy is important for giving you the sense of safety that helps you relax.

It can be difficult to keep people out of your room in a hospital, where nurses, doctors, and sometimes residents may freely walk in and out. Each time they do, your internal voice likely thinks, "Who is this person and what do they want?" Talk to your partner, birth coach, or doula about who they should and shouldn't let into the area where you're laboring.

One of the reasons privacy is so important is that it helps you keep any negative energy from other people out of your space. For this reason, it's also a good idea to talk to your partner about how important it is that they manage their emotions around you while you're in the throes of labor.

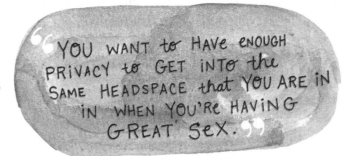

"YOU WANT to HAVE eNOUGH PRIVACY to GET INTO the SAME HEADSPACE that YOU ARE IN iN WHEN YOU'Re HAVING GREAT SeX."

They can give some thought to who they'll talk to if they have moments in which they need support (doulas are great for this). When you're in labor, you need their love and support—you don't want to have to support them while you're in your time of need. You also don't want their moments of panic or fear (which are perfectly normal for them to have) to spread to you.

Set the Mood

In addition to who is in the room, there are other aspects of your physical space that can help foster that sense of safety that allows you to relax. Some of the elements you want to think about in whatever room you labor in are sound, light, sights, and smell.

Sound

It doesn't need to be so quiet you can hear a pin drop, but you want to minimize stressful sounds, like TVs, loud music, machines beeping, phones dinging, and even people talking. You can use a white noise machine, or run a fan, to create a soothing background noise. Or make a playlist of music that gets you in a relaxed state—think more spa music than pop music. Noise-cancelling headphones can really help protect your mental space, too.

In a hospital setting, you can always ask them to turn the noises on the monitors that are in the room with you way down or off completely. Especially once you're in active labor, it's best to keep the screens off. Labor takes focus, and screens are focus hogs.

Light

Try to minimize the artificial light you're exposed to, especially at night. If it's dark when you're laboring, keep lights dim and use electric candles or even holiday lights to add ambient lighting. If you're laboring in the day, try to have some natural light in the room by opening the blinds or curtains. Your hormones are very sensitive to light exposure, and you want to keep your light levels lower at night and brighter during the day to help your hormones find their natural levels.

Sights

The things you can see have a big impact on your mental state, so know that you can always choose what you're looking at. You may want to make a poster board with your affirmations written on it so you can look at it during labor—that's what I did, and each time, there were one or two affirmations that I really latched onto and spent many contractions looking at, letting those words carry my attention away from the pain. You can also make eye contact with your partner or doula—being seen and sharing that space with another person can make you feel supported. And remember that you can always close your eyes—it's an instant way to give yourself privacy and darkness.

Smell

You might be super sensitive to smells, as your oxytocin will be running high and it can trigger nausea. Ask your partner, coach, or doula to move anything that might be smelly—like the laundry hamper—away from where you're laboring. And think about having some essential oils on hand (I make suggestions on which ones in the next chapter) to diffuse, sprinkle on a damp washcloth that you can keep around the back of your neck or on your forehead, or even just take a whiff of straight from the bottle.

Also remember that whenever there's something happening that you don't like or want—pressure that's coming either from outside or inside—you can always interrupt it by going to the bathroom. The privacy it gives you and the fact that you are trained to relax on the toilet can help shift things into a more favorable pattern.

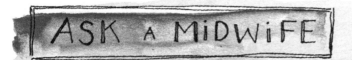

WHAT MENTAL STRATEGIES CAN HELP ME THROUGH THE PAIN?

from MARi MiKeL:

"The best thing you can do is stop trying to resist the pain. Remind yourself that moving through pain is the way out. After all: no pain, no baby. Be a noodle, go limp, and don't fight. You are safe.

"Also remember that there is a gift in the pain of labor, and that is transformation. You are being forever changed by this physical trial, by the bonding hormones that birth elicits, and by love."

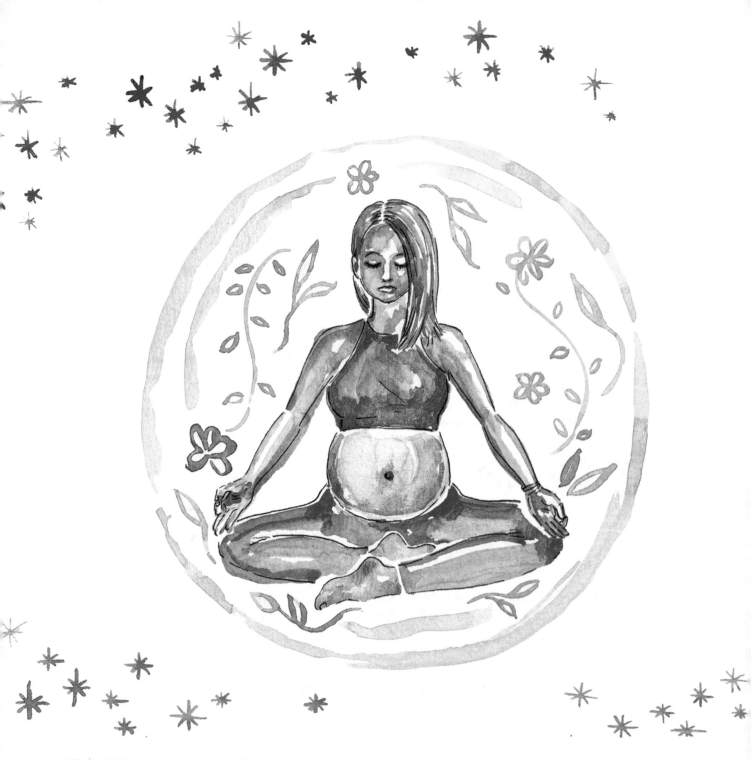

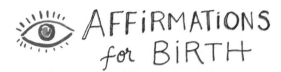

AFFIRMATIONS for BIRTH

I DESERVE THIS BIRTH.

MY BODY IS COMPLETELY RELAXED.

I TRUST my BODY.   I BELIEVE IN MYSELF.

ALL IS WELL.   I LISTEN to MY BODY.

I RELEASE STRESS EASILY.

MY BODY WAS MADE for THIS.

EVERYTHING IS GOING JUST GREAT.

SOFT, OPEN, RELAXED.

INHALE PEACE, EXHALE TENSION.

MY BODY WAS DESIGNED for THIS.

I AM LOVED.   MY BABY IS LOVED.

I LOVE my BODY.   I LOVE my BABY.

MY BODY and MY BABY ARE DOING JUST WHAT THEY SHOULD.

I AM AN AMAZING WOMAN.

I AM CALM.

CONTRACTIONS ARE MY FRIEND.

THE BABY and I ARE DOING BEAUTIFULLY.

ASK A DOULA

WHAT'S THE BEST WAY TO QUIET MY MIND DURING LABOR?

from KHRISTINa

"Just like you want to do squats and core exercises to strengthen the muscles you'll need for birth, you also want to train your mind to help you stay clear-headed once labor begins. As a Hypnobirthing instructor, I teach my clients to practice the things that quiet their mind and get them into a dreamy, relaxed state every day. If you haven't already, start reading and repeating your affirmations daily. Also think of a setting that's the most relaxing spot in the world for you—really imagine all the sights, sounds, and smells and tune into how your body feels when you're there. Then spend a few minutes each day visualizing yourself there—it will give you a place you can 'go to' in your mind during labor where you have a recent experience of being fully relaxed. Your imagination is so powerful; even if you've never done any visualizations before, you can elicit a very real sense of relaxation your first time trying it. When you practice your visualizations now, it will be easy for you to visit that relaxed state during labor."

HOW CAN I ADVOCATE FOR MYSELF DURING LABOR?

"It's so important that you think through how you'd like things to go in labor beforehand. You've got to expect the unexpected, especially when you're doing something as amazing as giving birth.

"Once labor starts, you're not going to be thinking as clearly. You're going to be more vulnerable. You decide that you don't want an epidural, for example, but if a nurse offers it to you when you're in active labor, it will be hard to turn it down—kind of like waving a milkshake in front of your face when you're starving but you're trying to avoid sugar.

"It's important to have someone in the room who can help you remember what's important to you and your wishes for labor, whether that's your partner or your doula or someone else you trust. If someone suggests turning on the TV in early labor and waiting for you to dilate, your partner or doula can ask you, 'What do you know about what helps you go into the zone?' Answering that question can help you remember that what you really need is privacy and quiet, so you can say, 'No, I want the TV off and I need some privacy, please.' Ideally your partner can handle being your intermediary, so all you have to do is go into the zone and stay there.

"Just remember that even though planning is important, you still need be able to roll with the unexpected. At my first birth, I had all these affirmations written out and I told my husband that I wanted him to read them to me when labor got challenging. Once we got to the hospital, got checked in, and got into the labor room, I got directly in the tub. My husband was holding my hand and I wouldn't let him leave my side to do any of the things we had talked about doing. That's why I like to call birth plans birth preferences—because you can't plan how labor is going to go. You can only stay connected to what you know to be true, and your partner (or doula) can help you do that.

"If you get to a point in your labor when you start to feel fear or doubt creep in, a powerful technique is to remember why you're in the room—that you're there to give life to your child, that you've been preparing for this day for at least nine months (and for many women, it's been a long journey to getting pregnant, so this is the culmination of something they've been working toward for years). You can always take just one second to get quiet and talk to your baby; tell them that you love them and you can't wait to meet them, assure them that everything is going to be fine, and even ask them what they need in this moment—you're already bonded to them on multiple levels, remember that they are your partner in this and it can help you have the strength to go on. (Also remember that feeling overwhelmed is a hallmark of transition, and that your feeling is completely natural and it means you are getting close!)"

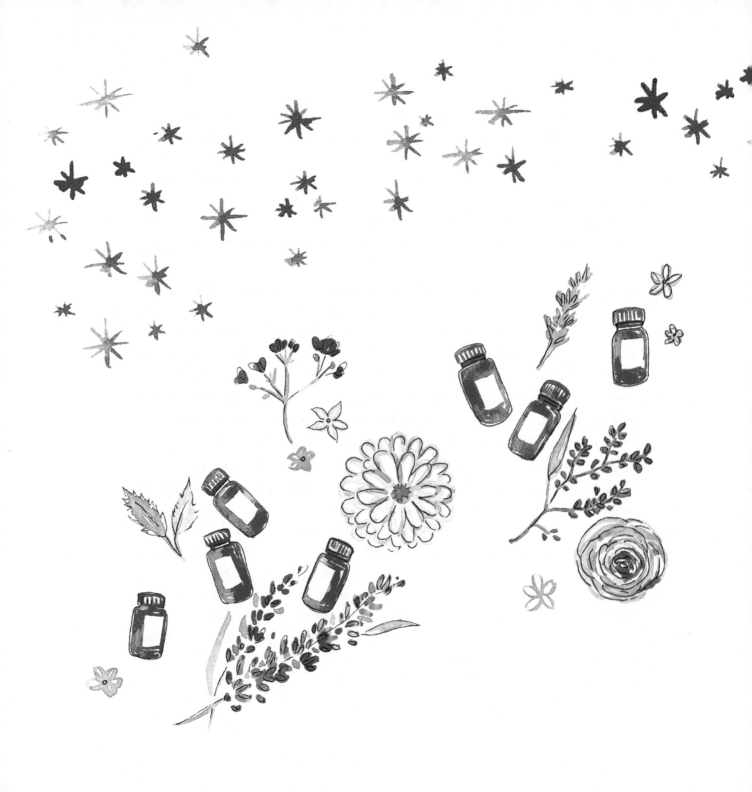

Chapter 21

NATURAL REMEDIES FOR LABOR AND DELIVERY

L abor is such an individual experience, one that you can prepare for but not truly plan for. You just can't know what will appeal to you (or repel you) until you're in it. There are a few tricks and products you can learn about and gather in advance, though, that may provide just what you need in the moment.

Here are a few of the things I found helpful during my labors, and that Khristina and Mari Mikel have used to great success with their clients.

Nausea Remedies

It's very common to feel nauseated or even vomit in labor. (You can thank cresting oxytocin levels for that.) One trick you can use is to keep a bowl with ice and a little bit of water nearby with a washcloth in it. When you feel nauseated, have someone hold that cold cloth on your throat. That will slow down the firing of your vagus nerve, which runs down your neck and into your abdomen and all its organs, and can help keep your nausea at bay. Heat, bright light, movement, and certain smells can all make it worse. Inhaling peppermint essential oil can also help. Khristina says she had a client who was feeling nauseated on her hour-long ride to the hospital; she held a bottle of peppermint essential oil up to her nose for the whole ride, and only threw up once she got out of the car. Sometimes you've just got to get it out and then you'll feel better.

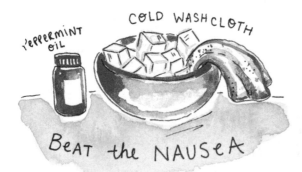

PEPPERMINT OIL · COLD WASHCLOTH

BEAT the NAUSEA

Helpful Tools

- Scalp massager. These are made out of wire and look a little like an octopus—your partner can use one on your hand between contractions to help you relax.

- Fine-tooth hair combs. There are a lot of pain receptors in the palms of your hands; when you squeeze the ends of the comb into your palm, you help override some of the pain signals that are coming from your contractions. We naturally clench our fists and squeeze our fingernails into our palms when we are stressed; this just intensifies that action. Have two combs, one for each hand, and as your contractions come on, you can curl your fingers around the comb and squeeze the tips of the teeth into your palms.

Essential Oils for Birth

You can use an essential oil a few different ways—you can add it to a diffuser for a more ambient effect; sprinkle a few drops on a warm washcloth and hold it up near your face; mix a couple drops with a teaspoon of neutral oil (like sweet almond or coconut) and massage it into the skin on the back of your neck, bottoms of feet, wrists, or ankles; or just hold the bottle up to your nose.

The following essential oils have been shown in studies to provide the benefit I've listed for women during childbirth. Just remember that it's important that the oil actually smell good to you in the moment, otherwise it might just be an irritant.

Pain relief
Lavender
Bitter orange (*Citrus aurantium*) [36]

Lowered stress/anxiety
Rose (*Rose centifolia*) [37]
Geranium (*Pelargonium graveolens*) [38]

Nausea
Peppermint

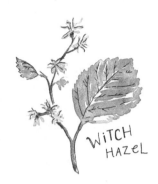

WITCH HAZEL

- **Witch hazel.** Witch hazel is a powerful anti-inflammatory derived from the witch hazel tree (maybe you've used it as an astringent on your face). It feels great on your pelvic floor—it's instantly cooling. Either keep some in a spray bottle, or pour a little bit on a cotton pad.

- **Large exercise ball.** One of these big rubber balls can give you a place to rest your body weight while still being upright; even when you're sitting on one, you can move around easily to find a comfortable spot. Also, if you're sitting on the floor or on all fours, the ball is a great to lean on and find a bit of rest.

How Your Chin Can Help You Push—Or Not Push

The position of your chin has a direct impact on the effectiveness of your contractions. When you are trying to push the baby out, lowering your chin toward your chest will help you bear down. The reverse is true too; if there's ever a time when you don't want the baby to move down just yet (say, you're in the car on the way to the hospital and you don't want the baby to be delivered en route), lifting your chin up into the air during a contraction will help the baby stay put.

Breathing Exercises for Pain Reduction & Mental Focus

Probably the most effective natural remedy for labor is to use your breath to give you and your baby plenty of oxygen, your mind something to focus on other than the pain, and your body something to do other than resist.

Mari Mikel teaches her clients three basic breaths, which are based on Lamaze techniques. The pant blow really helped me stay in the zone during both my labors.

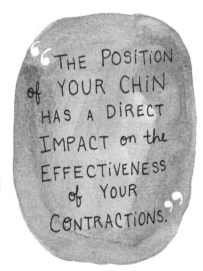

"THE POSITION of YOUR CHIN HAS A DIRECT IMPACT on the EFFECTIVENESS of YOUR CONTRACTIONS."

Deep Breathing

Works best during: Early labor

Breathe in through your nose and out through your mouth for equal amounts of time. Fully inhale, then fully exhale, and repeat. You can return to a normal breathing pattern between contractions.

Panting

Works best during: Active labor

When deep breathing stops being as helpful, switch to the pant—a breathing pattern that all animals do when they give birth. This breath is shallower than deep breathing. With each inhale and exhale, breathe through your mouth and make a whispery 'hee' sound as you do. Take a deep cleansing breath at the beginning of the contraction, then start panting, keeping it very light. Start out slow and speed up as the contraction intensifies. Then you can slow down as the contraction recedes and take another deep cleansing breath when the contraction is over. Breathe normally between contractions.

This breath will signal to you and to the people around you when the contractions begin, crest, and end. It helps you remember that they do end, and that you only need to focus on one at a time.

Pant Blow

Works best during: Transition and pushing

Like its name suggests, this breath builds on the pant and adds a more pronounced (although not longer) blowing out of air. The pattern is like this: hee (quick exhale); quick inhale; hee (quick exhale); quick inhale; hee (quick exhale); quick inhale; blow (longer exhale), all in the same rhythm—the blow is exactly the same length of the pant. Adding the blow forces you to concentrate a bit harder to keep the rhythm; it also separates each contraction up into manageable bits. Again, you can do a deep cleansing breath at the beginning and end of each contraction, and match the speed of your breathing to the intensity of the contractions. And then you still breathe normally between contractions. It's good to practice all the breaths beforehand, but the pant blow requires the most practice—it's worth the prep, though, believe me!

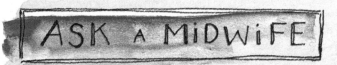

WILL VOCALIZING DURING LABOR HELP OR HURT THE PROCESS?

from MARI MIKEL:

"I know how tempting it is to want to moan or even scream during contractions—kind of like tennis players shout when they hit the ball. But in my experience, the more you vocalize, the more stress and anxiety you and your baby tend to feel. You really want to keep as much oxygen as you can circulating to you and the baby, and making sounds diverts oxygen outward. At births I've attended where the mother makes a lot of loud sounds, the baby tends to come out with a high heart rate; I think it stresses them out. It's not your voice that's going to get that baby out, it's your core and your pelvic floor. Staying quieter will help you send more of your focus and your breath to these key players.

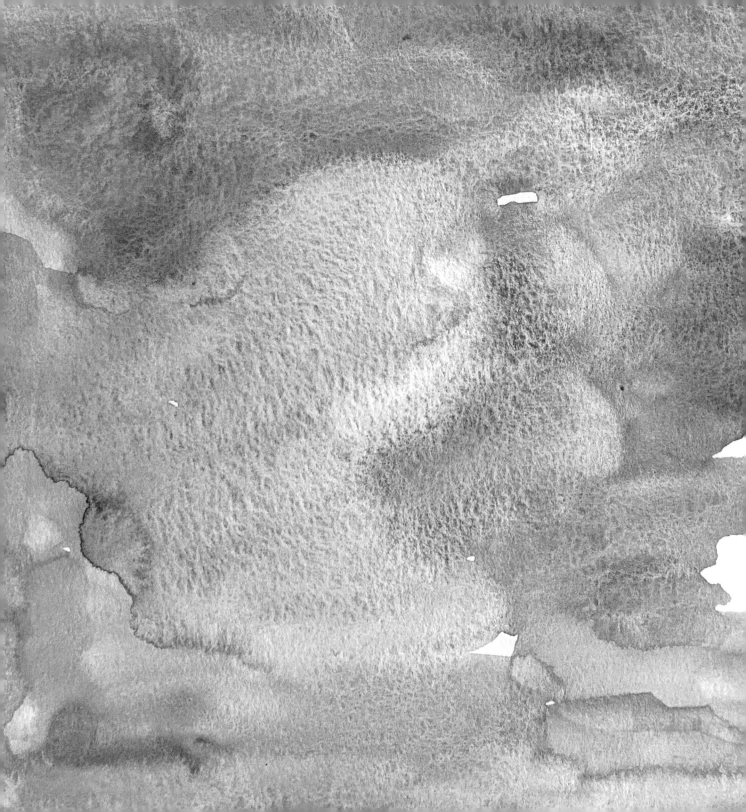

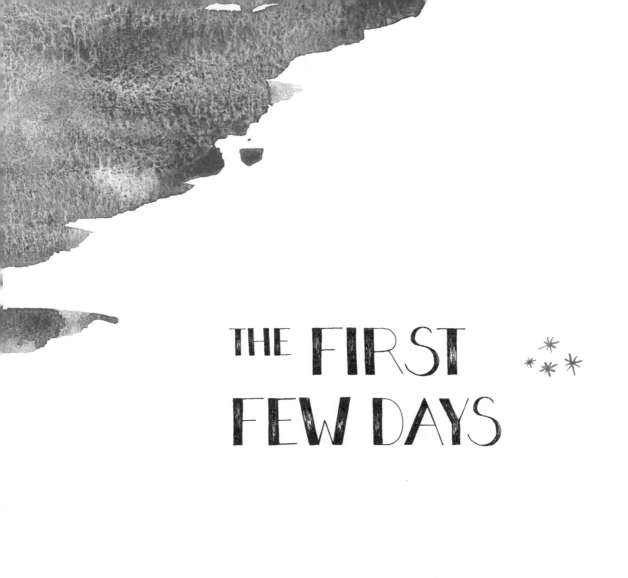

THE FIRST FEW DAYS

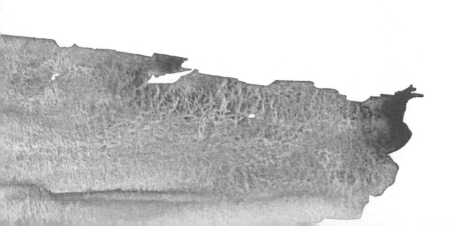

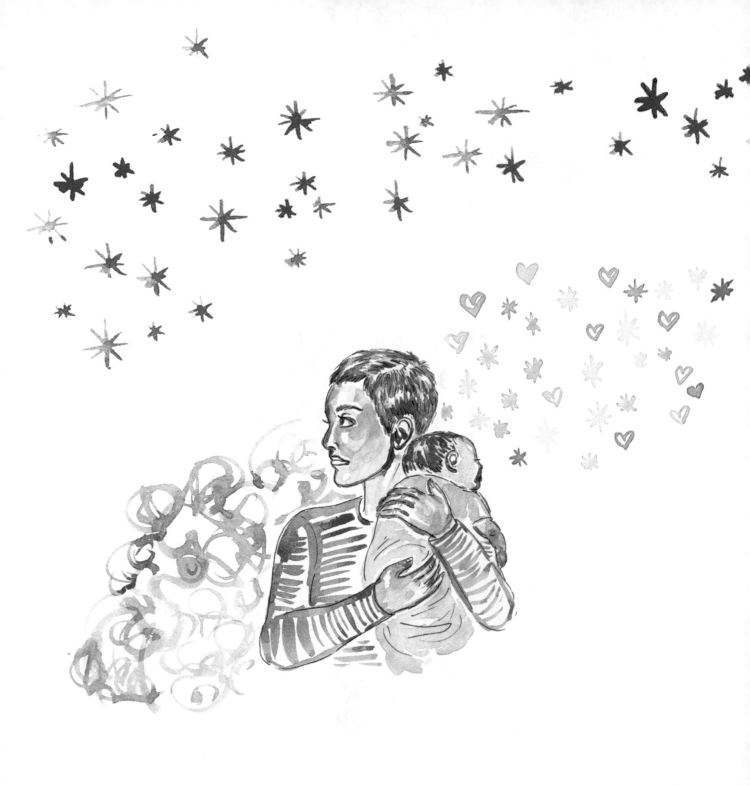

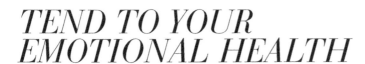

Chapter 22

TEND TO YOUR EMOTIONAL HEALTH

I n the first few days after your baby (or babies) is born, there are no two ways about it: You are on an emotional rollercoaster that is fueled by hormones. It's common to bounce between elation, overwhelm, and exhaustion, peppered with crabbiness and moments of just getting lost in love with your baby and feeling awe over how amazing they are.

You may ride on euphoria for a few days—I did—but at some point the crash comes. It's like you're living in a different dimension than everyone else. Your partner is more rested than you. You are in your own reality. After the twins were born, I barely left them for the first 10 days. Because they were born in mid-December, after 10 days it was Christmas, and even though then I was in the same room as our other family members, I felt like I was observing but not really a part of the gathering. And I wasn't even dealing with my milk coming in that time around! After my second son Legend was born, I remember being really mean when that was happening—there was a moment I remember clearly of standing in our closet and just hating my husband. I don't remember the specifics of why, now. It can be helpful to tell your partner that if you have moments of intense bitchiness, not to take it personally. You need time and space to feel your feelings so you can ultimately move past them. In this chapter, I'll share some ways to find—and protect—that time and space.

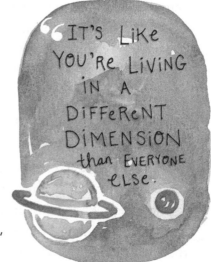

"IT'S LiKE YOU'RE LiViNG iN A DiFFeReNT DiMENSiON than EVERYONE eLSe.

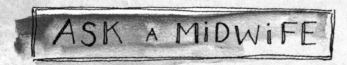

WHY AM I ALL OVER THE PLACE RIGHT NOW?

from MARi MiKeL:

"The amount of hormones it takes for your body to give birth are enormous. As soon as baby comes out, those hormones have to subside so that the hormones of breastfeeding and bonding can come to the forefront. That means your entire being is in flux. If you feel all over the place, it's because you're in the midst of a huge transition. Give over to it, and to the bonding that's happening now. It is sacred. The biochemical things that are happening in both you and your baby during these early days lead to a lifelong bond to each other and foster the baby's ability to connect with other people throughout their lifetime.

"Exhaustion has its own biochemistry, and after giving birth, no matter how it went, your body is tired and needs rest. It's hard to sleep after giving birth, too, because having lived through what is likely to be the biggest physical endeavor of your life is such a relief and holding your baby (or babies) is such a rush. You're also likely to be worried about whether the baby is breathing, and what if they can't latch properly, or what if they don't like you? Your mind is on hyperalert. By the time the third day hits you are super exhausted.

"You may also be coming down off of stress hormones, especially if you were in a hospital setting or your birth didn't go the way you had hoped. There's also a hormonal storm that happens when your milk comes in, which generally happens two to three days after birth.

"I tell my clients to expect being intensely crabby during these first few days. It's another reason not to have your mother there telling you not to pick the baby up that way, or saying things like, 'I didn't do it that way and you turned out just fine.' You'll want to bite her head off. Don't put yourself in a position in which you'll feel you have to try to be more than you can be. Give yourself the space to do less—physically, yes, but emotionally and mentally too."

Give Yourself the Gift of Space

The first few days after birth are sacred space. Really give some thought to who you want around you at this time. You may feel you should invite people over to meet the baby right away, but it takes energy to entertain people. Even if you don't plan to get out of bed or up off the couch while they're there, you will probably feel that you need to have the house tidy and your hair brushed. As much as is humanly possible, you want to give yourself the space to just be enthralled by your baby. That may even mean not seeing people who want to bring you food. Doing so is a lovely gesture; accept their offer, but have your partner ask them to leave it by the door.

Plus, you want to be able to nap whenever you get sleepy. If someone's just shown up at your house just as your eyes are starting to close on their own, you'll rouse yourself because you don't want to be rude.

When you don't have the distractions of other people around, you can devote all your energy to bonding, healing, and feeling your feelings. Dealing with people detracts from your bonding, your care of your baby, and your healing.

The one exception to this suggestion is any professionals you may want to bring in specifically for the purpose of supporting you now (see more about your options on page 347). If you or the baby needs care, absolutely get it. I'm just saying, think about how much socializing you want to do during this time, and be mindful of the people in your life who may say they want to help, but who in reality will take too much of your energy.

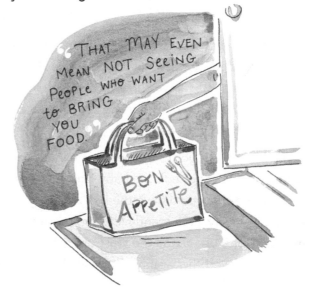

"THAT MAY EVEN MEAN NOT SEEING PEOPLE WHO WANT to BRING YOU FOOD."

BON APPETITE

For example, if one or both of your parents or in-laws are more takers than they are givers, stand your ground, ask them not to come right away, and give yourself a break. Have them hold off a bit until you have more energy to meet their needs.

For the people in your life you trust to honor your bubble and who truly want to help, some things they can do for you now include:

- Doing laundry
- Making meals
- Cleaning up
- Playing with older kids
- Running errands

You want to be the one holding the baby, at least in these first three days. There will be plenty of times when you will happily let someone else hold them in the weeks and months to come!

Newborn Support Options

If you are having any difficulties at all, please don't hesitate to get the support you need. You might not even think you need it. I know I didn't.

Before my first child was born, a friend suggested that we get a baby nurse. I thought it was ridiculous. In fact, I was really upset by it, as if she were suggesting that I couldn't take care of a baby. I was pregnant and pissed. I did agree to talk to a mutual friend of ours who had had a baby nurse. When I chatted with her, it sounded fine, but I was not at all convinced. My husband said, "Let's just try it. If you don't like it, we'll send her home."

The baby nurse got to us the day Hendrix was born. I remember looking at her like who is this woman? She took the baby from me, re-swaddled him, and told me to go take a shower and she would have the baby waiting for me right there. I noticed she swaddled him really nicely. I reluctantly left and came back 20 minutes later. I just watched her with my baby for a bit. It was the start of my building trust in others to care for my kids. Two weeks in, I loved this woman. I'm really happy I did it.

I didn't have a doula or a lactation consultant because Mari Mikel prides herself on performing those roles in addition to being a midwife. But if I hadn't had her, I certainly would have hired these professionals to benefit from their support. I didn't use a sleep consultant, but I have seen them change people's lives when they can't get their babies to sleep. I'm a big proponent of hiring professionals, because the chance of you having access to all this wisdom inside your family or friend group is so small. We don't grow up around extended family anymore, so we aren't exposed to babies and child-rearing throughout our lives. When we do have kids, our learning curve is steep. If you can't hire a consultant or a baby nurse, read the books and watch the videos on your subject on YouTube. Do what it takes to get support at whatever level you can manage, because the truth is, you need it. It's no failing on your part.

> "WE DON'T GROW UP AROUND extended FAMILY ANYMORE, SO We AREN'T EXPOSED to BABies and CHILD-REARING THROUGHOUT OUR LIVES. WHEN WE DO HAVE KIDS, OUR LEARNING CURVe is STEEP."

Whether you're a new mom—or a second-, third-, or fourth-time mom—if you need help in the postpartum period, I encourage you to seek it out and take it. All you can get, in fact. There's so much going on with your body and your mind, with your baby, in your household... It can be a difficult time, even if it's "old hat" for you. There's no need to just grin and bear it when there are a variety of really great support options available. It takes a village!

Here's a basic rundown of your options:

Breastfeeding Support

There are many ways to feel supported around your nursing efforts. You can talk to friends, family members, and neighbors who have breastfed their own children; you can hear their struggles to know you're not alone, and learn their tips and tricks for success. If you want more formalized help, consider the following avenues.

Lactation Consultant

You've heard over and over that "breast is best," and that you should exclusively breastfeed for your baby's first six months, and then continue for their first year or two, or even longer, depending on which experts and organizations you turn to for advice or which school of thought appeals to you. But just because you "should," doesn't mean it's easy. In fact, it's estimated that around 60 percent of moms stop breastfeeding before they intended to in part because of difficulties with the act itself.[39] That's a shame, because lactation consultants (specialists trained in all aspects of breastfeeding) can really help make the process smoother for both parties involved. In fact, one review of 16 studies on the subject, with more than 5,000 participants, found that lactation consultants and counselors not only helped women initiate breastfeeding, they also improved breastfeeding rates over time, as well as boosted rates of women exclusively breastfeeding their child.[40]

Exactly which types of breastfeeding problems can a lactation consultant help with?

- Trouble with latching

- Painful nursing (sore nipples, mastitis, engorgement)

- Low milk production

- Issues with weight gain

- Position difficulties

- Emotional blocks to breastfeeding

- And the list goes on

Truly, they're trained to tackle even the most complicated cases. In general, think of them as a partner there to help you meet your breastfeeding goals. Serious difficulties or not, they can advise you on continuing a breastfeeding routine when you return to work, as well as share advice on what breastfeeding equipment to use (and how to use it properly), how to safely store pumped breast milk, and much more.

Lactation consultants often work in hospitals and doctor's offices and clinics, although they may also work for themselves. Sometimes, your health care provider may provide one for you. If you're considering working with or hiring a consultant as part of your support team, be sure to interview them just as you did your doctor and/or midwife so that you can find someone you truly connect with that you trust to join you on your motherhood journey. It's always a good idea to ask those already on your care team for recommendations. I advise choosing someone who is an International Board Certified Lactation Consultant. Learn more at iblce.org.

Other Nursing Support Options

- **Postpartum doulas:** Postpartum doulas are specially trained in postnatal issues, including breastfeeding, and can often help with the nursing issues you're having. If they can't, they're a great resource for additional options. Read more about postpartum doulas on the next page.

- **La Leche League:** This international organization promotes breastfeeding as an important part of a baby's healthy development and provides educational resources and mother-to-mother support through online and in-person groups. Learn more and find groups near you at llli.org and by searching Facebook.

- **Other online resources, from videos and tutorials to support groups to podcasts:** La Leche League has lots of great online resources, as do many other groups and organizations; not to mention, much can be found on YouTube.

In writing this book, I came across the *New York Times* article "If Only Everyone Had a Postpartum Doula." The title alone speaks to the immense benefits these support team members provide! It goes on to discuss the void they fill in our medical system, providing important care for mom, baby, and the entire family during the critical postpartum period.

Postpartum doulas provide nonmedical physical, emotional, and educational support specifically in the days and months after you've given birth. As mentioned above, they can provide breastfeeding support, but they can help in so many other ways as well.

As are all doulas, postpartum doulas are a wealth of information and resources. They can educate you about normal newborn behavior, easing fears and providing practical advice to get you through what can be a harrowing time. They can teach you new techniques for soothing and comforting a fussy baby, as well as help make diapering and bathing as easy as possible. Of course, they also know what's normal for your health, and can assist in your healing and recovery process, including if you've had a Cesarean birth.

> " A POSTPARTUM DOULA iS OFTeN SAiD to NURTURE the ENTiRE fAMiLY, and TO HELP EVERYONE iNVOLVED EASE iNTO THEIR NeW LiFe WiTH A NeWBORN. "

And it doesn't end there. They can help around the house as well, with things like meal preparation and light housework, and they can even run your errands, all in an effort to help you (and the rest of your family; more in a minute) feel less overwhelmed and to give you more time to bond with your little one.

In other words, they're not just there for you and your baby's physical health, they're there for emotional support, too. Maybe that's by providing the information you need to feel relaxed and assured, or a hug, or a helping hand, or even by supporting the other people in your close circle. A postpartum doula is often said to nurture the entire family, and to help everyone involved ease into their new life with a newborn. They can comfort and share information with your partner and with your baby's siblings, as well as their grandparents, so that everyone adapts well to their new roles. Research shows that postpartum doulas can have beneficial impacts on the entire family, and that mothers and babies working with them have superior outcomes in postpartum adjustments, from greater breastfeeding success to higher self-confidence. Studies also suggest that when partners are supported, they can be better support systems for mom.[41]

To find a postpartum doula, or birth doula, visit www.dona.org.

Baby Nurse

Also called a night nurse, or sometimes night nanny, baby nurses are there to care for your baby at night so that you can get some much-needed rest. Unlike a postpartum doula, they're focused pretty much solely on your baby's needs. Of course, they're not relegated to only helping out at night—in the early days, baby nurses are typically at your house 24 hours a day, and help with pretty much all aspects of newborn care.

They can soothe your baby, change diapers and bathe your newborn, and help with nightly feedings, whether by bringing them to you for breastfeeding sessions or feeding them a bottle. With my girls, I did the midnight feeding and the baby nurse did the 4 am feeding; that way we could each get a good stretch of uninterrupted sleep. Depending on their credentials, they may be able to help with breastfeeding issues or newborn health issues like diaper rash or cradle cap. They help you navigate feedings—they weigh the baby and tell you how many ounces they should be eating per day based on weight. They can also tell you to move up to a bigger nipple because it's taking too long to feed. Often, they'll keep a log of sleeping, feeding, and changing times to help get you on a good schedule. They may help with baby-care specific chores, like preparing bottles and cleaning breast pumps, organizing the nursery, and doing the baby's laundry. If you have a gassy baby, they can teach you how to soothe them and burp them (my favorite was sitting them on the edge of the crib and holding their torso straight up—they'd burp three times in a minute). When my girls got the beginnings of a diaper rash, the baby nurse sent me to the store to get cornstarch and Mylanta. We whipped up a concoction out of it and by the next diaper change, all traces of rash were gone (I include a recipe for it on page 419). They can teach you how to give a bath and how to wrap the baby in a towel easily and safely when you get them out of the bath. Having a baby nurse is basically like a parenting coach living in your house, who is also hands-on so you can go take a shower.

I hired a baby nurse after each of my subsequent children were born; it's amazing how much I forgot each time. In order to find the right one, you'll need to do your homework here, as lots of people call themselves "baby nurses," meaning they can have all different types of training. They may, in fact, be a registered nurse with a true medical background. Or, they may or may not have other types of licenses or accreditations, or have any medical experience. Typically, they're certified in CPR and trained in feedings (they may or may not be a certified lactation consultant or a postpartum doula). The Newborn Care Specialist Association is a good place to start if you're looking to hire a qualified baby nurse (visit them at www.ncsa.international.)

Sleep Coach

It's just as it sounds: a coach to help you get your baby to, ahem, sleep like a baby. They're there to ultimately get your child to learn to fall asleep on their own—no pacifier or long car ride needed—and to stay asleep.

As with a baby nurse, you'll want to investigate before hiring. The industry isn't regulated, and you'll want to find a sleep coach whose philosophy matches yours. (There are lots of sleep training approaches out there.) They may provide in-home coaching or share their training strategies over the phone or a video call.

Of course, sleep coaches can come in handy as your child gets older as well, helping toddlers and preschoolers with nighttime sleeping and naps.

Depending on your individual postpartum experience, there are a variety of other resources that may prove beneficial to you. For instance, if you're experiencing postpartum depression or even post-traumatic stress disorder from a traumatic birth, there are a host of mental health providers who can assist you in healing and finding your way back to yourself. Postpartum Support International is a good resource regarding emotional postpartum changes; visit them online at postpartum.net.

If you're having pelvic floor issues after childbirth, and issues rekindling intimacy as a result, you may want to seek out a physical therapist, along with a couple's counselor specializing in sexual issues or an intimacy coach.

What's more, there are countless alternative health care practitioners, from nutritionists to acupuncturists to homeopaths, who can help balance your hormones as they change during the postpartum period and otherwise provide healing care and advice during this time.

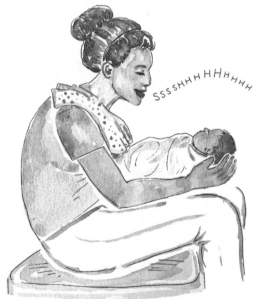

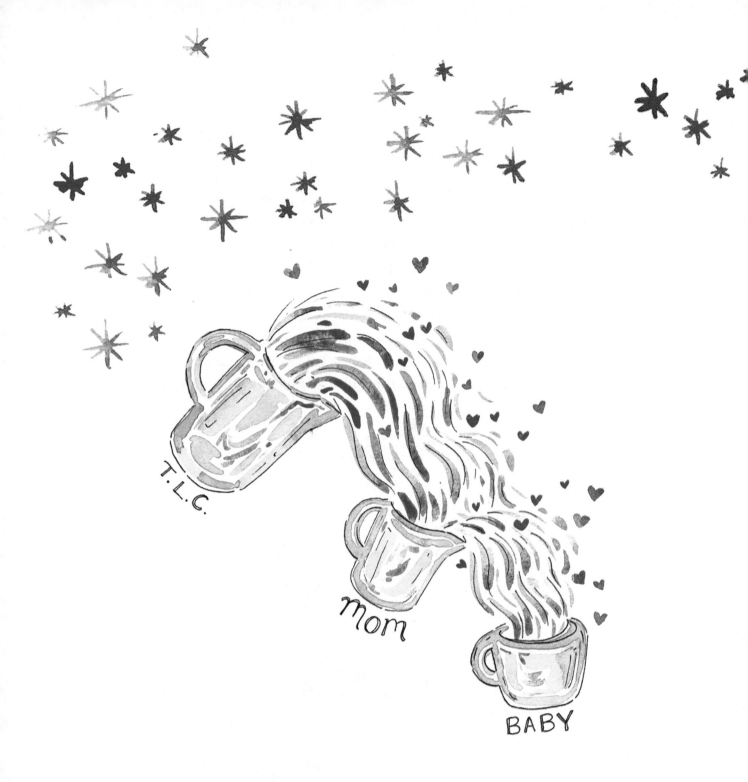

Chapter 23

THE TLC YOUR BABY AND YOUR BODY NEEDS NOW

W hen my first son, Hendrix, was born, I remember being so lost in surprise that he was a boy (we did not find out his gender beforehand) and that he was here that I was in a bit of a daze for the first hour or two of his life. In this chapter, I'll give you a preview of what to expect in these first heady moments so that you can be prepared to give yourself and your baby the conditions you both need to recuperate, bond, and get off to as solid a start as possible.

Baby's First Hours of Life

The temperature inside your uterus is 102 degrees, so once the baby comes out, even an 80-degree room is going to feel really cold. If you're home or in a spot where you control the temperature, you want to crank up the heat so that it's plenty warm.

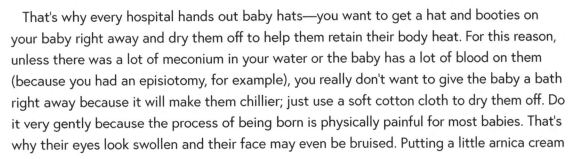

That's why every hospital hands out baby hats—you want to get a hat and booties on your baby right away and dry them off to help them retain their body heat. For this reason, unless there was a lot of meconium in your water or the baby has a lot of blood on them (because you had an episiotomy, for example), you really don't want to give the baby a bath right away because it will make them chillier; just use a soft cotton cloth to dry them off. Do it very gently because the process of being born is physically painful for most babies. That's why their eyes look swollen and their face may even be bruised. Putting a little arnica cream on their face and neck helps relieve the pain and reduce the swelling. It's also helpful to put some all-natural skin cream, like the one Weleda makes specifically for babies, on their skin. Because up until this point the baby has been immersed in water, it can get dried out when exposed to air, and the cream helps it retain moisture.

Consider waiting to cut the umbilical cord (or, more specifically, having your partner do it) until the placenta is born—as long as the placenta is inside you there's still a vital connection between you and the baby that you don't want to interrupt. You also want to wait to put the baby on the breast until you have delivered the placenta. Because breastfeeding stimulates oxytocin, and oxytocin can trigger uterine contractions, if you put the baby on the breast before the placenta is delivered, your cervix can close to the point that it makes it hard for the placenta to come out.

The placenta generally follows along quickly after the baby to the point that about 30 minutes after birth most babies are ready for the breast—Mari Mikel suggests letting them spend one hour on one breast and one hour on the other. (More on breastfeeding later in this chapter.)

While you don't need to worry about giving the baby a bath right away, you can wash their hair: Wrap them in a blanket, have your partner cradle the baby in their arms with their head angled slightly back, and very gently wet their head with warm but not hot water, rub a little baby shampoo over their scalp, then rinse. It's very soothing for the baby and a nice photo opportunity. It's a great thing to do after the baby has nursed on one breast for an hour and before you switch them to your other side.

As for you, it's a great idea to take a couple of ibuprofen right away to bring down any discomfort you might be feeling. An ice pack on your perineum can also be very helpful to get the swelling down.

As soon as you're ready—maybe even before you think you're ready—eat something. After Hendrix was born I didn't realize I was hungry until someone put a plate of food in front of me and I ate three huge helpings.

You want to keep this food easy to digest, both because it's easy for you to get constipated after birth (especially if you had a Caesarean birth and are on painkillers, which are notorious for slowing down your digestion), and because what you eat will show up in your breast milk and may be difficult for the baby to digest. Yogurt, eggs, applesauce, oatmeal, fish, chicken, and sweet potatoes are all good examples of nutrient-dense yet easily digestible foods that are good to eat now. You don't want to eat a huge hamburger because the red meat is hard to digest, or sulfur-containing vegetables like broccoli or cabbage, or beans (including chickpeas and soybeans), because they can cause gas in newborns (refer back to page 278 for more on which foods to avoid).

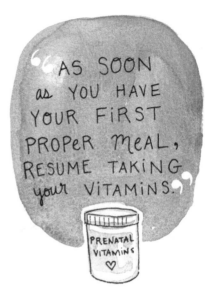

"AS SOON as YOU HAVE YOUR FiRST PROPeR meaL, RESUME TAKiNG your ViTAMiNS."

PRENATAL VITAMINS ♡

Drink lots of water now. You need to rehydrate after your physical exertion, and being hydrated helps with recovery and fatigue, too. As soon as you have your first proper meal, resume taking your vitamins. Your body gets really used to having all those nutrients delivered to it; it starts to create a new balance point with them. If you suddenly abandon ship at a point when you need all the nutrients you can get to help you recuperate from pregnancy and birth, feed your baby, and complete your transition to motherhood, it's a double whammy.

Skin for the Win

During the first minutes of the baby's life and throughout the first days and weeks, it is so important for the baby to have skin-to-skin contact with you and your partner. One reason this is so is that it helps expose them to the beneficial bacteria that live on your skin. They also get that exposure during a vaginal delivery and from breastfeeding, but friendly bacteria are so important to their overall health now and into the future that you want it coming from every source available. Skin contact is also crucial for bonding—it's one way babies learn to trust and love. The power of touch works on many levels, not all of which we fully understand, but what is absolutely clear is that babies need touch—those who aren't held enough will fail to thrive.

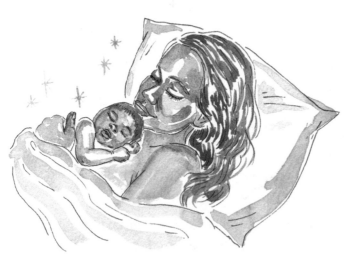

Once your baby is here, you really want them to be in full skin contact with you as much as possible. In these early days when the baby is primarily in bed with you or being held, have them as undressed as room temperature will allow—with a diaper on and then covered in a blanket—so that you can snuggle them up close to your skin. As I mentioned in Chapter 9, I loved the NüRoo shirts that let you place the baby right up against your chest and then strap them in so that they are secure and you are both covered. Either my husband or I had one of the girls in these shirts almost constantly in their first days of life—it lets you keep them close, hands-free.

Speaking of things that go directly on baby's skin, since their skin is so sensitive at first, in the first day or two of your baby's life, consider using cloth diapers. If you plan on using disposable diapers, you can switch to them after a couple of days (although I do recommend using a brand—such as Seventh Generation or Honest—that doesn't use bleach, has fewer chemicals, and is made in a more sustainable way than your standard diapers). This gives their skin some time to acclimate to the outside world before you start swaddling them in the rougher texture of disposables.

Another portion of their skin to consider not covering up is their hands. Many people put mittens over a newborn's hands because they can come out with long fingernails, and since they have very little motor control, they can scratch themselves with their nails. But since newborns can't see very far and their hearing can be muffled (the ear canals take a while to drain), their hands and skin are their primary sensory organs in those early days, and you don't want to impede them from acclimating to their new surroundings through their one mode of input.

"SINCE *their* SKIN is SO SENSITIVE AT FIRST, IN the FIRST DAY *or* TWO *of* YOUR BABY'S LIFE, CONSIDER USING CLOTH DIAPERS."

Making the Choice: Breast Milk or Formula?

You've heard over and over that "breast is best." Major health organizations promote breastfeeding as the best choice for feeding your baby and recommend it if at all possible. In particular, the American Academy of Pediatrics says breast milk is the most nutritious option for newborns and infants, and advises breastfeeding exclusively for six months, continuing even after other foods have been introduced in their diet and until they are at least a year old.

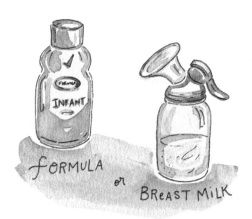

FORMULA *or* BREAST MILK

But there can be so much pressure that comes from the "breast is best" message that it starts to mess with your head. And, it doesn't mean formula isn't nutritious. In fact, it offers its own advantages for you and baby. So, which should you choose?

Ultimately, what you feed your little one is up to you. Let's explore the benefits of both breast milk and formula so you can make the decision that's right for your family.

Benefits of Breast Milk

Breast milk has been called "nature's perfect food," and with good reason:

- **It's abundant in immune-boosting antibodies.** These proteins help your baby's immune system fend off common illnesses and infections like colds, ear infections, respiratory infections, and urinary tract infections. They might also play a role in protecting them from developing asthma and allergies, and they may even be the reason that breastfed babies are less likely than formula-fed babies to develop much more serious diseases as well, such as childhood acute leukemia. Likely in part from the antibodies in breast milk, although scientists aren't entirely certain why, studies show breastfeeding reduces the risk of sudden infant death syndrome (SIDS), by anywhere from 36 to 50 percent! Other helpful immunity-improving substances in human milk? Prebiotics, or friendly bacteria. In particular, these good bacteria help keep your baby from having diarrhea. (Note: You may hear it said that a breastfeeding mom gives "passive immunity" to their child; that just means that your breast milk provides the benefits shared here.)

- **It's beneficial for the brain.** Breast milk is rich in long-chain polyunsaturated fatty acids, which are vital to brain development and growth. In fact, some studies show that breastfeeding raises a child's IQ, possibly up to 7.5 points.

- **It's easily digestible.** Breast milk contains only lactose, protein (whey and casein), and fat. As a result, newborns can typically more easily breakdown milk than formula, which includes additional ingredients. This is another reason why breastfed babies usually have less diarrhea, as well as less constipation, than those fed formula.

- **It provides a healthy start.** Research suggests that babies fed breast milk early in life may have a reduced risk of developing diabetes (types 1 and 2) and of being overweight as they get older and reach adulthood.

- **It's free and convenient.** These benefits may not be as important as those that directly affect your baby's health, but they can't be overlooked. Formula can be expensive, as can all the associated supplies, such as bottles. And breast milk is always fresh and readily available any time; it's always the right temperature too. Also, you can't forget it at home. Wherever you are, so is baby's food.

Benefits of Formula

Formula is the best alternative to breast milk and can be a nutritious choice for your baby.

- **It contains vitamin D, along with other important vitamins and minerals.** The US Food and Drug Administration oversees formula-making companies and ensures that their formulas provide the necessary nutrients your baby needs. One of these nutrients is vitamin D, which is not present in ample amounts in breast milk. (For this reason, breastfed babies need a vitamin D supplement.) Most formulas are also fortified with iron, which, as is the case with vitamin D, breast milk doesn't contain enough of; iron supplements are often recommended for breastfed and partially breastfed infants to help them avoid iron deficiency and iron deficiency anemia. As long as your baby gets the right amount of formula for them each day, you can rest assured they're getting all the vitamins and minerals they need as well.

- **It can be hypoallergenic.** Many brands of formula are processed to help babies avoid allergic reactions. Formula can be a lifesaver if your baby has an allergy and you're unable to entirely avoid that allergen in your diet.

- **It's available to other caregivers.** As above, this last bullet doesn't directly have to do with a beneficial impact on your baby's health, but it's important nevertheless. Your partner can help with feedings, as can the baby's grandparents and other care providers. (Although, if you breastfeed, you can always pump so that someone else can feed the baby your breast milk via a bottle.)

More Pros to Consider

There are benefits to the act of breastfeeding in addition to the milk itself, just as there are benefits in choosing to feed formula and not just in the formula on its own—for your baby and you!

Breastfeeding...

- Provides lots of skin-to-skin contact, which enhances bonding and connection with your baby.

- Helps you out: It actually burns calories, so you may return to your prepregnancy weight quicker if you breastfeed than if you feed formula. What's more, studies show that breastfeeding lowers your risk of breast, uterine, and ovarian cancer; diabetes; heart disease; hypertension; and osteoporosis.

- Means fewer dental issues for babies, like overbites and misaligned teeth.

- May help your baby adjust to solid foods, since your breast milk tastes like what you've eaten.

Formula Feeding...

- Usually equals more rest for mom. Babies fed formula stay full longer, meaning they need to eat less often. You may be able to better set a schedule that works for you than if you were to breastfeed.

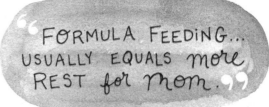

"FORMULA FEEDING... USUALLY EQUALS *more* REST *for mom*."

- Means you don't have to adjust your diet: You don't have to avoid foods your baby may have a hard time tolerating or be allergic to, and you can have a glass or two of alcohol without worry.

All this said, there are also drawbacks to consider. As mentioned above, breast milk does lack significant vitamin D and iron, so supplements are likely necessary. If you're breastfeeding, you do need to be aware of what you're eating and drinking and may need to alter your diet, as well as possibly your medications. It can also be painful and difficult for some women and requires a significant time commitment; if you're going to work or otherwise need to be away from your child for longer than a few hours, you'll need to purchase a breast pump and pump breast milk to have available.

On the other hand, formula doesn't contain beneficial antibodies and can't match the magical contents of breast milk. It can also make your baby gassy and cause them to experience other tummy troubles. Feeding your baby formula can be quite expensive and requires a great deal of preparation: You need to always have formula and clean bottles and other supplies on hand and at the ready. What's more, formulas can be recalled, so you need to pay careful attention to the news and what you're buying.

> BREAST MILK HAS BEEN CALLeD 'NATURE'S PERFECT FOOD,' and WITH GOOD REASON."

If you go the formula route—whether exclusively or as an adjunct to breastfeeding—I definitely recommend choosing an organic formula, since it won't have ingredients that have been exposed to pesticides or derived from genetically modified organisms, and one that doesn't contain corn syrup, since it has a high glycemic index and can get baby hooked on an overly sweet taste right from the start of their life. Some also contain soy or ingredients derived from soy, like lecithin, that can be problematic. The biggest concern with soy in babies is that soybeans contain compounds known as isoflavones that mimic the effects of estrogen, and could potentially disrupt baby's delicate hormonal balance. Definitely talk to your pediatrician and do your research to find the right formula for your baby. The brand I used the most was Baby Organics.

As for me, I breastfed both my boys, and our surrogate provided breast milk for our girls for their first six months. I made it to about three months with Hendrix and five months with Legend. It was painful both times. While it was important to me to breastfeed, I wasn't one of those women who had a wonderful breastfeeding journey; it often felt like a struggle. That being said, it was important enough to me to keep going even though it was painful. (The only thing that helped me make it as long as I did was silicon nipple covers.) I ultimately stopped both times because my supply wasn't enough to keep the babies full and thriving.

Honestly, I felt a huge relief once I gave up on doing what I felt like (and was told) I was supposed to do and switched to formula. I knew that while breast may be best, formula isn't bad. I think if women could head into breastfeeding completely relaxed, knowing that whatever happens the baby will be OK, it would alleviate a lot of guilt, angst, and difficulty. If breastfeeding works for you, great; if it doesn't, that's OK too.

We think that breastfeeding should be instinctual and therefore easy, but the truth is, it's neither. We don't grow up seeing women breastfeed throughout our lives. It's no longer a behavior that we can absorb through modeling.

If breastfeeding is important to you, it's really essential to prepare—take a breastfeeding class, read books on breastfeeding, seek out a La Leche League meeting in your area that you can attend in person, hire a lactation consultant if you encounter difficulties. For most women, it takes perseverance and grit to establish and maintain breastfeeding; I hope the breastfeeding information in this book will help make it easier.

> "I THINK iF WomeN COULD HEAD INTO BREASTFeeDiNG COMPLeTeLY ReLAXeD, KNOWiNG that WHATeveR HAPPENS the BABY WiLL BE OK, iT WOULD ALLeViATe A LOT of GUiLT, ANGST, and DiFFiCULTY."

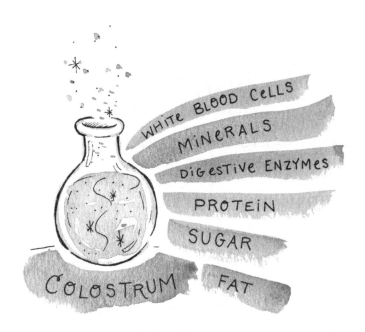

When Your Milk Comes In

It takes an average of three days for your full milk supply to come in. Although the baby can nurse and gain sustenance as soon as they are born, what is coming out of your nipple isn't technically breast milk—it's colostrum, a fluid that contains a high amount of white blood cells to lend your baby some immunity to the outside world. It also contains minerals, digestive enzymes, protein, sugar, and fat. And, it acts as a laxative, helping your baby clear the meconium from their digestive tract, which helps to prevent jaundice (something I talk more about on page 374). The exact components of colostrum change every 12 hours or so. At first it's high in sugar in order to replenish baby after birth. Then it gets more protein to help with repairing any tissue that may have been bruised during birth. Then it gets fattier to give the baby more calories and help them gain weight. It truly is a miraculous substance—and your body is just as miraculous for producing it.

At any point in your milk-making journey, if you are concerned the baby isn't getting enough, know you can always weigh the baby before and after feeding them. That way you can see exactly how much they consumed.

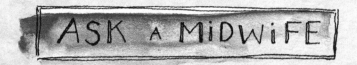

WHAT'S THE BEST WAY TO SET MY BABY AND ME UP FOR BREASTFEEDING SUCCESS?

from MARI MIKEL:

"As soon as your placenta has been delivered, it's time to initiate nursing. There is a magical learning curve in the first two hours after birth. If you can get a good connection now, the baby will never forget.

"I advise that you do these initial breastfeeding sessions lying down: It's better for your bottom, which has just been traumatized and doesn't need the pressure, and will help slow your bleeding. It's also better for the baby, because when you hold the baby in your arms there are parts of their spine that aren't supported, no matter how well you cradle them. When they're lying down on the mattress, all their bones and vertebrae are supported. You can lie on your side with the baby next to you, tummy to tummy with you so that they don't have to turn their head to reach the breast.

"Line the baby's mouth up with your nipple, taking care that their chin isn't tucked down toward their chest, and make sure their head is lying on the bed, not your arm. Typically babies come out of the birth canal with a very tucked chin. This orientation is good for helping them penetrate the cervix, but not as helpful to your nipple. If your baby tries to nurse with a tucked chin, it will put their top gum in direct contact with your nipple, which doesn't feel great for you. Lifting their chin up will also move their nose back away from your breast so that they can breathe easier.

"You want to be sure that you get the baby's mouth wide open. To do that, brush the baby's mouth with your nipple, which will initiate the baby's rooting reflex and cause them to turn their head toward your breast. You may also want to use your thumb (or have your partner help you) to pull the baby's chin down just for a moment so that their mouth opens wider—you really need to get as much of your areola as you can in the baby's mouth, because although the milk comes out of the tip of the nipple, it's the compression on your breast tissue that comes from the work of your baby's jaw opening and closing slightly as they suckle that helps release the milk.

"You can also hold the back of baby's head (or have your partner do it) so that they aren't moving their head back and forth, which is a natural part of the rooting reflex but not very helpful for effective nursing. You can use one hand to stabilize the baby's head and the other hand to guide the nipple into baby's mouth, using your index finger and thumb, as if you were holding a teacup.

"If they're having a hard time getting a good latch, you can stimulate their sucking reflex by putting your clean pinkie finger, with the pad up and the fingernail on their tongue, inside their mouth. Once they get a good sucking rhythm going, you can take your finger out and quickly insert your nipple—all the way up to the areola—in its place.

"After an hour on one breast, the baby can have its newborn exam, and perhaps you can wash their hair and re-swaddle them, then put them on the other breast for an hour.

"I recommend to my moms that they breastfeed lying down as much as possible during the first two weeks—it removes a lot of variables from the equation, like different holds—and means you only need to concentrate on getting a good latch. If anything isn't going well—your nipples hurt, the baby doesn't seem to be getting enough, start pumping and give yourself and the baby a rest. The pump will not hurt you, and your number one priority is to make sure the baby is fed.

"If the baby loses more than 10 percent of their body weight in the first 24 hours, especially if they weighed seven pounds or less at birth, give them a little formula or some diluted coconut water (diluted with filtered water) using a medicine spoon or eye dropper. No matter how devoted to breastfeeding you may be, the number one rule, especially now, is to feed the baby. If it's not happening with the breast it has to happen some other way.

The Importance of Resting as Much as Possible

Staying in bed as much as you can for the first two weeks of the baby's life makes a huge difference in your own recovery, your bond to the baby, and even how comfortable you feel breastfeeding. I know how strong the urge is to get up and move about; no one wants to be the slacker mom who doesn't care for her baby.

But right now, your primary job is to bond with the baby, feed the baby, and heal. Those things are all a lot harder when you're trying to 'get things done.' Breastfeeding can be hard; it is even harder when you're trying to figure out how to hold the baby. If you're in bed, you can lie down every time. It lets you just focus on the latch. And if you're tired, you can doze off while the baby nurses.

It was easy for me to stay down with my first child; it was a lot harder with the second one because now I had two children to care for. I tried, I really did, but I was walking all over the place. But just knowing that the most productive thing I could do was to rest with the baby helped me talk myself out of the urge to get up and make a meal or do a load of laundry. This is why I say the best baby gift anyone can give you is some precooked food that someone only needs to heat up for you—your partner can do that (and the dishes too, for that matter). Just for these two weeks, don't try to do more. Do less.

Circadian Rhythms Are Your Friend

Newborns typically want to stay up all night and nurse and sleep all day. After all, they had no exposure to light in the womb. The motions you made while you were awake often lulled them to sleep, and once you were still, at night, they had to move around more to get comfortable.

To start to get your newborn adjusted to being awake during the day and sleeping at night, you want to be very careful of the light you expose them to and when. You want them exposed to as much natural light as possible—open the curtains in your rooms as soon as you're awake and use natural light during the day as much as you're able. Then, dim your electric lights as the sun goes down and keep the room where you and the baby sleep as dark as possible at night—no night-lights. Because blue light (which is found in sunlight, most electric lights, and the light emitted from screens) is stimulating, and red light is calming, if you need a light in the middle of the night to see (such as for a diaper change), use a red light bulb. If you have an electronic clock in your room, it's better for those numbers to be red than green or blue. That will help your baby's internal clock set itself properly and help them naturally be more awake when the sun is up and sleepy when it is down. And guess what? It will also help do the same for you.

Since my second son and two girls were born, I've only used blue-light-blocking night-lights in the kids' rooms or during nighttime diaper changes. And those three kids all started sleeping 12 hours a night when they were three months old. With my first son, I didn't know to make these changes. I would turn on a regular light in the room when I changed his diaper in the middle of the night. And it took him seven months to sleep through the night. I also made sure that my girls got all their recommended calories during the daytime, so that they were less likely to be hungry at night.

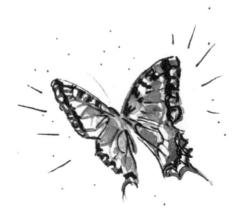

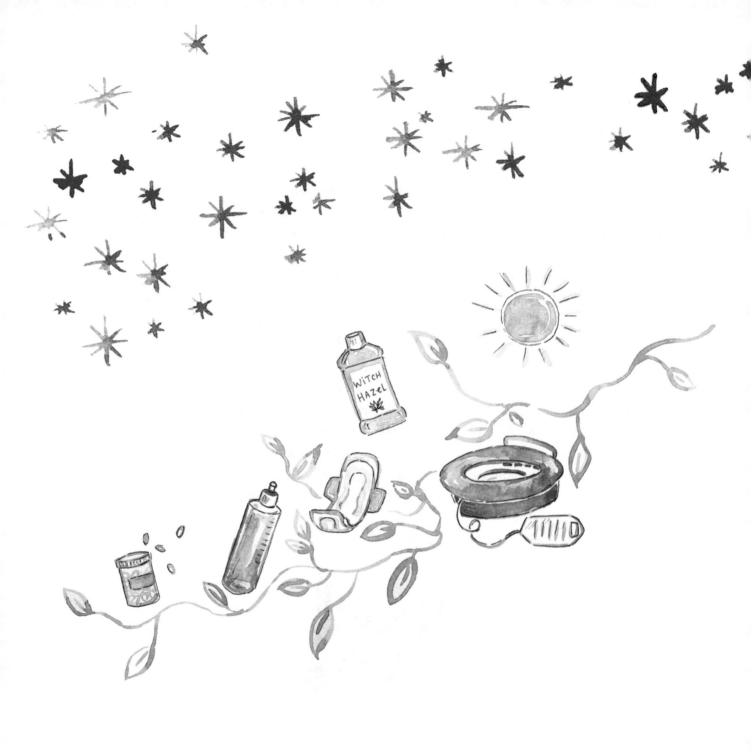

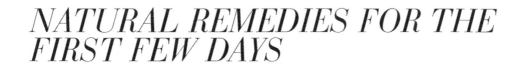

Chapter 24

NATURAL REMEDIES FOR THE FIRST FEW DAYS

After birth, you might feel like your entire body aches—and so might your baby! Here are some remedies that can help ease your recuperation and the baby's transition into being out in the world.

Body Aches and Pains

Just like it can take 24 hours to feel sore after a workout, the first day or two after you give birth is a common time for you to notice increasing discomfort that peaks around day three. To relieve soreness and reduce inflammation right from the start, take two ibuprofen every four hours for the first three days. It helps with so many things—vaginal pain, nipple pain, breast pain, and muscle soreness from holding the baby. It can even help prevent hemorrhoids.

Arnica gel is also great to use on sore muscles, and even a little on the baby's face, head, and neck—the areas that really get compressed during birth. You can also put it right on your pelvic floor; just don't put it directly on or in any stitches or wounds.

Vagina Care

After a vaginal delivery, your perineum can really sting when you urinate, whether you have actual tears or micro-tears. A great way to take away the pain and keep the area clean is to get a few peribottles—empty squeeze bottles—and fill them up with water that you've added enough of an antiseptic iodine solution (such as povidone/Betadine) to so that it looks like iced tea. Then, while you're urinating, squirt the antiseptic water on your pelvic floor, but don't touch the bottle to your perineum, only the stream of water.

I kept my peribottles on a heating pad right in the bathroom so the water would be nice and warm (because it's hard to pee when you're exposed to cold water). I used mine for a good 10 days until I was urinating comfortably without them.

For even more healing, purchase a sitz bath—a plastic mini tub with just enough room for your bottom that goes over the toilet. You can add a few inches of warm water to it that you've dissolved about a tablespoon of Epsom salts in, and if you have any red raspberry leaf tea leftover from pregnancy you can put that in there too, and then sit down in it to bathe and soothe that whole area. If you don't want to buy an actual sitz bath, you can also use one of those under-the-bed plastic storage containers: fill it with about three inches of water and do the same thing. You just don't want to get directly in your bathtub because it has too many germs for you to be exposed to right now, while you're still healing.

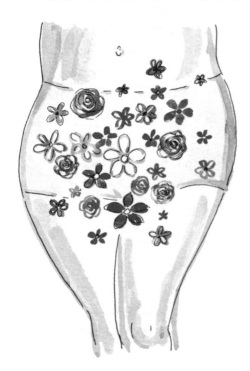

If you have stitches in your perineum, douse them in a half capful of hydrogen peroxide every day to keep them clean.

You can also soak a menstrual pad with witch hazel (that you can buy at the drugstore) and keep it in the freezer—the coolness can feel amazing. Just be sure to spend some time each day if you can without a sanitary pad on, just lying on a disposable absorbent pad (you can take some from the hospital or they will be in your at-home birth kit) so that your vagina is exposed to some air, because moistness creates a great breeding ground for bacteria.

Sore or Cracked Nipples

Here's the deal: Breastfeeding is hard—really hard—on nipples. You want to take great care of them.

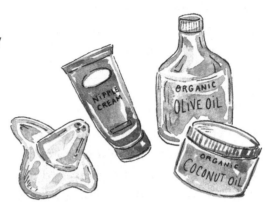

The thing that worked best for me was a silicon nipple cover that still lets the milk out but puts a barrier between your areola and the baby's gums. Nipple cream is also helpful to keep the skin moist yet also allow it to breathe to prevent any cracking, or help any cracking that has already occurred to heal. Mari Mikel recommends Lansinoh, which includes lanolin—a waxy substance that is a component of sheep's wool. But if your nipple cream has lanolin in it (as Lansinoh does), you're supposed to wipe it off before the baby nurses. So that I didn't have to take that step, I used an organic lanolin-free nipple cream—two great examples are by The Honest Company and Earth Mama. You can also use unrefined organic coconut oil, organic olive oil, or, once your milk comes in (which generally takes about three days), you can rub a little of the fatty hindmilk into the nipple and then let it air dry.

To help your nipples heal and strengthen up a bit, expose them to the sun if you can. Not enough to get a sunburn, of course, just five to 10 minutes a day.

Umbilical Cord Care

To keep your baby's umbilical cord stump free of germs and bacteria as it heals, put a little alcohol on a cotton ball to dab it with once or twice a day. Goldenseal is an herb that is great for speeding healing—Mari Mikel taught me to dip a Q-tip lightly into an open capsule of goldenseal to get just a tiny bit on the tip, then lightly apply it to your baby's cord stump. Goldenseal is antibacterial and helps keep the area germ-free and healing beautifully. It's also okay to completely leave it alone. Your doctor or midwife will be there to guide you.

Jaundice

After a baby is born every red blood cell in their body has to be replaced, to allow the baby to derive their oxygen from breathing air instead of breathing amniotic fluid. The liver is responsible for breaking down all those old red blood cells into bilirubin (a yellowish substance that contains the waste products of those old red blood cells) and ushering it into the digestive tract where it can be excreted through the baby's poop. (That's why the baby's first few poops are so dark—as anyone who has had to take iron supplements will tell you, when the body is excreting high amounts of iron it turns your stool dark, and bilirubin contains a lot of iron.)

Because the liver is still a little immature at birth, it can get behind on the job. That's when bilirubin will build up in the baby's skin, giving it a yellow-ish cast, in what's known as jaundice. Jaundice is a completely natural occurrence—it usually starts on day two and peaks on day three.

The best way to treat jaundice is to prevent it, and you do that by making sure the baby is hydrated enough to soil (pee and/or poop) one to two diapers in the first 24 hours, two to three diapers in the second 24 hours, and three to four in the third 24 hours. If the baby isn't producing this many dirty diapers because your milk hasn't come in yet, Mari Mikel suggests diluting some coconut water with filtered water and feeding it to the baby using a medicine spoon or eye dropper—it will deliver electrolytes and a tiny bit of sugar in addition to the fluids to help the baby stay hydrated and get some calories. If you see that your baby is becoming too jaundiced or jaundice is occurring too early, give the baby a little bit of cow's milk formula. It doesn't mean you have to give up on breastfeeding; this can just be a short-term measure until your milk comes in and your baby's skin is less yellow.

Also, placing the baby in direct sunlight helps their liver break down the bilirubin. After the first 24 hours of the baby's life (because that first day is sacred time that should be spent resting and bonding), undress the baby and lay them down on a disposable pad in the sunshine—outdoors is best, as glass filters sunlight and only some of the rays get through—for five minutes on each side. If it's cold where you live, you can get in the car, position the car so the passenger seat is getting a nice amount of direct sunshine, run the heater, and roll down the window while holding the baby in your lap.

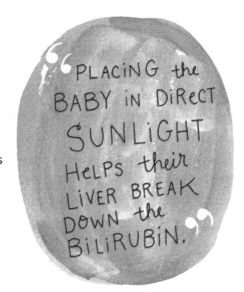

"PLACING the BABY in DiReCT SUNLiGHT HeLPS their LiVeR BREAK DOWN the BiLiRUBiN."

When you lay the baby on their stomach (because you want both their front and their back to be exposed to the sun), turn their head to one side for two minutes, then to the other side for two minutes so that they don't get a crick in their neck. You want to do it at a time when the baby has just eaten, otherwise they may try to root (meaning, look for a nipple) and bury their face in the blanket when they're lying on their stomach. You also want to do it a time when you haven't recently applied cream to their skin so that there's nothing impeding their skin's absorption of sunshine. And to ensure that they don't get sunburned, give your baby their sunbath before 10 am and after 3pm (later if it's summer and super hot where you are) so there are fewer rays that can cause sunburn.

Fatigue

Keep drinking as much water and taking all of your supplements that you were taking when you were pregnant. You still need extra support to help replenish yourself after pregnancy and delivery; and breastfeeding requires extra hydration and nutrients from you, too. If you stop taking them cold turkey after you give birth, it will add to your fatigue.

Another option is to have your placenta encapsulated and take it as a supplement. I realize that can sound pretty 'out there,' and there's a definite yuck factor, but your placenta contains iron as well as hormones such as progesterone and estradiol (a form of estrogen). Anemia (low levels of iron) has been linked to fatigue and postpartum depression, as has the sudden drop in hormones that happens after birth. Ingesting the placenta is also believed to promote milk production. Studies have found some mild benefit in preventing postpartum depression and little to no risk—so even if the benefit comes from the placebo effect, there's no reason not to do it.[42]

I encapsulated my placentas after my sons were born. Someone came to the house and used a dehydrator to dry it out, then ground it up and put it in capsules. The process of dehydrating it does diminish the iron and hormone levels in the placenta—if you really want to maximize those, it's better to only lightly cook the placenta before eating it. But encapsulating it helps it last longer—you just want to take several capsules a day to help get higher amounts of iron and hormones. I knew it was controversial, but I wanted all the help I could get. Some famous moms who have talked about encapsulating their placentas are Kim Kardashian, Chrissy Teigen, and Alicia Silverstone.[43]

Everyone will tell you to nap when the baby naps and you will resist that advice, because you'll want to 'get something done' while the baby is napping. Especially in these first few days, just stay in bed with the baby nearby so that you can doze off whenever you need to. You are recuperating now, you need rest. Sleep as much as possible (although remember to open your curtains during the day, as the light will help regulate your baby's internal clock and help them make the transition to being up during the day—with naps, of course—and sleeping at night).

To me, I felt like nothing really helped with my fatigue after Hendrix was born, but I didn't realize that I had come down with an autoimmune disease at the same time. I learned that postpartum is a common time for autoimmune conditions to present themselves, so if everything you do to address your fatigue—napping, self-care, going to bed early, etc.—doesn't help, talk to your doctor about it. Be prepared to advocate strongly for yourself because they will likely tell you it's normal for a new mom to be tired, which is true, but only you know how deep your fatigue really is.

Engorgement

When your milk comes in your boobs can get so big and so rock hard that they're painful for you and difficult to latch onto for the baby. A trick that can really help is wrapping raw red cabbage leaves around each breast and putting a bra on. (Change them every four hours.) The cabbage leaves contain some powerful anti-inflammatory compounds.

Icing your breasts (over your bra, not directly on the skin) can also help. To make this easy, have four packages of frozen peas or corn on hand. Break up any clumps within the bag and they will mold perfectly to the shape of your breast. You need two bags to use on the breasts and two bags ready to go in the freezer when the others start to thaw.

To help prevent over-filling in the first place, make sure you put a bra on in the first 24 hours after birth so that your breasts don't swell to their full potential.

And when your breasts are super full, you want to gently massage from the outside of the breast toward the nipple; it will force out some milk and soften the nipple and the areola so that the baby can latch easier.

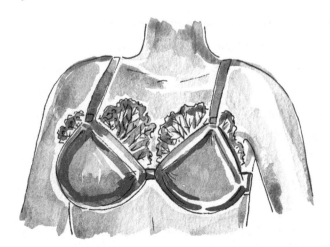

My Second Birth Story

By the time my second son, Legend, was born, I thought I knew exactly how his birth would go (although, as with my older son, my husband and I opted not to find out his gender until he was born). But I'd soon find out that even with the same parents, same gender, and same circumstances (I also had Legend at home), each birth is as unique as the baby it brings into this world.

Dear Legend,

I loved being a mom so much that I didn't waste any time getting pregnant with you. When I married your Dad only the two of us knew I was pregnant. I declined having my grandfather or stepfather walk me down the aisle because I always wanted to be able to tell you that you walked me down the aisle. You weren't even the size of a raspberry but it was you that shared that special moment with me.

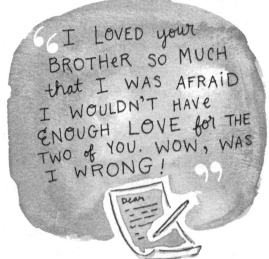

"I LOVED your BROTHER SO MUCH that I WAS AFRAID I WOULDN'T HAVE ENOUGH LOVE for THE TWO of YOU. WOW, WAS I WRONG!"

The pregnancy flew by and you were healthy and so was I. I couldn't wait to meet you even though I was scared. I loved your brother so much that I was afraid I wouldn't have enough love for the two of you. Wow, was I wrong! My heart expanded to places beyond my imagination.

The day you were born I worked out and then went for a smoothie with your Dad and Hendrix. When we got home, I started feeling light contractions but didn't say anything because I didn't want to complain and honestly didn't think you were going to come anytime soon. I was only 39 weeks and four days, and I didn't deliver your brother until 41 weeks.

I rocked Hendrix to sleep and continued to time my contractions. After laying him down I told your Dad, "I think this is it. I may really be in labor!" He called the midwife and she said she was on her way.

As she began to set up her 100+ pounds of equipment, I walked the halls. You were very high so I wanted to help encourage you to drop down lower in my pelvis. As the contractions intensified I got into the warm bathtub so I could continue to labor there. Even though I had loved being in the tub when Hendrix was born, this time it was so uncomfortable, and only intensified the pain from the contractions! Instead your Dad and I spent most of the evening in the shower. He sat on the bench and I sat on a stool with the running hot water on my back and asked him to apply pressure with his hands. This went on for hours.

I really wanted to meet you so I stayed upright and walked around as much as I could. I remember walking outside during transition; it was dark and the lights outside were so beautiful. The world felt safe and warm. Eventually it was time to push. We went to the bedroom and the midwife and her team helped me onto the bed. I pushed for 17 (excruciating) minutes, and there you were, crying with the loudest and deepest cry I've ever heard. You were beautiful and had so much hair it could've been a wig! Thick, black, straight hair like silk, and I loved it!

You were perfect. Seven pounds, eight ounces, and 20-3/4 inches long. I really think if I had carried you as long as I carried Hendrix you would've been much bigger than he was.

You are the sweetest addition to our family; a piece that can never be replaced and before you were here that was always missing. Years before I met your Dad I wanted kids more than anything. I had to wait for the right man and when I found him I wasted no time. Thank you for choosing me to guide you through these magical beginnings. It is my life's honor to watch you grow. You are everything I've ever dreamed of in the most pure package. I love you. *Mommy*

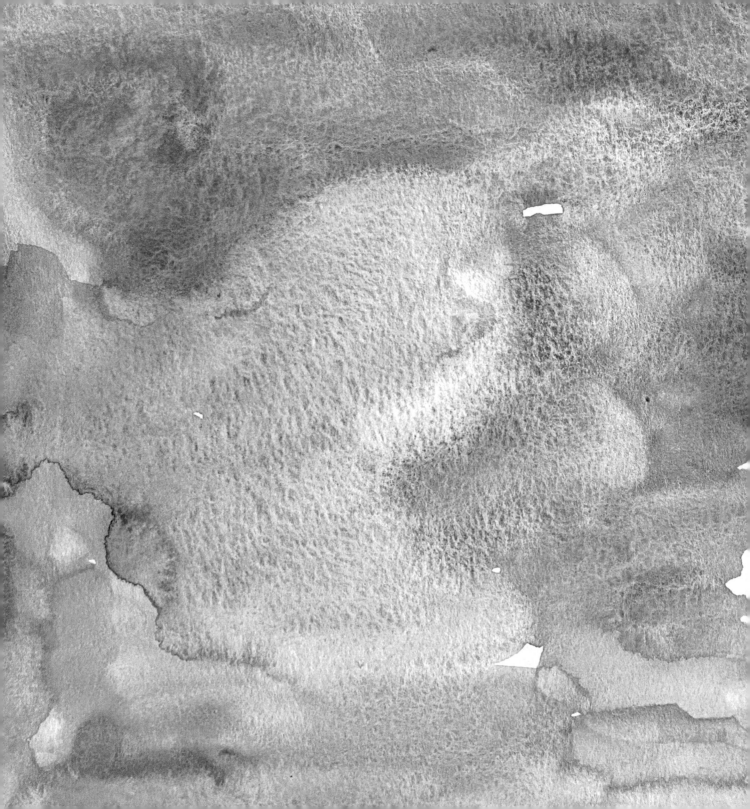

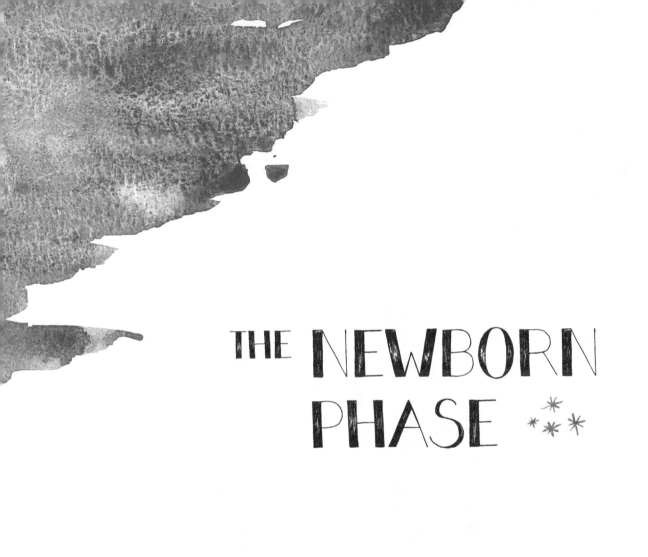

THE NEWBORN PHASE

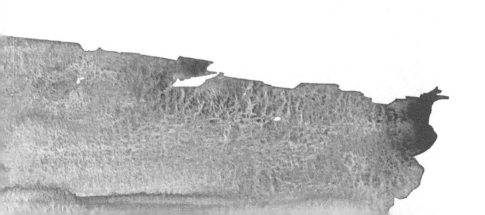

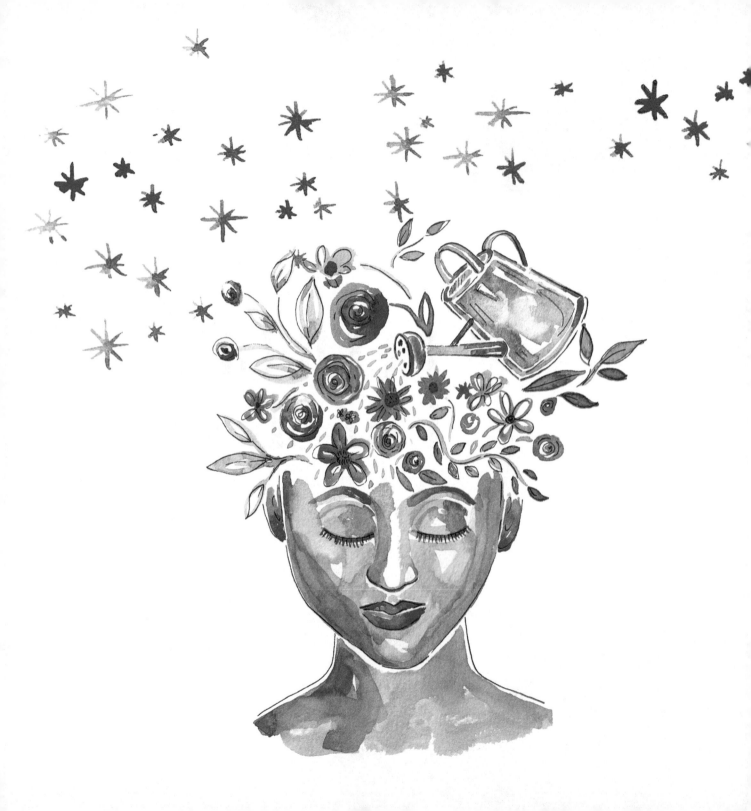

Chapter 25

MOTHER YOUR MENTAL HEALTH

The weeks following the birth of your baby (or babies) are an understandably emotional time. It's so important to remember that while of course your baby needs mothering now, so do you. You are, after all, a whole new version of yourself. You're a mother. Maybe you're a mother for the first time, or now you're a mother of two, or three, or four, or more. However many children you have, you're in a new reality. Couple that with hormones and exhaustion, and it's too easy to lose sight of the emotional transformation you're going through now. I hope that the topics I cover in this chapter will help make this transition go as smoothly as possible for you.

You Deserve—and Require—Self-Care

We do so many things for our children that we neglect for ourselves. You may be giving your baby a bath whenever they need it, but what about you? You deserve the same care that you give to your baby. (That's why at my skincare company, we say, "We MUTHA you like your own MUTHA would.")

It's so important to have someone who can give you two hours to yourself and give you the peace of mind that the baby will be fed, changed, and held, whether that's your partner, your mother, a friend, or a postpartum doula. You don't need to leave the house, or even your bedroom. Have a cup of tea, take a long shower, paint your nails, sleep, read, or lie in bed and do nothing. (If you don't have someone to watch the baby and you need a shower, the Dockatot or a vibrating chair can go into the bathroom with you and keep the baby safe so that you can have your time.) I used to consider self-care to be going to the gym or the spa, but now I recognize that just having time to myself *is* self-care.

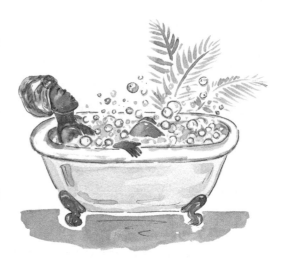

At the same time, sometimes self-care means letting something go—even if that thing is a shower. You *still* require and deserve time to yourself, however. And of course, self-care also includes eating well and doing all your wellness routines, like taking your vitamins (which I'll cover in the next chapter) and anything that makes you feel well cared for.

Navigating the Emotional Ups and Downs

Birth is a major life experience that's also coupled with a tsunami of hormones, so *of course* it is going to affect you emotionally. (Perhaps especially if your birth didn't work out in the way you had hoped, something I cover in just a bit.) Up to 80 percent of new moms experience intensified moodiness, known as the baby blues, that typically starts a couple days after the baby is born and can last a week or two. Or maybe you're euphoric after the baby is born—and realizing what a badass you are for having given birth—but the dip in mood comes later, after your tiredness kicks in and you fully recognize that your life is never going back to the way it was. Either way, the baby blues are characterized by mood swings—one minute you're filled with love for your baby, then you're crying the next, only to then get angry, all within the span of a short time.

Sometimes the baby blues can linger and intensify into postpartum depression. You are more prone to having postpartum depression if you've experienced depression before.

Is It the Baby Blues or Postpartum Depression?

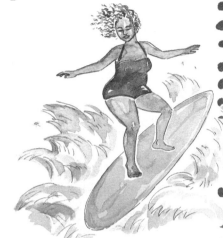

Symptoms of the Baby Blues

- Fast-moving mood swings

- Super tired, don't feel like taking care of yourself

- Irritable, overwhelmed, anxious

Symptoms of Postpartum Depression

- Feelings of deep sadness and frequent crying

- Feelings of hopelessness and/or worthlessness

- Doubt in your ability to be a good mom

- Not feeling bonded to your baby

- Unable to take care of yourself because you're too overwhelmed

- Possible anxiety or panic attacks

- Possible thoughts of harming your baby

- Possible thoughts of harming yourself

- Sleeping too little or sleeping too much

You may dismiss the idea altogether that you're experiencing either the baby blues or postpartum depression, or perhaps not think much about it, because who wouldn't feel tired and unconcerned with their own self-care while taking care of a newborn? Now, when I look back to the newborn phase with each of my sons, I can clearly see that I had the baby blues. If I could have recognized that I was having a very normal, to be expected dip in mood, I think it would have helped me be easier on myself. It also would have inspired me to share more of the caretaking with my husband, which would have been good for him, for me, for the babies, and for our relationship.

If you're feeling down now, it's so normal. There is nothing wrong with you and you're not weak. You are essentially reconfiguring your whole identity, and your hormones are having their way with you. Please don't forget to mother yourself, too. You deserve it. After all, you are a magical creature capable of creating life.

If you are feeling anything on the list of symptoms for the baby blues or for postpartum depression, talk to your care provider about it. They can help you with some perspective on what you're feeling, and a skilled care provider will also be able to validate your experience.

Consider that part of what's going on with your emotions right now is grief. To become a mother and give new life your old identity and way of life have to die. It's the natural cycle of death and rebirth, like the trees that lose their leaves every fall and then re-bud in the spring. To move through grief, you need time and space to feel your feelings and to treat yourself very gently. Know that the more time you spend in that bubble of bonding with and nursing your baby the more your hormones will kick in—particularly oxytocin and prolactin—to help you feel loving, lovable, and content.

> "Consider that part of what's going on with your emotions right now is grief. To become a mother and give new life your old identity and way of life have to die."

Maternity Leave Is Not a Vacation

A lot of women head into their maternity leave, if they're lucky enough to have one (it's horrible that I even have to say that, as paid and extensive maternity leave should be the right of every mother), thinking that they will have a lot of free time on their hands to do as they please—catch up on reading, organize the closet, or whatever activity they've been hungry for an opportunity to dive into. A lot of partners and co-workers think you're going to be taking it easy, too. You might have that same expectation. But taking care of a newborn is a lot more work than your typical 9-to-5 job—and it's work that you don't get paid for.

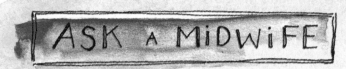

ASK A MIDWIFE

AM I NORMAL IF I FEEL BLUE?

from MARI MIKEL:

"Most of the moms I work with experience an elation period where they think, *I did it! And the baby is beautiful and I'm so in love*. Then the relentlessness of fatigue and nursing kicks in, and their hormones shift and they feel down; it's so easy and common to feel this way. If you know it's coming you're not going to be overwhelmed by it. This is just another reason to stay in bed and rest as much as possible during the first two weeks of baby's life. Trying to take care of anything other than the baby and yourself is just too much right now.

"You do think differently once the baby is born. Your brain is hotwired to keep the baby alive. Focusing on the survival of the baby can take over your self-survival drive. Also, it's a big deal to create and nurture this new being; it naturally pulls some energy away from your brain. But just like your sex drive, it will come back.

"Now is the time to dramatically lower your expectations for yourself and what you think you ought to be doing or accomplishing. Ask for the help you need, and if at all possible, get your partner to do all the meal planning, cooking, and cleaning. If you're struggling, get yourself some support immediately, whether that's a therapist or a new mom's group you connect with online. There's a reason why you have to put your own oxygen mask on first: You cannot take care of the baby if you don't take care of yourself, and the baby's need for you right now is immense. If you aren't motivated to give yourself the care you need for your own self, do it for the baby."

> "TAKING CARE of A NEWBORN is A LOT *more* WORK THAN YOUR TYPICAL 9-TO-5 JOB – AND iT's WORK *that* YOU DON'T GET PAID *for*."

It's tempting to think that you'll get things done around the house or in your work while you're taking care of a newborn, but in reality, you probably won't. It is so easy to stay busy all day while taking care of a baby. Between feeding, changing diapers, changing their clothes, putting them down for a nap, giving them a bath, and putting them to bed it can feel a little bit like you're in baby jail—you can't escape their need for your attention and care. And yet, at the end of the evening, even though you've been busy all day, it might feel like you didn't truly 'accomplish' anything.

The truth is, our culture does not value rest, or doing less. And we don't put a lot of value on childcare—as evidenced by how little childcare workers are typically paid. You've got to consciously remind yourself that taking care of the baby is 100 times more important than any household task. The clothes don't need to be folded and the dishes done for you to feel good about yourself. You have to decide to either let that stuff go, hire someone to help you do it, or change your living situation (my Mom moved in with us after the twins were born, for example, so there would always be another set of hands to help care for them).

You have to change your mindset; bonding with your baby and doing what it takes to keep them well-fed and gaining weight is your new top priority. You can't do it all. Plus, this time is going to go by so fast; put everything else you can on hold. Remember that giving birth is a big accomplishment. You just created life! You don't have to do anything extra right now.

When my girls were three months old, we entered the lockdown phase of the COVID-19 pandemic. It made me realize that all my kids' newborn phases felt a lot like the lockdown. My best advice for making this time that can feel so isolating more manageable is to develop a daily rhythm. Have your morning coffee at about the same time every day, and get the baby outside for sunning at a regular time (if it's not freezing where you live, exposure to morning light is great for helping to set their internal clock). Have a regular lunch break and a regular rest period when you get into bed in the middle of the day (even if you don't fall asleep, resting helps you feel less fatigued). Try to get to bed at the same time each night.

And then add little rituals into your routine—I like to light candles at dinnertime that I keep on until bedtime, just to make nighttime feel more special. Or you can put fresh flowers in a vase next to the chair where you have your coffee or where you breastfeed. Little things like these make you feel more in control of your day during a time when your main job is to be responsive to someone else's needs all day and night.

I found it really helpful to get off social media during the early weeks, just so I wouldn't see or read about anyone else's accomplishments. You're in a different space than everyone else; you don't need to see influencers posting about things that are worlds away from where you're at right now. You can go back in a few weeks—the outside world isn't going to go anywhere.

Leaving the House: When, How, and Why

I talked about this in Chapter 23, but in the first two weeks after birth you want to rest as much as possible—it helps you recover from birth and gives your uterus a chance to shrink up a bit and your pelvic floor a chance to come back together so that you heal well. It also guarantees you plenty of bonding time with baby. And it keeps you home, which is good for the baby since their immune system isn't fully online yet.

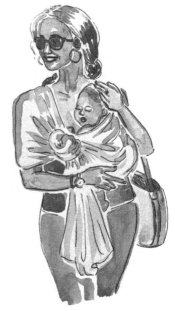

It's really just for two weeks, which sounds like a long time until you're living it and you realize just how fleeting it is.

Your Resting Schedule for the First Month

First 3 days: Stay down as much as possible, except to use the bathroom and shower; even eat in bed if you're able

Second 3 days: Get up for 4 or 5 10-minute periods throughout the day

Second week: Get up for 5 or 6 10-minute periods throughout the day

Third week: Now you can leave the house; just plan to take a 2-hour rest in the morning and in the afternoon (4 hours total of rest per day)

Fourth week: Take one 2-hour rest in the middle of the day

After two weeks you can start leaving the house. Because the baby's immune system is still developing, stick to places where you can easily maintain a physical distance from other people so that your potential exposure to germs stays low. Just keep in mind that you're still going to need a lot of rest—see the list just above to gauge how much downtime you need during each week of the newborn period. Giving yourself a nice long stretch in the middle of the day to be home and resting is also good practice for respecting the baby's nap schedule that will develop in the weeks to come.

Once you do start going places, the first time you leave the house it can feel like you have packed enough stuff to fill a suitcase. Gradually you'll pare that down to the essentials and know how to roll with anything that you forget.

The list on the next page can help you prepare for anything that might come up on those early outings.

(And here's one little pro tip: Don't ever leave the car seat in the car, as it can easily get too hot or too cold. Bring it in with you so that it stays room temperature.)

What to Bring With You When Leaving the House With Baby

- At least one change of clothes for baby
- Formula or breast milk
- Pacifier and a spare pacifier (if you use them)
- An extra layer for baby if it's cold— a coat or a blanket
- Bottle of water for you
- Snack for you
- Changing pad
- Swaddle blanket
- Clean burp cloth or two
- Diapers

- Diaper cream
- If it's hot, a travel-sized bottle of corn starch to prevent heat rash
- Wipes
- Mask (for you, if it's a pandemic)
- Empty plastic bag for soiled clothes

It's also a good idea to keep a change of clothes for yourself in your car and/or in the bottom of your stroller, because at some point the baby will pee, poop, or vomit on you and you will be so happy to be able to change into something clean.

Staying Connected to Your Partner

In these early weeks when you and the baby are in a love bubble—especially when you're breastfeeding—I think it's hard for partners. They can feel like a third wheel. Also, because you are being so wholly responsive to the baby now, and often have the baby physically on or right next to your body, it's natural for you to feel less of a desire to be physically close with your partner. I'm not even talking about having sex (which I'll cover more in Chapter 26). I mean just snuggling in bed or even sometimes being in the same room. Especially if you're an introvert, the lack of alone time can deprive you of solitude that maybe you never truly realized just how much you needed before.

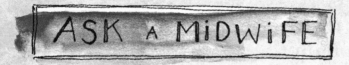

ASK A MIDWIFE

DO I REALLY NEED TO LIE DOWN AS MUCH AS POSSIBLE AFTER GIVING BIRTH?

from MARI MIKEL:

"Before you got pregnant, your uterus was the size of a plum and weighed six to eight ounces. All those contractions your uterus had during pre-labor, labor, and birth built its muscle mass to the point that after the baby comes out, the uterus weighs approximately four and a half pounds and is the size of a large cantaloupe. On top of that, your pelvic floor and pelvic muscles had to basically turn to mush to allow the baby to come out, so if you are back on your feet the day after birth your uterus is going to hang down with nothing to hold it up, and as you heal your uterus will be too low in your body. There is a condition called uterine prolapse, where the uterus presses on or can even start coming out of the vagina, that a full 50 percent of women endure; this has a lot to do with our 40 percent rate of full hysterectomy.

"And yet so few women hear the advice to stay lying down in bed—not even sitting up in bed, but fully lying down—for as much as possible during the first two weeks after birth. I see tiny little babies who are only a couple days old out with their moms at Target. And while I make it a point not to judge women for their mothering, I do worry, because at that point the baby has no immune system and the woman's uterus is hanging awfully low.

"Once the baby is here, and I know this is hard to do, for your sake and your baby's sake, stay lying down as much as possible for two full weeks. When you're bored and losing your mind, write letters, read books, finish off magazines, do paint by number, call people you always mean to call but haven't, or make a scrapbook. You can always go lie down in another room. Wherever you are reclining, just gaze adoringly at the baby, which aids in bonding so much and opens your heart more and more every moment. I know it sounds crazy, but once you're living it, you get it. Just plan on it.

"After two weeks have gone by you can start to get up and about more and more. And yes, even go to Target (so long as it's not flu season or a pandemic, in which case I'd stick to less populated places)."

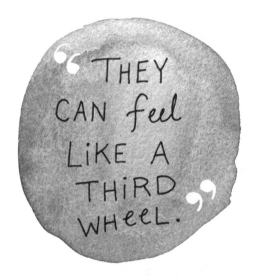

"THEY CAN *feel* LiKE A THiRD WHeeL."

It can also be hard for new moms to allow others to take care of their babies. I know I was convinced that I was the only one who could put Hendrix down for a nap, for example, so I would kind of shoo my husband away from taking over. I'm glad to say I've learned from my past mistakes! Now that we have four children, he's very hands on. Thank God I learned my lesson, as it's been so much better this time around. Don't wait until baby number three to figure this out, please! It's better for you, for your partner, and for the baby.

The best way to keep your partner involved during the newborn time is to have them be responsible for certain duties or times of day. It could be a certain feeding (which means, if you're breastfeeding, you'll have to pump), or if they're back to work they can take over

> **"A CRUCIAL factor in ALL THiS iS LeTTiNG YOUR PARTNER DO WHATeVeR THeY'RE DoiNG THeiR WAY."**

on their days off. Or they can be in charge of bath time, changing diapers, burping the baby, giving the baby skin-to-skin contact, or taking care of you by bringing you something to drink while you're nursing.

A crucial factor in all this is letting your partner do whatever they're doing their way. This can be hard to do even when you're talking about something mundane like loading the dishwasher; when you're hormonal and every cell in your body is on high alert for anything that might harm the baby, you may have to exert a lot of willpower to keep from making comments. Otherwise, they'll assume that you're going to do it better.

The fact is, you and the baby are having a great love affair, and you want to make sure your partner feels like a part of it.

Processing Your Birth Story

It's very rare that a woman's birth experience exactly aligns with her birth plan. In these weeks when the experience is so fresh, you may be having a hard time processing some aspect of how your birth went down.

If you had a traumatic birth experience, you were treated poorly, or you didn't get the birth you had planned and hoped for, it's important to advocate for yourself. When you're ready, talk to someone who was in charge, whether that's your midwife or a hospital administrator. After my girls were born (read more about that experience on page 423), I spoke to the hospital administrator and told them that it was unacceptable for laboring women to be treated the way our surrogate was. I didn't get huffy or up in their face. I remained calm, but direct. But if you don't speak up for yourself at some point, you're likely to beat yourself up later. Also, the mother-friendly changes to the typical American birth experience that we so desperately need won't happen if we women don't share our points of view. Someone else can do it on your behalf, too; what's important is that you feel your voice is heard.

If you're feeling bad that you didn't speak up when you were in labor, remember that you were vulnerable and in the throes of one of the biggest physical challenges of your life. Cut yourself some slack. You can still advocate for yourself now. Have a meeting with somebody to get it off your chest and help change future births.

You have a choice about how you think about things. It's a choice to decide that your birth sucked. You can just as easily decide that what happened was the perfect birth. I believe that life provides us exactly what we need—not necessarily what we want, like, or think is good, but what teaches us and shapes us in ways that make us better. Sometimes it's hard to see in the moment what the positive side of your birth experience might be; in those moments, even just telling yourself that one day you'll be able to look back and see the benefit can help you not feel like a victim.

Remember that this is your baby's birth, not yours, and that the baby has their own path that will foster their spiritual growth. You can expect the best, visualize your most ideal birth, and then you have to surrender. This is really extra hard for Type A go-getters, of which I am one, so I get it; we think we can make things be the way we want them to be out of sheer will. Surrender is a big challenge. But parenthood requires surrender on a daily basis. You have to surrender to your kids all the time. They won't go to sleep when you need sleep more than anything in the world, for example. If nothing else, a difficult birth experience is teaching you how to let go of expectations.

> "The mother-friendly changes to the typical American birth experience that we so desperately need won't happen if we women don't share our points of view."

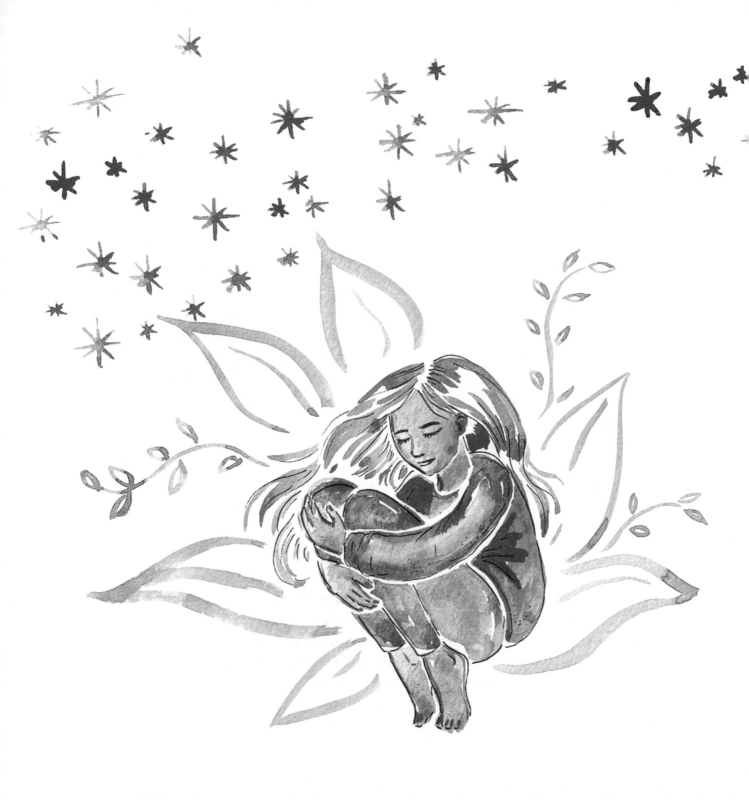

Chapter 26

BABY YOUR BODY

I know it can feel like everything in your life and all your awareness has reoriented toward taking care of the baby. Just remember that you need loving care, too. In this chapter, I outline the ways you can nurture your body even as you're nurturing your baby.

Your Body Never Left

It drives me crazy to see headlines about how to 'get your body back' after giving birth. Um… it never left you. It carried you through every single second of your pregnancy and your baby's birth. In fact, it only got more magical than it was before because *your body created a new life.*

I don't even like the term 'bounce back,' because it implies that you're somewhere that you shouldn't be and you need to go back to somewhere else. When people say, "Are you ready to get your body back?" or "How long did it take you to bounce back?" I suggest you say, "It never left! It's right here and it's healthy as ever." And, of course, remind yourself of that too.

I know it's not popular for a woman to love her body; I know how tempting it is to look at it and see its so-called 'flaws' and not appreciate it. But take a split-second to remember: You just built a baby. (Maybe more than one baby!) I've heard it said about birth that you were given a nail and you built a house. However it went down, you performed a miracle.

Please don't let your thoughts about your body now have anything to do with wanting to get back into your prepregnancy jeans. Put your focus on reverence for all that your body has done—how strong and powerful of a being you are.

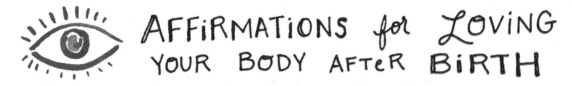

AFFIRMATIONS *for* LOVING YOUR BODY AFTER BIRTH

I AM PERFECT and COMPLETE JUST AS I AM.

I APPRECIATE MY BODY, I RESPECT MY BODY, I TRUST my BODY, I LOVE my BODY.

MY BODY CAN DO AWESOME THINGS.

I DESERVE to FEEL GOOD.

I AM PROUD of MY BEAUTIFUL, POWERFUL, MAGICAL BODY.

THANK YOU, BODY, for SUPPORTING ME and MY BABY.

Rehab Your Core and—Ultimately—Return to Exercise

I'm not going to lie. Bringing your core back together can be hard. The muscles have moved and stretched so far that it feels like you're piecing it back together. I found even sitting up in bed to be a challenge at first—I had to roll to my side and use my hands (all the more reason to follow Mari Mikel's advice to stay reclined as much as possible those first two weeks!).

I also found Brooke's guidance on rehabilitating the core so helpful. Following her advice after both of my pregnancies truly did help my core come back even stronger than before. I'll let her take it from here.

ASK A FITNESS PRO

HOW CAN I TAKE CARE OF MY CORE NOW?

from BROOKE

"It's vital that you honor what you have just accomplished through rest, grace, and a gentle reconnection to your physical body, specifically the core and pelvic floor. With a focus on breathing and physical awareness, I think of it as spending quality time with your body. In addition to helping you physically heal, it also provides space for mental and emotional rest, too.

"This reconnection period can begin whenever you feel ready. For some, this will be immediate, and for others, waiting three weeks or more feels more in line with their needs. If you choose to begin your rehabilitation in the first week, please remember to start slow. You won't be moving a ton and you most definitely won't be breaking a sweat.

"While you're lying in bed, even with the baby in bed with you, you can begin to re-implement your diaphragmatic breathing and gentle belly pumps. When you feel ready you can also start gentle pelvic floor contractions, trying to hold those for 10-20 seconds at a time with an equal amount of rest before your next contraction. Don't worry about how many you've completed or how long you hold them. Just remember that after pushing your baby out through these muscles, it's common for your contraction to be slightly more difficult to access—this will pass as you continue your reconnection phase of rehab.

"If you like to follow a prescribed routine, here's one for the first one to weeks after birth. You can refer back to pages 40 and 41 for instructions for these exercises if you need a refresher."

The Bloom Method's Early Postpartum Circuit (for the 1st and 2nd weeks after birth)

Diaphragmatic Breaths

Duration: 1 minute

Diaphragmatic Breaths, feeling the movement of the pelvic floor

Duration: 1 minute

Belly Pumps

Duration: 1 minute

Belly Pumps, feeling the slight contraction and release of the pelvic floor

Duration: 1 minute

Pelvic Floor Contractions (About 15)

Duration: 1 minute

Diaphragmatic Breathing, feeling the movement of the

Duration: 1 minute

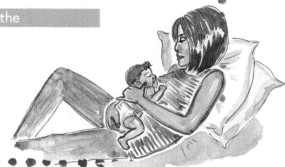

"From the start, it's important to enroll your core and pelvic floor muscles to support you through your everyday movements. Doing so will better prepare your body for more traditional exercises whenever you are ready for them. At Bloom, we call this rebuilding the foundation, and you can begin to do it during the typical movements that you're doing now, including:

- *Reclining to nurse or bottle feed baby, and then sitting up from nursing or bottle feeding baby.* Your core and pelvic floor should engage to guide you back into the reclining position and help you sit up. Practicing this will not only help ensure that your core is firing appropriately during your daily movements but will also begin to prep you for moves like sit-ups and crunches after you've moved out of the six-week postpartum phase.

- *Picking up your little one and placing them down (in a crib, on the bed, handing them to a partner, etc.).* This action changes the distribution of the load you're carrying (meaning, your baby) and requires help from your core and pelvic floor. Prior to picking up your baby, try to gently engage the pelvic floor followed by a subtle activation of the inner core (much like the exhale component of the belly pump), and then keep it engaged as you lift. The same goes for when you are standing for a long period of time while holding your little one. The level of core engagement shouldn't feel like you are squeezing the muscles with all your might, instead it's as if this new core- and pelvic-floor-based awareness simply provides an element of stability that you wouldn't have if you hadn't called on these muscles.

"Once you feel as though you have moved through a decent amount of reconnection techniques and are feeling the inner core come back online, you are ready to perform a gentle rehab circuit to continue building and restrengthening your core. This usually happens between three and five weeks, depending on you, your birth, and how you are healing. Remember this is your journey, so you write the script!"

The Bloom Method's Postpartum Circuit (for the 3rd to 6th weeks after birth)

As you perform this same circuit over the course of a month, try to increase how long you perform each exercise by 15 seconds each week, working up to one minute total per exercise.

Supine Leg Marches

Duration: 30 seconds

Directions: Lying supine with feet flat on the floor, knees up towards the ceiling, exhale as you engage your pelvic floor and deep core and bring one knee up towards your chest. Maintain your core engagement as you inhale and guide the leg back down until your foot meets the floor, then repeat on the other side. Keep the core engaged the entire time.

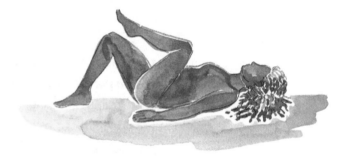

Supine Pelvic Tilts

Duration: 30 seconds

Directions: From the same starting position, exhale as you engage your pelvic floor and deep core and tuck your pelvis (roll your hip bones towards rib cage). Inhale as you untuck the pelvis and release it back to starting position. Keep going, allowing your core activation to guide the movement of the pelvis.

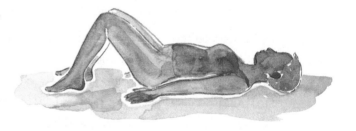

Supine Inner Thigh and Deep Core Squeezes

Duration: 30 seconds

Directions: In the same starting position, place a yoga block, foam roller, or inflatable ball between your knees. Exhale as you squeeze the object and simultaneously engage your pelvic floor and deep core. Inhale as you release the squeeze and core engagement. Repeat.

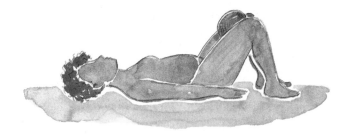

Supine Upper Body Squeezes

Duration: 30 seconds

Directions: Building on the previous exercise, this time exhale as you squeeze the object and press palms together while simultaneously engaging your pelvic floor and deep core. Inhale as you release. Repeat.

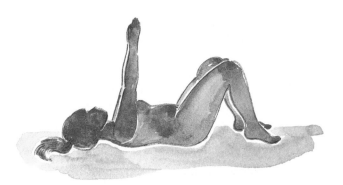

Booty Bridge with Inner Thigh and Deep Core Squeeze

Duration: 30 seconds

Directions: In the final exercise in this position, exhale as you squeeze the object, engage the pelvic floor, deep core, inner thighs, and glutes, and press down through your heels to lift your hips up towards the ceiling. Make sure that your rib cage doesn't flare out—keep it in line with your hip bones. Inhale as you lower while maintaining your core engagement to guide the hips back down. Repeat and try to match your inner thigh squeeze with your core contraction so that everything works together.

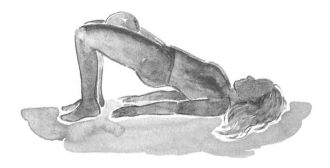

Spinal Balance with Holds

Duration: 30 seconds

Directions: Come onto all fours. Exhale and engage your deep core as you lift and extend your right arm and left leg away from the mid-line. Allow your core engagement to drive the lift and maintain the core contraction as you lower back to neutral. Repeat on the other side keeping your hips level (be sure not to let the non-working hip dip down). After 30 seconds of alternating spinal balances, finish with a 15-second lift and hold on each side. During the hold, stay engaged in your core the entire time while continuing to breathe.

Superman

Duration: 30 seconds

Directions: Lying on your stomach (if this is uncomfortable you can roll a small towel up and place underneath your breasts to support them in this position), extend your arms and legs out long. As you exhale, engage the front of your core (think about lifting it away from the floor beneath you) as you lift your arms and legs up using the back side of your core muscles to create the movement. Inhale as you lower and repeat.

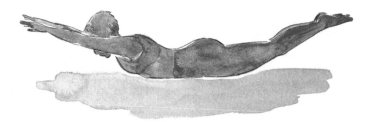

Having Sex Again

Really, as soon as sex sounds like a good idea, you are ready. Mari Mikel cleared me for having sex again about four weeks after my first birth, and it did not sound like a great idea, so I waited. Generally, it takes somewhere between six to eight weeks for women to feel ready to have sex again.

You don't want to keep your sexuality on a shelf for too much longer than that, because sex will help you and your partner feel connected, and it is a great stress reliever. Afterward, you will be glad you did it.

> *"Generally, it takes somewhere between six to eight weeks for women to feel ready to have sex again."*

Just be sure to use a condom if your partner is a man, for two reasons: 1) normal bacteria that's found on the penis could potentially lead to a uterine infection while your womb is still healing, and 2) you could get pregnant right away, even if you're breastfeeding exclusively and even if your monthly period hasn't returned yet. Most women start getting periods somewhere between six and 12 months after birth if they're breastfeeding, but you just can't be sure. Some get it after a few weeks. And even the resumption of your period isn't a good indicator of your return to fertility, because you will always ovulate before your period resumes. Unless you're ready to have another infant in nine months, use birth control every time. Condoms are easy, and they have the benefit of shielding you from bacteria. You can also get fitted with a cervical cap, but not until three months have passed because that's how long it takes for your cervix to finish healing and recuperating.

You may experience vaginal dryness when you are postpartum, so have some lube on hand. Also, a lot of women are not that orgasmic while breastfeeding—it's nature's way of preventing you from getting pregnant again so soon. Don't panic, though, as they're not gone forever: When your period comes back, so will the intensity of your orgasms.

Postpartum Nutrition: What to Eat Now

You've paid careful attention to what you've put on your plate for more than nine months. As tempting as it may be to loosen the reins now that your little one has arrived, your first few weeks (and even months) postpartum isn't the time to throw in the towel and binge on chips, cookies, and other junk foods. That said, it's okay to let yourself indulge in many of the healthful whole foods and beverages that were off the list while you were pregnant, such as freshly pressed juice, fresh sprouts, and soft cheeses (remember, though, choose full-fat dairy and do consume in moderation). Bad bacteria like *salmonella* and *listeria* can still make you sick, of course, but you don't have to worry about them passing into your breast milk and harming your child.

Even though breastfeeding does burn up to 500 calories a day, you still want to keep 80 to 90 percent of your diet very clean. Don't limit your intake of healthy foods—wild salmon, nuts, smoothies, soups, salads will all help you recover from pregnancy and birth and nourish your baby. And if you want a hamburger, have it, but make it organic and grassfed beef, for example. (For some reason my comfort food postpartum was peanut butter and jelly sandwiches.)

The last nine months put a great deal of stress on your body. You want to nurture it through nutrition now, to help it recover, not tax it further with a lot of unhealthy foods. And if you're breastfeeding, you want to do what you can to help your body make milk and maintain a steady milk supply. What's more, studies suggest a link between low levels of certain nutrients and postpartum depression, including vitamin D, folate, fatty acids, iron, calcium, selenium, and zinc. Researchers think this is because pregnancy and lactation can deplete levels of these nutrients, which are critical to the production of neurotransmitters that play major roles in mood and mood regulation.[44] Research also indicates that inflammation in the body may play a role in depression in general, and specifically in postpartum depression, and that many foods can help put out the internal fire that inflammation causes.[45] While healthy eating may not necessarily be able to keep the blues away all on its own, it's a great place to start to reduce your risk.

General Guidelines for Eating—and Supplementing— in the Postpartum Period

Here are the basic things you want to keep in mind when it comes to giving your body what it needs to fully recuperate and nourish your baby.

Watch Your Water Intake

I've talked a lot about the importance of hydration during pregnancy, and it remains vital postpartum. Water helps your body recover. It also supports breastfeeding and helps you avoid constipation, which is common for many moms at this point (fiber-rich foods help too—I would add a tablespoon of chia seeds to eight ounces of water and let them sit long enough to form a thicker consistency, then drink it down, to help with constipation; I also kept up my morning shot of apple cider vinegar).

I've seen different recommendations, ranging from six to 15 glasses of water a day, depending on if you're nursing or not. I think the best way to tell if you're hydrated is to pay attention to the color of your urine: You'll know you need to drink more if it's dark, or if you're not going to the bathroom regularly; it should be a pale, almost clear yellow. If you get tired of plain water, other fluids count too. Avoid sodas and, for the most part, caffeine and alcohol (more on the latter two on page 411), and instead opt for herbal teas or unsweetened or low-sugar fruit juices or sparkling waters.

Be Conscious of Calories

If you're not breastfeeding, you may be able to return to your prepregnancy diet, at least calorie-wise—aiming for around the average recommended daily intake, somewhere between 1,800 and 2,200 calories. But if you are nursing, in the months after birth you'll need to consume up to 500 more calories per day to compensate for the calories and nutrients your baby takes through breastfeeding. If you're back to working out a lot or are breastfeeding multiples, you may need even more than an extra 500 calories per day. Talk to your care provider about the amount of calories you should be consuming. You'll know you're not eating enough if your milk supply dries up, if your baby isn't gaining weight, or if you lose weight too rapidly.

Focus on Whole, Nutrient-Dense, Anti-Inflammatory Foods

The same general healthy eating advice I've shared all along applies now: Think the entire rainbow of fresh fruits and vegetables and healthy fats like those found in fish and olive oil, lean meats, and seafood. If you keep eating as you have been over the next few weeks and months, you'll be doing wonders in helping your body and mind feel their best, and ensure your baby gets the nutrients they need. Although your grocery cart will look similar, and if you continued to eat the same foods you'd be on a great path, I still want to highlight the specific nutrients that play important roles in the postpartum period, and the foods rich in them. There may be a few new foods to add to your basket now that you hadn't enjoyed before.

Specific Nutrients to Focus on Now

In general, it's a good idea to continue taking your prenatal vitamin while you're breastfeeding. That way you can make up for any deficiencies in the following that may occur in your diet (even though you're eating a wide array of healthy, whole foods). Know that the recommended daily intake for some nutrients may increase as much as 50 percent during lactation. Even if you aren't breastfeeding, you'll still need to focus on a few specific nutrients.

- **Iron.** I'm starting with iron, because it's especially critical in the first week after you've delivered. You may have lost a significant amount of blood during childbirth, so you'll want to replenish your red blood cells, and eating iron-rich foods is just the way to do that. Plus, your breast milk provides iron for your baby to support their development. Recommendations vary widely, from around 10 mg a day while breastfeeding up to 30 mg a day, depending on your specific situation. But you don't want to overdo it, so talk with your doctor about the iron intake that's right for you. Foods rich in iron include red meat and poultry, tofu, and beans. If you have twins or don't consume animal products, you may need to consider a supplement.

- **Protein**. Lactation increases the body's need for protein. Recommendations vary, but typically range from 65-80 grams of protein a day, which is around 25 extra grams of protein beyond normal recommendations daily during the postpartum period. You should easily be able to meet these needs through foods alone; think of having a generous serving or two of protein with each meal or at least your larger, main meals. Protein helps your body bounce back from the stress of pregnancy and childbirth. It repairs your cells and helps build baby's cells too, as they're growing rapidly. Great sources include lean meats, eggs, fish, beans, nuts, full-fat dairy, and whole soy foods like tofu.

- **Calcium**. When you were pregnant, you needed more calcium than normal because your body took calcium from your bones to support your baby's growth. In the weeks and months postpartum, your body still pulls calcium from your bones into your breast milk to continue to aid in baby's growth. In other words, both your body and your baby are counting on you to get adequate calcium—you want them to grow big and strong, and you want to prevent bone loss and osteoporosis for yourself later on. (Estrogen is low during nursing, making your bones at extra risk for brittleness and deterioration.) During this time, you need about 1,000 milligrams (mg) a day. Good sources include dairy (remember, I recommend full-fat dairy, in moderation); sesame seeds; leafy greens; tofu; and plant-based milks (if they're fortified with calcium; read the label carefully).

- **B Vitamins**. Recommended intakes of folate and vitamin B6, in particular, increase during lactation and the postpartum period. And as I have mentioned before, low levels of folate may play a role in the development of postpartum depression. In general, the B family of vitamins are involved in so many important bodily processes, affecting your brain functioning (hence the role in mood), energy levels, and much more. Folate-rich foods in particular include leafy greens and other green veggies like broccoli, asparagus, and Brussels sprouts; avocado; and black-eyed peas. To get a boost of all the Bs, enjoy nuts, beans, eggs, yogurt, animal foods, and nutritional yeast, which you can sprinkle on salads, popcorn, you name it.

- **Choline**.   If you're breastfeeding, your choline needs increase a good bit, as large amounts are found in breast milk. Like folate, choline is absolutely crucial for your baby's brain development. Eggs are rich in choline (just remember to eat the whites and the yolk); as are meat; poultry; fish; and dairy products. The recommended intake for breastfeeding moms is 550 mg daily.

- **Vitamin D**.   Vitamin D supports so many bodily processes. And as I've covered, low levels of vitamin D have been linked to postpartum depression, and depression in general. Although the best way to get vitamin D is from the sun's rays, there are foods that are more rich in this nutrient than others. Focus on eggs (again, you need to eat the yolks here); fatty fish (which are also rich in omega-3s, discussed next); and fortified dairy or fortified nondairy alternatives. If you don't get out much in the sun, or you've given birth during winter when you can't get outside regularly, or at least not for long enough for your body to synthesize D, you may also want to try a supplement, or just continue taking a supplement if you started during pregnancy. Look for a high-quality product providing vitamin D3, or cholecalciferol, and talk to your health care provider about the right amount for you.

- **Omega-3s**.   These fatty acids are perhaps the most important nutrient of all those discussed so far for helping reduce your risk of postpartum depression. In fact, studies show a diet rich in omega-3s can go a long way toward reducing inflammation in the body and boosting mood, not to mention helping with many essential systems and functions.[46] In addition, babies whose mothers have high concentrations of the omega-3 DHA, in particular, in their breast milk show improvements in vision and cognition.[47] Good food sources include coldwater, fatty fish like salmon; fortified eggs; and dairy products. Since many moms don't get enough omega-3s in their diet, you may also want to consider a supplement that contains both EPA and DHA and is certified to be free of contaminants like mercury.

- **Selenium and Zinc**.   Low levels of these minerals have also been implicated in postpartum depression. Meats, legumes, seeds, nuts, and dairy products can up your zinc levels. Brazil nuts are one of the best single sources of selenium; you can also get selenium from seafood (especially tuna, sardines, and shrimp); meats and poultry; brown rice; and cottage cheese.

*A **word of warning**.* Fish are great sources of almost all of the nutrients covered here. But just as you were while pregnant, you still want to be mindful of the types of seafood you eat during the postpartum period, taking care to avoid fish high in mercury, which can pass to your baby through breast milk and is extremely harmful to them. Refer back to pages 196–197 for healthy options that are low in this toxin.

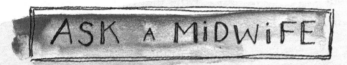

ASK A MIDWIFE

DO CAFFEINE AND ALCOHOL AND BREASTFEEDING MIX?

from MARI MiKeL:

"Caffeine is more problematic than alcohol. One glass of wine doesn't warrant pumping and dumping—any alcohol that does find its way to the baby is relaxing. So long as you are keeping it very moderate—no more than two drinks with plenty of food and time in between glasses, and only on a truly as-needed basis to reduce stress—you are okay to breastfeed.

"If you want something more definitive than that, you can purchase test strips that measure the alcohol level in your breast milk and clearly show if it's suitable for giving to your baby or if you should toss it out.

"Caffeine, on the other hand, is a stimulant and can really mess with your baby's sleep. You don't want to learn this the hard way. So long as you are breastfeeding, I advise that you keep your consumption limited to two caffeinated beverages a week. It's also better for you, because if you don't try to manipulate your energy with caffeine, you'll be much more able to doze when the baby dozes and address your fatigue via what your body truly needs—sleep. I love the ritual of making and drinking coffee so I know it's not easy to go without. Just make decaf coffee instead."

What's Happening Now: Postpartum and Newborn Phases

The postpartum period typically spans the first six weeks after you have given birth, although some experts believe it actually lasts up to six months; you may even see it referred to in books and articles as the first year after delivery. Why the discrepancy about an "end date"? Because the postpartum period refers to the time it takes for the physiological shifts that occurred during pregnancy to shift back to their nonpregnant state, or at least for the most part. And that timeline may look different for different women. Note that I'm not talking about weight here, rather the other changes that took place—i.e., your uterus expanding—to help you bring a baby into this world.

This is the space for you to heal, as well as adjust to the new demands and realities of motherhood. Over these six weeks, you'll notice many things happening with your body as well as your mood, thanks to the hormonal swings and rebalancing occurring now. Of course, there's also so much going on with your little one in terms of their growth and development over this time. Here's what to look out for.

With Baby

Your baby will grow and change at a rapid pace in their first six weeks. In fact, they may even outgrow an outfit or develop an adorable new skill literally overnight! Stay tuned for these exciting developments:

- **Putting on the pounds.** It's totally normal for your newborn to lose weight in the first week of their life. But usually in their second week, by around day 10, they'll be back up to their birth weight or even weigh in a little heavier. As a general guideline, they'll gain around two-thirds of an ounce a day initially, and then typically between five and seven ounces a week until they're around six months old.

- **Growth spurt.** If your baby is eating more (and waking up more often to eat) or acting a tad fussier, they may be telling you that they're going through a growth spurt. The first spurt usually happens around week two—additional growth spurts then typically occur at three months, six months, and then nine months. From birth to six months, a baby will typically grow between a half inch to inch a month, although they may grow even taller that first month. During this time, your baby's head is also growing, an indicator of brain development. If their head appears a little misshapen after birth, it will take its normal shape soon, so it may appear slightly smaller at first before you notice the growth. Your newborn's head circumference will increase to about 15 inches in their first month of life and continue to grow about two centimeters monthly for their first year. Your health care practitioner will share growth charts and average height, circumference, and weight percentiles with you to help you track your baby's growth and development.

- **The skin they're in.** Around four weeks or so, you may notice that your baby has developed baby acne. This is common, so don't panic. You can wash their face gently once a day with a mild soap formulated especially for babies. They may also have harmless white dots on their nose, called milia. Their skin can also look blotchy and range in color from pink to blue based on their temperature, and their face may turn a very bright red when they cry. Again, this is all A-OK. They may also lose the fine little baby hairs on their head, or develop a temporary bald spot where they sleep; the hair will grow back in the first few months.

- **Get motoring.** Over the first few months of their life, you'll watch your baby's motor skills develop. They'll go from looking like a bobble-head doll to being able to control and lift their head first for a few seconds then few minutes, and they'll also be more able to control the movements of their arms and legs. They'll be able to stretch and kick while lying on their back as well as open and close their hands, even grabbing onto objects briefly.

- **Listen up.** Your baby will start responding to the sound of your voice and other noises during this time. When you talk or sing, they may smile (around one or two months old), and they may begin turning toward the direction of noises.

- **Have a look-see.** Their eyes may wander, sometimes even in different directions and sometimes appearing crossed or as if they're rolling back in their head. And that's OK, I promise. When they're a very new newborn, you may also notice broken blood vessels in the whites of their eyes or scratches or bruising of their eyelids from delivery. Again, don't panic; all will disappear after a few weeks. As they get older, their eyes will become more coordinated. They'll be able to focus on your face while they're feeding. By around two months old, they'll be able to track objects.

With You

Again, this is your time to heal. Be patient, as you may still be experiencing some bodily discomfort, and things won't just go back to 'normal,' poof, in the blink of an eye.

- **Look out for lochia.** Lochia is the bleeding and vaginal discharge that you experience after birth. It may last for two to four weeks or longer, say closer to six weeks. Usually, it starts as heavy bleeding, but eventually the bleeding gets lighter and appears more pink or pale brown in color, and later it should turn yellow and then clear. The vaginal soreness and discomfort may be worse if you had an episiotomy.

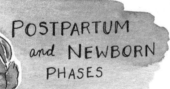

POSTPARTUM *and* NEWBORN PHASES

- **A pain in the abdomen.** You may have what feels like cramps for a bit of time. And coupled with the lochia, you may think you're having a period. (According to the science, on average, a woman's first period after pregnancy happens around 74 days postpartum.)[48] Your uterus is shrinking back to its normal, not pregnant size and shape, and sometimes you're going to feel that contraction as it's happening in your low belly. You may hear these cramps called "after pains." Sometimes they increase while you're breastfeeding, as oxytocin is released when you're nursing and it can trigger the uterus to contract. The pain should ease as time passes, typically over the first two weeks, and with a little helpful heat from a hot water bottle.

- **Shedding weight.** Most women lose up to 12 pounds with childbirth. But how much you lose after delivery depends on lots of aspects about you as an individual, including how much weight you gained during pregnancy as well as if you're breastfeeding or not.

In full hormone swing. Lots of shifts are happening with your hormones now, affecting these areas:

- **Hair.** Estrogen stimulates the growth of your hair. When you were pregnant, high levels of estrogen gave you a thick, gorgeous mane and kept all that hair from falling out and going through its normal shedding cycle. After you give birth, however, estrogen levels fall pretty sharply, which may cause you to experience significant hair thinning or loss postpartum. Try not to worry too much, although I know it's disconcerting. Once your estrogen levels increase again and level out, your hair will return to its normal state, typically within six months to a year.

- **Sweating.** Low levels of estrogen postpartum may also cause you to sweat more, especially at night while you sleep. Night sweats should stop after about two weeks. In the meantime, experiment with different strategies to stay cool, and consider sleeping with a water-resistant pad or absorbent towel underneath you.

- **Swelling.** During pregnancy, an increase in progesterone caused water retention, leading to swelling. While your hormones are settling back to prepregnancy levels, your body may continue to hang onto that pregnancy swelling for a little while, usually in your hands, legs, and feet. But it shouldn't last much longer than a week or so.

Know that while most of the discomfort you may feel or changes you may notice in the first few weeks after birth are normal, there may be others that are signs or symptoms of something more serious that needs medical attention. Be sure to attend your postpartum checkups, and to mention anything you may have noticed, even if you think it's no big deal, to your health care practitioner.

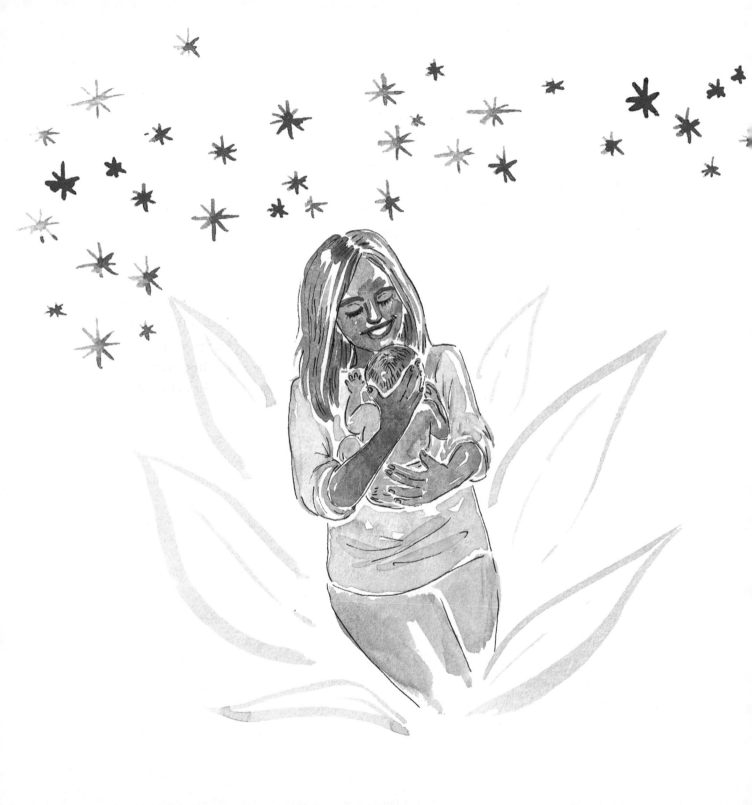

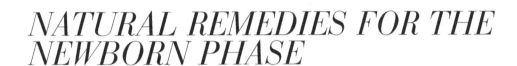

Chapter 27

NATURAL REMEDIES FOR THE NEWBORN PHASE

R ight about now, when you're still recuperating and probably sleeping less than you ever have, it's easy for every thing to feel urgent, whether that's something little like diaper rash or something big like mastitis or colic. I hope these tips will help you feel empowered to take great care of your baby and yourself. Because I'm a strong advocate for mothering yourself, I'm listing the remedies that moms need first.

Fatigue

My favorite way to relieve fatigue is going after it via the body. Exercise is great to boost your energy as well as your spirits—of course, take your time with getting back to true fitness pursuits until you are feeling healed and ready to move more. Until (and after) that time, stretching is a great way to boost circulation and just help you feel better overall. Using a foam roller can turn a stretching session into a DIY massage. Massaging devices like the Theragun or the Hypervolt are more of an investment (they run anywhere between $200 and $600), but are worth every penny because they really get into your muscles to relieve aches and pains. And breastfeeding, bending over your baby, looking down at your baby all the time, and your body recalculating its alignment after being pregnant can all take a toll on your muscles. Seeing a massage therapist is also wonderful; if you have access to that, I definitely recommend it.

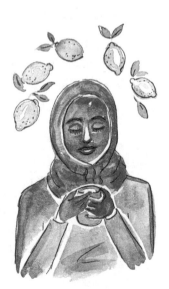

I also find that having a cup of hot water with lemon is invigorating (I have one every day about an hour before I have my coffee). And so are eucalyptus and peppermint essential oils—you can put them in a diffuser, or add a few drops to your bath or even the floor of your shower before you start running the water, as the hot water will naturally diffuse them while you bathe.

Milk Production

One of my biggest concerns with breastfeeding was that I wasn't making enough milk. I found mother's milk tea (various companies make a blend meant to support breastfeeding; I liked the Traditional Medicinals version). You can also pump after the baby nurses for 15 minutes per breast. Even if nothing comes out, you are signaling to your body to make more milk. In two days, you should see an increase in supply.

And of course, you also want to be sure you're drinking enough water.

Mastitis

Mastitis is inflammation in your breast tissue that often occurs as the result of a clogged milk duct. It can be very painful (I can attest—it happened with both my boys) and be accompanied by redness, swelling, and even fever and chills. It can also lead to a bacterial infection that requires medical treatment, and so deserves your immediate attention.

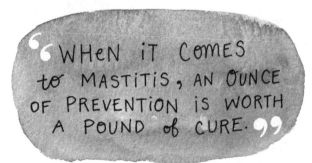

"WHeN iT CoMES to MASTiTiS, AN OUNCE OF PREVENTiON iS WORTH A POUND of CURE."

When it comes to mastitis, an ounce of prevention is worth a pound of cure. Make sure you nurse until your breast is completely empty and stay well hydrated and nourished, as this will help the area stay healthy.

The first sign of mastitis is usually a sore spot. It may feel hard to the touch and be a little red. Should you notice this has happened, fill up a water bottle, take two ibuprofen, and go get in bed so that you can rest and stay hydrated. You can also apply heat to that spot with a heating pad or hot water bottle and massage the spot to make sure there's not milk clogged in the ducts surrounding the area. Nurse the baby on the affected breast as much as possible, and even pump afterward to keep the breast as empty as you can. Continue taking ibuprofen every four hours for 24 hours. If the spot hasn't gone away, go to the doctor.

My lactation consultant also advised me to put the baby on the ground and get over him on my hands and knees and nurse him that way to help encourage as much milk as possible to drain out of the ducts. It did help.

Diaper Rash

No matter how reactive you are to your little one's dirty diapers, at some point every baby will develop a diaper rash. For every day, use a white diaper paste that has zinc oxide in it. I like the diaper creams from Weleda and Beautycounter as well as Boudreaux's Butt Paste. If your baby is extra sensitive, look for a concentration of 40 percent zinc oxide and use it for every change. Of course, I also make my own. If you're up for a DIY project, see the recipe on the following page. These are great preventatives and help keep this whole area protected and moisturized.

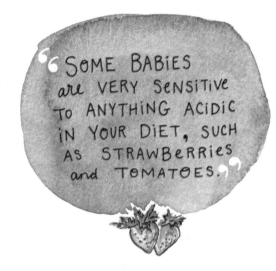

"SOME BABIES are VERY SENSITIVE TO ANYTHING ACIDIC IN YOUR DIET, SUCH AS STRAWBERRIES and TOMATOES."

Some babies are very sensitive to anything acidic in your diet, such as strawberries and tomatoes, so if your baby develops a recurring diaper rash, take these foods out of your diet and see if it helps.

For an emergency diaper balm—say, they poop in the middle of an epic nap and get really red—blend equal parts Phillips Milk of Magnesia or Maalox and cornstarch in a small glass jar. You want it to be thick enough to adhere to their skin. Then use it until the rash clears up.

Baby Bottom Cream

Here's the diaper cream I made for my babies. You don't have to add the lavender essential oil—I just had it in my drawer so I added it. It does give it a lovely scent and is good for calming you and baby both when you smell it. Apply this cream liberally to diaper rash and cover all nearby areas as well. It has a shelf life of three months.

Ingredients

2 ounces ivory shea butter

2 tablespoons argan oil

1 ounce aloe vera gel

2 tablespoons non-nano zinc oxide powder

10 drops organic lavender essential oil

Directions:

Add all oils to a glass mixing bowl. Using low speeds to start, use a hand mixer to blend all ingredients together. Once combined, turn up to medium and continue to whip the oils until peaks start to form and you have a light, fluffy consistency. With mixer off, add the zinc oxide powder slowly then put the mixer back on low to combine. Using a small spatula or spoon, pack it in small glass jars for future use. I found my jars on Amazon and preferred glass over plastic, but you could use either.

Thrush

Thrush is basically a yeast infection in the baby's mouth; you can tell they have it if they have a white coating on the tongue. (It won't wipe off and may even bleed if you try...so don't try.)

In a clean glass jar with a tight-fitting lid, mix a half-cup of water and a teaspoon of baking soda. Dip a cotton swab in the mixture and swab baby's tongue and mouth from back to front after every feeding. You should also dip a cotton ball in the mixture and wipe off your nipples after each feeding.

Typically babies also have a bright red diaper rash at the same time. Try the emergency diaper cream I mentioned on page 419. If that doesn't help, try applying Monistat cream (that you buy for vaginal yeast infections).

This overgrowth of yeast can be triggered if you eat too much sugar and too many carbs. (All the more reason to keep your diet really clean!)

Eczema

Many babies develop eczema because their skin is still balancing. My girls had eczema when they were infants. Their doctor gave them a cream, but it didn't really help and I hated the list of ingredients. So I made my own, and it has really helped clear their skin and keep it moisturized and smooth. The recipe for it is at the right.

Colic

Technically, colic is when an otherwise healthy baby cries for more than three hours a day for three days a week. No matter how long your

Hope for Eczema in a Jar

When my daughters developed eczema as babies, I used this recipe on them. It cleared right up, and I loved not having to worry that I was exposing them to any potentially harmful chemical ingredients.

Ingredients

½ cup organic soy oil

¼ cup beeswax pastilles

2 tablespoons oatmeal, ground up in a coffee grinder or food processor

20 drops vitamin E

10 drops rosemary essential oil

Directions:

Melt the soy oil and beeswax in a double boiler over low heat. Stir in the oatmeal, vitamin E, and rosemary oil. The texture will be very thick. Store in a nine-ounce glass jar and apply twice a day—in the morning and after the bath.

baby's cries last, it is really challenging, as a baby's cries are designed to grab your attention and inspire you into action.

One thing to try is laying them on their tummy either in your lap or over your shoulder. You can also lay them on their back and then bicycle their legs, which moves their digestive organs around and can help dispel gas. Then roll them from side to side. You can also take them outside, as sometimes a change in scenery from indoor to outdoor can shift a baby's whole demeanor.

> "IF YOU'RE BREASTFEEDING, COLIC OFTEN IS RELATED to SOMETHING YOU'RE EATING THAT UPSETS the BABY'S DiGestive SYSTEM."

If you're breastfeeding, colic often is related to something you're eating that upsets the baby's digestive system. One of the bigger problems can be carbs—wheat and even rice seem to be some of the major culprits. Beans and legumes can also be problematic (this includes hummus, which is made from chickpeas), as can cruciferous vegetables (such as broccoli, cauliflower, cabbage, and Brussels sprouts) and dairy products. It can be helpful to eliminate all these foods from your diet for three to five days and see if it makes a difference. Then you can experiment with adding them back in, one by one, to see which foods your baby truly reacts to. Just experiment in the morning so that if a food doesn't agree with the baby, you have a bad day instead of a bad night.

You can also make a tea out of fennel seeds and chamomile that you sweeten a tiny bit with sugar (not honey, maple syrup, or agave nectar, as you're not supposed to give these unpasteurized sweeteners to babies less than a year old because of a risk of botulism) and give to the baby via a spoon or a bottle.

Generally, babies outgrow colic by four months. Hang in there!

Our Surrogacy Journey

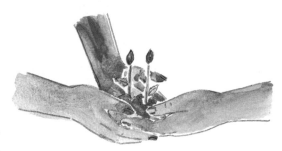

Now that we've come to the end of the book, I want to share the story of how our twins, Zuri and Zya, came into this world thanks to our amazing surrogate. Their story shows three hugely important things: just how different the hospital setting can be from a home birth, how special surrogates are, and how even if you don't carry the baby in your womb, you are still your baby's (or babies') mama from their very first breaths.

This is the letter I wrote to the girls to chronicle their births.

Dear Zuri and Zya,

Because I knew that I wouldn't be able to carry any more babies after I was diagnosed with my autoimmune condition, your Dad and I went through the process of in vitro fertilization in the hopes of finding someone who would be able to carry you in her womb instead of mine. We used an agency that helped us find just the right surrogate. The woman who carried you and birthed you is an amazing woman; she has kids of her own and is a highly trained doula. I felt such a connection to her right away, and she couldn't have been a better home for you. She and I developed a special relationship—I followed her pregnancy even more closely than I had followed my own!

We were all shocked and thrilled when we learned that the one embryo had divided into two and we would be having twins! It was too good to be true. I always said that I'd have three or four kids. I know I manifested two of you because at every first ultrasound from when I was pregnant with your brothers I looked for twins and felt a slight disappointment when I didn't see twins. I was there with the doctor and our surrogate when we did the embryo transfer. I saw you on the microscope before you were placed in her womb. One embryo. I was sure as science you'd remain one embryo. But the Universe had other plans and so did the two of you.

When I received the call from the surrogate and she shared that there were two of you I was cutting up an apple for your brother Hendrix. I started screaming, "What do you mean there are two?! We put only one in." Hendrix immediately looked up at me and said, "Mom, I said I want two babies and you said we are only getting one baby so the babies *aren*'t yours they are mine because I created them with my words." I was speechless. I remembered Hendrix telling me that he and Legend each wanted a baby and that we were going to have two babies and not one. I argued with him and was so sure of myself. You two are the miracle I was sure I wouldn't get but always dreamed of.

Five weeks before your due date, I got a call at 6:15 am from our surrogate, telling us that her water had broken. We told her we would get there as soon as we could. We were in Austin and she was out of state. We had made a plan for that day, and we activated it and immediately went to get on the plane.

I was the meanest person from that point until we were on her floor at the hospital. I was mean to your Dad, your brothers, my mother (who came with us), the pilot, the rental car person… I didn't know how fast you were coming, and I just wanted to be there so badly to greet you. I had to be there. No one could move quickly enough for me.

> "MOM, I SAID I WANT TWO BABIES AND YOU SAID WE ARE ONLY GETTING ONE BABY so the BABIES AREN'T YOURS THEY ARE MINE BECAUSE I CREATED THEM WITH MY WORDS."
> – HENDRIX

I couldn't think clearly. Once we arrived, even though I had done the hospital tour, I couldn't remember where anything was. When we finally made our way upstairs, it was 11 am and I relaxed a bit.

As soon as I got into the room where your surrogate was, we hugged and cried. Later she would tell me, "It was like our souls were talking to each other while we couldn't have words to say." The energy in the room was so strong and so healing.

When the surrogate's water broke, you two were lying cross-ways (also known as transverse), and the doctors told her that if you remained that way, she'd need to have a Cesarean. When she got to the hospital and things were a little further along, the doctor checked her and you were head down—meaning she could have a vaginal birth—and she cried with relief.

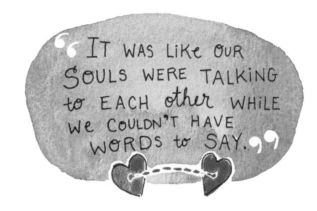

"IT WAS LiKe OuR SOULS WERE TALKING to EACH other WHiLe We COULDN'T HAVE WORDS to SAY."

She labored with you two for 13 hours. During this time, I acted as her doula. I made her drinks, lit candles, turned the lights down, applied counter pressure on her back during her contractions, massaged her, and helped in any way I could. The hospital experience was less than ideal. The nurses kept telling her to get out of the bathroom, where she felt most comfortable, and they kept checking on her every 20 minutes so that it was hard for her to go into the zone and stay calm. After laboring all day and into the night—with many disrespectful interruptions from some of the nurses—the surrogate felt the need to push.

Although she had done an incredible job of keeping her focus and helping her body get you two into position, the pushing caused her terrible pain—she had birthed her own babies before so she knew what pushing felt like, and this time felt different. She needed an epidural to give her some relief and help you two come into the world.

The doctor told her she needed to get the epidural in the operating room, because that's where she'd need to deliver the babies. Those many minutes of waiting for the epidural to kick in were so hard to witness; she was clearly in a lot of pain and scared. There comes a time in every birth when the laboring woman wonders if she can really do it; that was our surrogate's moment, and I felt like my heart was on the OR table with her.

> "THERE COMES A TIME IN EVERY BIRTH WHEN the LABORING woman WONDERS iF SHe CAN REALLY DO iT."

It was a huge distraction to go from a dark room with an essential oil diffuser running and tea lights lit, where she could have her noise cancelling headphones in, to the bright lights, cold temperatures, and busy OR, where it felt like there were 20 people running around. The anesthesiologist seemed angry and unhappy to be there and was very rough with her while he prepared to give her the anesthesia.

Finally the epidural started working and she started to push. After an hour of pushing, the doctor said, "I think we need to do an ultrasound, because I don't think what I just felt was a head." Our hearts went into our throats. It turns out you two had turned again and there were no other options but Cesarean (thankfully, the hospital staff let us stay in the OR with her—they didn't have to).

Watching all this, I was flooded with emotions that I still feel—I couldn't help her, and she was going through all of this for me and our family. It was heartbreaking and beautiful and made me feel immense gratitude and also guilt. I just kept telling her how great she was doing and that soon it would all be over.

While they scrubbed her up, the nurses started talking to each other, saying, "Why can't there ever be a normal birth shown on TV? Why do they always show someone bleeding out on the table, or dying?" My surrogate, her husband, and I all looked at each other, in utter shock that they were having this conversation as our surrogate was literally on the table.

There was nothing I could do in that moment; I had to step back and wait to meet you. When you emerged, I couldn't believe the primal sounds that came from my body—they weren't like any noise I had ever made before. I was so emotional—relieved, happy, angry at the hospital, worried for the surrogate. All those emotions came out through my voice.

The biggest emotion of all was happiness. It came out as uncontrollable screaming, laughing, and crying, then more screaming. Later I received a message on Instagram from a nurse who was in the OR. She said, "I've attended thousands of births and your birth was my favorite. I saw this most incredible gift of love this woman gave to you, and I got to see your reaction and the joy you felt. I'll never forget your screams when you first saw the babies."

Zya, when you came out, you were quiet and super calm, which is still your personality. And Zuri, you came out screaming and fighting, just like your personality now. As soon as you were born, and I saw that you were both five and a half pounds of healthiness, our surrogate felt at ease and OK. Even though she had just been through the most traumatic experience, she felt proud and thankful.

It was the most special love triangle between you, me, and your surrogate. Your Dad and I held each of you as soon as you were born. After we had a chance to bond, we gave each of you, one at a time, back to your surrogate so that she could breastfeed you. She told me, "I would do it all again in a heartbeat to see you meet your babies for the first time."

Zuri and Zya, I waited so long for you. I've always known I would have a girl and I was blessed with two. I couldn't be happier to be able to watch the two of you grow into the incredible women you will one day be. I am so proud of the two of you. Zya, you make us smile everyday at how you examine what's around you and are determined as ever to hit each milestone and more. You were by far my sweetest baby. Zuri, you make us smile daily. You love to play, dance, and laugh. You're the spokesperson for the two of you, and we love hearing what you have to say.

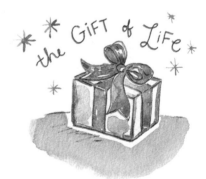

You have both made our family's world so much brighter. I cannot imagine life before you came and feel incredibly lucky that we are sharing **this** journey. I look forward to what's ahead. I love you. *Mommy*

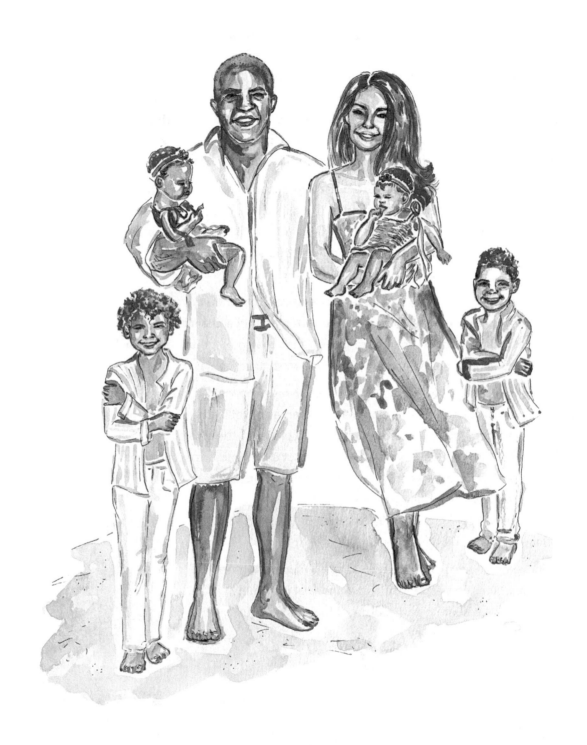

This book has turned out to be my fifth baby. I want to thank the following people for helping me bring it into the world:

Kate Hanley, you held my hand and listened to story after story and walked me through this book chapter by chapter, making sure we said everything I wanted to say and then some. You've been my light during this process!

Kimothy Joy, your illustrations moved me before ever working with you and I am so proud to have your women-empowering work here in this book.

Khristina Helmich, you've given me more than anyone else on earth and I forever love you for that. You also happen to be an amazing doula. Thank you.

Lauren Spicijaric, you give me more hours in a day and that's priceless! You keep my inbox and calendar organized so I can focus on things like this book or MUTHA or my own children. You're organized and on top of everything in our world. In fact when you aren't involved I doubt the outcome. I don't want to live a day without you (except when you're on one of your well deserved vacations somewhere in the world). You are the MVP.

Mari Mikel Potter, you filled me full of both information and confidence that led to my decision to have a home birth, which changed me in ways I never imagined it would. Thank you.

Jocelyn Foye, you turned this book into a masterpiece that I am very proud of. Thank you.

Brooke Cates, for the many training sessions and teaching me what my body was capable of while pregnant and how to fully heal my core. Also thank you for making it available to anyone everywhere online through The Bloom Method.

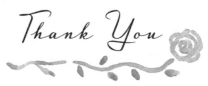

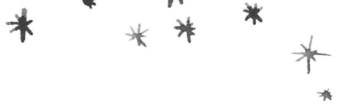

ENDNOTES

1 Jennings, V. (2014, April 2). *Fertility Awareness: Birth Control and Beyond!* Institute for Reproductive Health, Georgetown University. https://irh.org/blog/fertility-awareness-birth-control-and-beyond

2 *Miscarriage.* (Reviewed 2017, November). March of Dimes. https://www.marchofdimes.org/complications/miscarriage.aspx

3 Chavarro, J.E., Willett, W.C., & Skerrett, P.J. (2009). *The Fertility Diet.* McGraw-Hill.

4 Ben-Meir, A., Burstein, E., Borrego-Alvarez, A., Chong, J., Wong, E., Yavorska, T., Naranian, T., Chi, M., Wang, Y., Bentov, Y., Alexis, J., Meriano, J., Sung, H.K., Gasser, D.L., Moley, K.H., Hekimi, S., Casper, R.F., & Jurisicova, A. (2015). Coenzyme Q10 Restores Oocyte Mitochondrial Function and Fertility During Reproductive Aging. *Aging Cell*, 14(5), 887-95. https://doi.org/10.1111/acel.12368

5 Akarsu, S., Gode, F., Isik, A.Z., Dikmen, Z.G., & Tekindal, M.A. (2017). The Association Between Coenzyme Q10 Concentrations in Follicular Fluid with Embryo Morphokinetics and Pregnancy Rate in Assisted Reproductive Techniques. *Journal of Assisted Reproduction and Genetics,* 34(5), 599-605. https://doi.org/10.1007/s10815-017-0882-x

6 Ruder, E.H., Hartman, T.J., Reindollar, R.H., & Goldman, M.B. (2014). Female Dietary Antioxidant Intake and Time to Pregnancy Among Couples Treated for Unexplained Infertility. *Fertility and Sterility*, 101(3), 759-66. https://doi.org/10.1016/j.fertnstert.2013.11.008

7 Kesari, K.K., Agarwal, A., & Henkel, R. (2018). Radiations and Male Fertility. *Reproductive Biology and Endocrinology*, 16(1), 118. https://doi.org/10.1186/s12958-018-0431-1

8 Agarwal, A., Deepinder, F., Sharma, R.K., Ranga, G., & Li, J. (2008). Effect of Cell Phone Usage on Semen Analysis in Men Attending Infertility Clinic: An Observational Study. *Fertility and Sterility*, 89, 124–128. https://doi.org/10.1016/j.fertnstert.2007.01.166

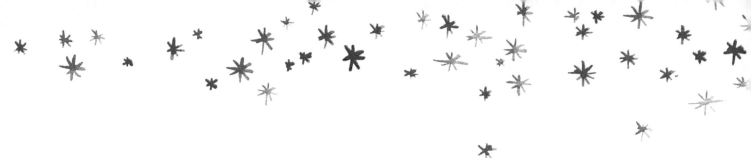

9 Li, D.K., Yan, B., Li, Z., Gao, E., Miiao, M., Gong, D., Weng, X., Ferber, J.R., & Yuan, W. (2010). Exposure to Magnetic Fields and the Risk of Poor Sperm Quality. *Reproductive Toxicology*, 29(1), 86–92. https://doi.org/10.1016/j.reprotox.2009.09.004

10 Agarwal, A., Desai, N.R., Makker, K., Varghese, A., Mouradi, R., Sabanegh, E., & Sharma, R. (2009). Effects of Radiofrequency Electromagnetic Waves (RF-EMW) from Cellular Phones on Human Ejaculated Semen: An in Vitro Pilot Study. *Fertility and Sterility*, 92(4), 1318–25. https://doi.org/10.1016/j.fertnstert.2008.08.022

11 Gorpinchenko, I., Nikitin, O., Banyra, O., & Shulyak, A. (2014). The Influence of Direct Mobile Phone Radiation on Sperm Quality. *Central European Journal of Urology*, 67(1), 65–71. https://doi.org/10.5173/ceju.2014.01.art14

12 Friedrich, M.J. (2015). Unraveling the Influence of Gut Microbes on the Mind. *JAMA*, 313(17), 1699–1701. https://doi.org/10.1001/jama.2015.2159

13 Reis, D.J., Ilardi, S.S, & Punt, S.E.W. (2018). The Anxiolytic Effect of Probiotics: A Systematic Review and Meta-Analysis of the Clinical and Preclinical Literature. *PLoS One*, 13(6), e0199041. https://doi.org/10.1371/journal.pone.0199041

14 Kilgallon, S.J. & Simmons, L.W. (2005). Image Content Influences Men's Semen Quality. *Biology Letters*, 1(3), 253–255. https://doi.org/10.1098/rsbl.2005.0324

15 Committee on Obstetric Practice. (2017, April, reaffirmed 2018). *Planned Home Birth*. The American College of Obstetricians and Gynecologists. https://www.acog.org/Clinical-Guidance-and-Publications/Committee-Opinions/Committee-on-Obstetric-Practice/Planned-Home-Birth

16 Chuck, E. (2020, January 30). The U.S. Finally Has Better Maternal Mortality Data. Black Mothers Still Fare the Worst. *NBC News*. https://www.nbcnews.com/health/womens-health/u-s-finally-has-better-maternal-mortality-data-black-mothers-n1125896; Villarosa, L. (2018, April 11) Why America's Black Mothers and Babies Are in a Life-or-Death Crisis. The New York Times. Retrieved from https://www.nytimes.com/2018/04/11/magazine/black-mothers-babies-death-maternal-mortality.html

17 Cheyney, M., Bovbjerg, M., Everson, C., Gordon, W., MPH, Hannibal, D., & Vedam, S. (2014). Outcomes of Care for 16,924 Planned Home Births in the United States: The Midwives Alliance of North America Statistics Project, 2004 to 2009. *Journal of Midwifery & Women's Health*, 59, 17-27. https://doi.org/10.1111/jmwh.12172

18 Centers for Disease Control and Prevention/National Center for Health Statistics. (2017, January 20). *Births—Method of Delivery*. Retrieved February 6, 2020 from https://www.cdc.gov/nchs/fastats/delivery.htm

19 Johnson, K. & Daviss, B. (2005). Outcomes of Planned Home Births with Certified Professional Midwives: Large Prospective Study in North America. *BMJ (Clinical Research Ed.)*, 330(7505), 1416. https://doi.org/10.1136/bmj.330.7505.1416

20 May, L., Meacham, C., Gustafson, K., & Glaros, A. (2011). Gestational Exercise Effects on the Infant Heart. *FASEB Conference Paper*, 25, 1108.5. https://www.researchgate.net/publication/235992173_Gestational_Exercise_effects_on_the_Infant_Heart

21 McMillan, A., May, L., Gaines, G., Isler, C., & Kuehn, D. (2019). Effects of Aerobic Exercise During Pregnancy on 1-Month Infant Neuromotor Skills. *Medicine & Science in Sports & Exercise*, 51(8), 1671-1676. https://doi.org/ 10.1249/MSS.0000000000001958

22 Vogt, M.C., Paeger, L., Hess, S., Steculorum, S.M., Awazawa, M., Hampel, B., Neupert, S., Nicholls, H.T., Mauer, J., Hausen, A.C., Predel, R., Kloppenburg, P., Horvath, T.L., & Brüning, J.C. (2014). Neonatal Insulin Action Impairs Hypothalamic Neurocircuit Formation in Response to Maternal High-Fat Feeding. *Cell, 156*(3), 495–509. https://doi.org/10.1016/j.cell.2014.01.008

23 Yelland, L. N., Gajewski, B. J., Colombo, J., Gibson, R. A., Makrides, M., & Carlson, S. E. (2016). Predicting the Effect of Maternal Docosahexaenoic Acid (DHA) Supplementation to Reduce Early Preterm Birth in Australia and the United States Using Results of Within Country Randomized Controlled Trials. Prostaglandins, Leukotrienes, and Essential Fatty Acids, 112, 44–49. https://doi.org/10.1016/j.plefa.2016.08.007

24 Beckmann, M.M. & Stock, O.M. (2013). Antenatal Perineal Massage for Reducing Perineal Trauma. *Cochrane Database of Systematic Reviews, 2013*(4), CD005123. https://doi.org/10.1002/14651858.CD005123.pub3

25 Owings, M., Uddin, S., & Williams, S. (2015, November 6). *Trends in Circumcision for Male Newborns in U.S. Hospitals: 1979-2010*. National Center for Health Statistics. https://www.cdc.gov/nchs/data/hestat/circumcision_2013/circumcision_2013.htm

26 Task Force on Circumcision. (2012, September). Circumcision Policy Statement. *Pediatrics,* 130(3), 585-586. https://doi.org/10.1542/peds.2012-1989; American College of Obstetricians and Gynecologists, Committee on Obstetric Practice. (2001). ACOG Committee Opinion. Circumcision. Number 260, October 2001. *Obstetrics & Gynecology, 98*(4), 707-708; Morris, B., Krieger, J., & Klausner, J. (2017). CDC's Male Circumcision Recommendations Represent a Key Public Health Measure. *Global Health: Science and Practice,* 5(1), 15-27.

27 Maternal and Child Health Bureau of the Health and Resources and Services Administration. (2010, September 3). *Newborn Screening for Critical Congenital Heart Disease: A Summary of the Evidence and Advisory Committee Decision.* https://www.hrsa.gov/sites/default/files/hrsa/advisory-committees/heritable-disorders/rusp/previous-nominations/cchd-27-june-2018.pdf

28 National Institute on Deafness and Other Communication Disorders. (2017, June 19). *Your Baby's Hearing Screening.* National Institutes of Health. https://www.nidcd.nih.gov/health/your-babys-hearing-screening

29 Terreri, C. (2015, January 21). *Hormones & Healthy Birth: Letting Labor Begin on Its Own.* Lamaze International. https://www.lamaze.org/Giving-Birth-with-Confidence/GBWC-Post/hormones-healthy-birth-letting-labor-begin-on-its-own

30 Condon, J., Jeyasuria, P., Faust, J., & Mendelson. C. (2004). Surfactant Protein Secreted by the Maturing Mouse Fetal Lung Acts as a Hormone that Signals the Initiation of Parturition. *PNAS,* 101(14), 4978-93. https://doi.org10.1073/pnas.0401124101

31 Sanchez-Ramos, L., Bernstein, S., & Kaunitz, A.M. (2002). Expectant Management versus Labor Induction for Suspected Fetal Macrosomia: A Systematic Review. *Obstetrics and Gynecology, 5*(1), 997-1002; Leaphart, W.L., Meyer, M.C., & Capeless, E.L. (1997). Labor Induction with a Prenatal Diagnosis of Fetal Macrosomia. *The Journal of Maternal-Fetal Medicine, 6*(2), 99-102. https://doi.org/10.1002/(SICI)1520-6661(199703/04)6:2<99::AID-MFM7>3.0.CO;2-K; Horrigan, T.J. (2001). Physicians who Induce Labor for Fetal Macrosomia Do Not Reduce Cesarean Delivery Rates. *Journal of Perinatology,* 21(2), 93-96. https://doi.org/10.1038/sj.jp.7200500

32 Butwick, A., Wong, C., & Guo, N. (2018). Maternal Body Mass Index and Use of Labor Neuraxial Analgesia: A Population-based Retrospective Cohort Study. *Anesthesiology, 129*(9), 448-58. https://doi.org/10.1097/ALN.0000000000002322

33 Kumar, M., Chandra, S., Ijaz, Z., & Senthilselvan, A. (2014). Epidural Analgesia in Labour and Neonatal Respiratory Distress: A Case-Control Study. *Archives of Disease in Childhood - Fetal and Neonatal Edition, 99*(2), F116-F119.

34 *Evidence on: Premature Rupture of Membranes.* (2017, July 10). Evidence Based Birth. https://evidencebasedbirth.com/evidence-inducing-labor-water-breaks-term; Robock, K. (2014, November 10). What to Expect When Your Water Breaks. *Today's Parent.* Retrieved from https://www.todaysparent.com/pregnancy/when-your-water-breaks-pregnancy; (2016). Ruptured Membranes: When the Bag of Water Breaks. *Journal of Midwifery & Women's Health,* 61, 545-546. https://doi.org/10.1111/jmwh.12509

35 Kaviani, M., Azima, S., Alavi, N., & Tabaei, M.H. (2014). The Effect of Lavender Aromatherapy on Pain Perception and Intrapartum Outcome in Primiparous Women. *British Journal of Midwifery,* 22(2), 125-128.

36 Namazi, M., Amir Ali Akbari, S., Mojab, F., Talebi, A., Alavi Majd, H., & Jannesari, S. (2014). Effects of Citrus aurantium (Bitter Orange) on the Severity of First-Stage Labor Pain. *Iranian Journal of Pharmaceutical Research: IJPR, 13*(3), 1011–1018.

37 Kheirkhah, M., Vali Pour, N.S., Nisani, L., & Haghani, H. (2014). Comparing the Effects of Aromatherapy with Rose Oils and Warm Foot Bath on Anxiety in the First Stage of Labor in Nulliparous Women. *Iranian Red Crescent Medical Journal, 16*(9), e14455. https://doi.org/10.5812/ircmj.14455

38 Rashidi Fakari, F., Tabatabaeichehr, M., Kamali, H., Rashidi Fakari, F., & Naseri, M. (2015). Effect of Inhalation of Aroma of Geranium Essence on Anxiety and Physiological Parameters during First Stage of Labor in Nulliparous Women: A Randomized Clinical Trial. *Journal of Caring Sciences, 4*(2), 135–141. https://doi.org/10.15171/jcs.2015.014

39 Odom, E.C., Li, R., Scanlon, K.S., Perrine, C.G., & Grummer-Strawn, L. (2013). Reasons for Earlier than Desired Cessation of Breastfeeding. *Pediatrics, 131*(3), e726–e732. https://doi.org/10.1542/peds.2012-1295

40 Patel, S. & Patel, S. (2016). The Effectiveness of Lactation Consultants and Lactation Counselors on Breastfeeding Outcomes. *Journal of Human Lactation, 32*(3), 530–541. https://doi.org/10.1177/0890334415618668

41 *Position Paper: The Postpartum Doula's Role in Maternity Care.* (2018). DONA International. https://www.dona.org/wp-content/uploads/2018/03/DONA-Postpartum-Position-Paper-FINAL.pdf

42 Johnson, S.K., Pastuschek, J., Rödel, J., Markert, U.R., & Groten, T. (2018). Placenta - Worth Trying? Human Maternal Placentophagia: Possible Benefit and Potential Risks [published correction appears in Geburtshilfe Frauenheilkd. 2018 Sep;78(9):e1]. *Geburtshilfe Frauenheilkd, 78*(9), 846-852. https://doi.org/10.1055/a-0674-6275

43 Blei, D. (2019, December 27). *Opinion: Placenta-Eating Went Mainstream When Many Doctors Stopped Listening*. NPR. https://www.npr.org/sections/health-shots/2019/12/27/791556565/opinion-placenta-eating-went-mainstream-when-many-doctors-stopped-listening

44 Sparling, T.M., Henschke, N., Nesbitt, R.C., & Gabrysch, S. (2017). The Role of Diet and Nutritional Supplementation in Perinatal Depression: A Systematic Review. *Maternal & Child Nutrition, 13*(1), 10.1111/mcn.12235. https://doi.org/10.1111/mcn.12235

45 Achtyes, E., Keaton, S.A., Smart, L., Burmeister, A.R., Heilman, P.L., Krzyzanowski, S., Nagalla, M., Guillemin, G.J., Escobar Galvis, M.L., Lim, C.K., Muzik, M., Postolache, T. T., Leach, R., & Brundin, L. (2020). Inflammation and Kynurenine Pathway Dysregulation in Post-partum Women with Severe and Suicidal Depression. *Brain, Behavior, and Immunity*, 83, 239–247. https://doi.org/10.1016/j.bbi.2019.10.017; Kendall-Tackett, K. (2007). A New Paradigm for Depression in New Mothers: The Central Role of Inflammation and How Breastfeeding and Anti-inflammatory Treatments Protect Maternal Mental Health. *International Breastfeeding Journal, 2*(6). https://doi.org/10.1186/1746-4358-2-6

46 Kendall-Tackett, K. (2007). A New Paradigm for Depression in New Mothers: The Central Role of Inflammation and How Breastfeeding and Anti-inflammatory Treatments Protect Maternal Mental Health. *International Breastfeeding Journal, 2*(6). https://doi.org/10.1186/1746-4358-2-6

47 Guesnet, P. & Alessandri, J.M. (2011). Docosahexaenoic Acid (DHA) and the Developing Central Nervous System (CNS) - Implications for Dietary Recommendations. *Biochimie, 93*(1), 7–12. https://doi.org/10.1016/j.biochi.2010.05.005; Judge, M.P., Harel, O., & Lammi-Keefe, C.J. (2007). Maternal Consumption of a Docosahexaenoic Acid-Containing Functional Food During Pregnancy: Benefit for Infant Performance on Problem-solving but Not on Recognition Memory Tasks at age 9 mo. *The American Journal of Clinical Nutrition, 85*(6), 1572–1577. https://doi.org/10.1093/ajcn/85.6.1572; Zielinska, M.A., Hamulka, J., Grabowicz-Chądrzyńska, I., Bryś, J., & Wesolowska, A. (2019). Association between Breastmilk LC PUFA, Carotenoids and Psychomotor Development of Exclusively Breastfed Infants. *International Journal of Environmental Research and Public Health, 16*(7), 1144. https://doi.org/10.3390/ijerph16071144

48 Jackson, E. & Glasier, A. (2011). Return of Ovulation and Menses in Postpartum Nonlactating Women: A Systematic Review. *Obstetrics & Gynecology, 117*(3), 657–662. https://doi.org/10.1097/AOG.0b013e31820ce18c

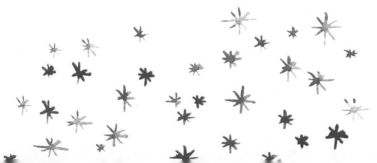

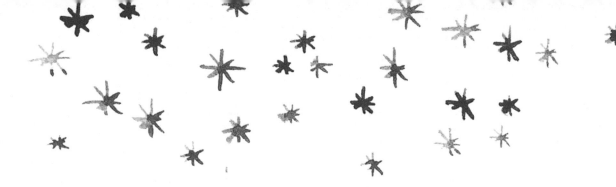

INDEX

C

diaper rash remedies, 419–420

diaphragmatic breathing, 39–41, 201, 202, 223

diastasis recti, 203

dilation of cervix, 310–312, 313–315

disinfecting spray for home birth, 297

dizziness, 75, 169

DONA International Birth Doula Training Workshop, 152

doulas, 93, 152, 153, 349, 350–351

Dual-Purpose Green Tea Toner (skin care recipe), 50, 51

due date debate, 253–261

E

eating. *See also* nutrition

    food aversions in first trimester, 108

    preparing food and drink for labor, 287–288

    preparing meals for after birth, 277–287

    small, frequent meals, 121, 232

echinacea, 126

eczema remedy, 421

effacement of cervix, 310, 316

elderberry syrup, 126

electromagnetic frequencies, fertility impact, 34–35

embryonic stage of development, 73–74

emergency plan, 301

emotional and mental self-care. *See* mental and emotional preparation and self-care

endorphins, 35, 46, 171–172, 292

Energizing Smoothie (recipe), 106

engorgement, breast, 377

epidural anesthesia, 90, 144, 261

episiotomy, 260, 414

Epsom salts, 126, 372

essential oils

O

P

protein, 22, 193–194, 229, 408

PTFE (polytetrafluoroethylene), 31

pumping breast milk, as labor stimulation strategy, 293

pushing phase of labor, 309, 315, 323

Made in the USA
Las Vegas, NV
09 July 2023

74416350R00260